Orthopedic Emergencies

Guest Editor

MICHAEL C. BOND, MD

EMERGENCY MEDICINE CLINICS OF NORTH AMERICA

www.emed.theclinics.com

Consulting Editor
AMAL MATTU, MD

November 2010 • Volume 28 • Number 4

SAUNDERS an imprint of ELSEVIER, Inc.

W.B. SAUNDERS COMPANY

A Division of Elsevier Inc.

1600 John F. Kennedy Boulevard • Suite 1800 • Philadelphia, Pennsylvania 19103-2899

http://www.theclinics.com

EMERGENCY MEDICINE CLINICS OF NORTH AMERICA Volume 28, Number 4
November 2010 ISSN 0733-8627, ISBN-13: 978-1-4377-2445-5

Editor: Patrick Manley
Developmental Editor: Jessica Demetriou

Emergency Medicine Clinics of North America (ISSN 0733-8627) is published quarterly by Elsevier Inc., 360 Park Avenue South, New York, NY, 10010-1710. Months of issue are February, May, August, and November. Business and Editorial Offices: 1600 John F. Kennedy Boulevard, Suite 1800, Philadelphia, PA 19103-2899. Customer Service Office: 6277 Sea Harbor Drive, Orlando, FL 32887-4800. Periodicals postage paid at New York, NY, and additional mailing offices. Subscription prices are $133.00 per year (US students), $264.00 per year (US individuals), $455.00 per year (US institutions), $189.00 per year (international students), $379.00 per year (international individuals), $549.00 per year (international institutions), $189.00 per year (Canadian students), $326.00 per year (Canadian individuals), and $549.00 per year (Canadian institutions). International air speed delivery is included in all *Clinics'* subscription prices. All prices are subject to change without notice. **POSTMASTER:** Send address changes to *Emergency Medicine Clinics of North America*, Elsevier Periodicals Customer Service, 11830 Westline Industrial Drive, St. Louis, MO 63146. Customer Service (orders, claims, online, change of address): Elsevier Periodicals Customer Service, 11830 Westline Industrial Drive, St. Louis, MO 63146. Tel: 1-800-654-2452 (U.S. and Canada); 314-453-7041 (outside U.S. and Canada). Fax: 314-453-5170. E-mail: journalscustomerservice-usa@elsevier.com (for print support); journalsonline support-usa@elsevier.com (for online support).

Reprints. For copies of 100 or more of articles in this publication, please contact the Commercial Reprints Department, Elsevier Inc., 360 Park Avenue South, New York, NY 10010-1710. Tel.: 212-633-3812; Fax: 212-462-1935; E-mail: reprints@elsevier.com.

Emergency Medicine Clinics of North America is covered in *MEDLINE/PubMed (Index Medicus), Current Contents/Clinical Medicine, EMBASE/Excerpta Medica, BIOSIS, SciSearch, CINAHL, ISI/BIOMED,* and *Research Alert.*

Printed and bound by CPI Group (UK) Ltd, Croydon, CR0 4YY
Transferred to Digital Print 2011

Contributors

CONSULTING EDITOR

AMAL MATTU, MD, FAAEM, FACEP
Program Director, Emergency Medicine Residency; Professor, Department
of Emergency Medicine, University of Maryland School of Medicine,
Baltimore, Maryland

GUEST EDITOR

MICHAEL C. BOND, MD, FACEP, FAAEM
Assistant Professor; Assistant Residency Program Director, Department
of Emergency Medicine, University of Maryland School of Medicine,
Baltimore, Maryland

AUTHORS

MICHAEL K. ABRAHAM, MD, MS
Clinical Assistant Professor, Department of Emergency Medicine, University
of Maryland School of Medicine, Baltimore; Attending Physician, Department
of Emergency Medicine, Upper Chesapeake Medical Health, Bel Air, Maryland

MICHAEL C. BOND, MD, FACEP, FAAEM
Assistant Professor; Assistant Residency Program Director, Department of Emergency
Medicine, University of Maryland School of Medicine, Baltimore, Maryland

JOSE G. CABANAS, MD
Associate Medical Director Wake County EMS; Associate Director Clinical Research Unit,
Emergency Services Institute, WakeMed Health and Hospitals, Raleigh; Adjunct Assistant
Professor, Department of Emergency Medicine, University of North Carolina at Chapel Hill,
Chapel Hill, North Carolina

CHRISTOPHER R. CARPENTER, MD, MSc, FACEP, FAAEM
Assistant Professor; Director, Evidence Based Medicine, Division of Emergency Medicine,
Barnes Jewish Hospital, Washington University in St Louis, St Louis, Missouri

ROSE M. CHASM, MD, FAAEM, FACEP
Assistant Professor, Department of Emergency Medicine, University of Maryland
School of Medicine; Co-Director, Combined Emergency Medicine/Pediatrics Residency,
University of Maryland Medical Center, Baltimore, Maryland

GEORGE CHIAMPAS, DO
Assistant Professor, Department of Emergency Medicine, Feinberg School of Medicine,
Northwestern University; Medical Director, Bank of America Chicago Marathon;
Assistant Team Physician, Northwestern University Athletics, Chicago, Illinois

LISSANDRA COLON-ROLON, MD, FACEP
Assistant Professor, Department of Emergency Medicine, Ponce School of Medicine/
Hospital San Lucas, Ponce, Puerto Rico

BRIAN N. CORWELL, MD, FACEP
CAQ Sports Medicine, Assistant Professor, Department of Emergency Medicine,
University of Maryland School of Medicine, Baltimore, Maryland

MOIRA DAVENPORT, MD
Assistant Professor of Emergency Medicine; Faculty, Department Orthopedic
Surgery, Allegheny General Hospital, Drexel University College of Medicine,
Pittsburgh, Pennsylvania

LAURA DIEGELMANN, MD
Senior Resident, Department of Emergency Medicine, University of Maryland School
of Medicine; Department of Emergency Medicine, University of Maryland Medical Center,
Baltimore, Maryland

JORGE L. FALCON-CHEVERE, MD
Associate Program Director; Assistant Professor, Department of Emergency Medicine,
University of Puerto Rico School of Medicine, Hospital UPR Dr Federico Trilla, Carolina,
Puerto Rico

CARLOS F. GARCÍA-GUBERN, MD, FACEP, FAAEM
Associate Professor; Program Director and Chair, Department of Emergency Medicine,
Ponce School of Medicine/Hospital San Lucas, Ponce, Puerto Rico

CARL A. GERMANN, MD, FACEP
Department of Emergency Medicine, Maine Medical Center; Assistant Professor,
Tufts University College of Medicine, Portland, Maine

DENNIS P. HANLON, MD, FAAEM
Associate Professor of Emergency Medicine; Vice Chairman, Operations, Allegheny
General Hospital, Pittsburgh, Pennsylvania

EDUARDO LABAT, MD
Chief Resident, Department of Diagnostic Radiology, University of Puerto Rico School
of Medicine, Rio Piedras, Puerto Rico

HEATHER LEONARD, MD
Resident Physician, Department of Emergency Medicine, Feinberg School of Medicine,
Northwestern University, Chicago, Illinois

SANJEEV MALIK, MD
Assistant Medical Director, Department of Emergency Medicine; Clinical Instructor,
Feinberg School of Medicine, Northwestern University, Chicago, Illinois

DANA MATHEW, MD
WakeMed Health and Hospitals, Emergency Services Institute, Raleigh; Adjunct Assistant
Professor, Department of Emergency Medicine, University of North Carolina at Chapel
Hill, Chapel Hill, North Carolina

ANDREW D. PERRON, MD, FACEP, FACSM
Program Director, Department of Emergency Medicine, Maine Medical Center; Associate
Professor, Tufts University College of Medicine, Portland, Maine

LAURA PIMENTEL, MD
Clinical Associate Professor, Department of Emergency Medicine, University of Maryland School of Medicine; Vice President and Chief Medical Officer, Maryland Emergency Medicine Network, Baltimore, Maryland

SARA SCOTT, MD
Clinical Assistant Professor, Department of Emergency Medicine, University of Maryland School of Medicine; Attending Physician, Department of Emergency Medicine, Mercy Medical Center, Baltimore, Maryland

MICHAEL E. STERN, MD
Assistant Professor; Co-Director, Geriatric Emergency Medicine Fellowship, Department of Emergency Medicine, New York-Presbyterian Hospital, Weill Cornell Medical College, New York, New York

SHARON A. SWENCKI, MD, FACEP
Assistant Professor, Department of Emergency Medicine, University of Maryland School of Medicine, Baltimore, Maryland

HAROLD WATSON, MBBS, MSc, DM (Emergency Medicine)
Lecturer and Residency Program Coordinator, The University of The West Indies; Faculty of Medical Sciences, Cave Hill Campus and Queen Elizabeth Hospital, Bridgetown, Barbados, West Indies

ERIC WILLIAMS, MBBS, MSc, DM (Emergency Medicine)
Associate Lecturer; Consultant Emergency Physician, Emergency Medicine Division, Department of Surgery, Radiology, Anaesthesia and Intensive Care, University of The West Indies and the University Hospital of The West Indies (Mona), Kingston, Jamaica, West Indies

JEAN WILLIAMS-JOHNSON, MBBS, MSc, DM (Emergency Medicine)
Lecturer and Residency Program Coordinator; Medical Director, Emergency Medicine Division, Department of Surgery, Radiology, Anaesthesia and Intensive Care, University of The West Indies and the University Hospital of The West Indies (Mona), Kingston, Jamaica, West Indies

Contents

The evaluation and management of cervical spine injuries is a core component of the practice of emergency medicine. This article focuses on evaluation and management of blunt cervical spine trauma by the emergency physician. Pertinent anatomy of the cervical spine and specific cervical spine fractures are discussed, with an emphasis on unstable injuries and associated spinal cord pathology. The association of vertebral artery injury with cervical spine fracture is addressed, followed by a review of the most recent literature on prehospital care. Initial considerations in the emergency department, including cervical spine stabilization and airway management, are reviewed. The most current recommendations for cervical spine imaging with regard to indications and modalities are covered. Finally, emergency department management and disposition of patients with spinal cord injuries are reviewed.

This article provides a review of the evaluation and treatment of common injuries to the shoulder, humerus, and clavicle in the emergency department (ED) setting. In addition to a focused review of the shoulder's physical examination, topics include common emergent injuries such as glenohumeral dislocations, proximal humerus fractures, and acromioclavicular separations as well as less common, but important injuries including pectoralis and biceps tendon injuries and sternoclavicular dislocations. Accurate recognition and management of these injuries is essential in the optimal care of patients in the ED.

Orthopedic injuries to the upper extremity are frequently seen in the emergency department (ED). The emergency medicine practitioner must be proficient in recognizing these injuries and their associated complications, and be able to provide appropriate orthopedic management. This article highlights the most frequent forearm and elbow injuries seen in the ED.

The anatomy of the hand is complex, which allows for the dexterity, strength, and adaptability of the most functional aspect of the musculoskeletal system.

The evaluation and management of injuries to this area can be time consuming and pose a significant medicolegal risk to the emergency physician. Improperly diagnosed and managed injuries can lead to chronic pain, inability to perform activities of daily living, and even seemingly minor injuries can lead to missed work causing a significant cost to the individual and society. The purpose of this article is to review injuries to the hand and wrist and discuss diagnostic studies and treatment plans that the emergency physician can use to treat patients effectively and minimize their exposure to risk.

Back pain is one of the most common symptom-related complaints for visits to primary care physicians and is the most common musculoskeletal complaint that results in visits to the emergency department (ED). With recent national health care initiatives moving toward universal coverage, an increasing number of patients with common complaints such as back pain will visit the ED. The first goal of ED assessment of patients with back pain is to evaluate for potentially dangerous causes that, if not promptly recognized, could result in significant morbidity and mortality. This article focuses on the essential elements of an efficient and effective evaluation, management and treatment of patients with back pain in the ED, with special emphasis on epidural abscess, epidural compression syndrome, malignancy, spinal stenosis, and back pain in children.

The management of pelvic fractures and hip injuries requires a multidisciplinary approach and begins in the prehospital setting. With the current advances in various investigative modalities along with the use of algorithms, the morbidity and mortality from these injuries has improved. This review discusses an outline of the current recommendations along with treatment strategies and options in the emergency department, which may vary from institution to institution based on the availability of expertise and resources and because no two trauma patients are alike with regard to the pathophysiology and injury patterns.

The knee plays a significant role in ambulation and the activities of daily living. During the course of these activities and its role in weight bearing, the knee is susceptible to a variety of different forces and the emergency physician should be familiar with the diagnosis and treatment of the injuries that result. In addition to following basic trauma protocols, thorough neurovascular and musculoskeletal examinations should be performed and supplemented with appropriate imaging. Emergency physicians should also consider recent developments in knee anatomy and function when evaluating the patient with an acutely injured knee.

The emergency provider (EP) must be aware of the anatomy of the leg, ankle, and foot. The varied presentation of common injuries must be recognized as well as the unique presentations of uncommon injuries. The astute EP must rely on a focused history and a precise examination to avoid the pitfalls and missed injuries from an over-reliance on radiographic studies. In some cases, emergent orthopedic consultation is required. Potential complications associated with these injuries must be anticipated and avoided if possible.

Many well seasoned emergency physicians often find it challenging to assess and treat pediatric patients regardless of the complaint. Because of anatomic and physiologic differences, pediatric patients experience orthopedic injuries that are both unique and specific to this subset of the population. Emergency physicians must be aware of these nuances to properly diagnose and treat these injuries. An understanding of fractures unique to growing bone, such as buckle/torus and greenstick types, will provoke clinicians to have a keener eye when reviewing pediatric radiographs. The Salter-Harris classification provides a proven, generally accepted stratification of injury to describe and properly disposition pediatric fractures. Emergency physicians must also recognize a distal radial fracture, because it is the most common pediatric fracture, and the many complications of the supracondylar fracture. Nursemaid's elbow and ankle injuries are further common presenting complaints that are discussed. Recognition of child abuse and the work-up of the child presenting with a limp are additional areas that the Emergency physician should feel comfortable evaluating.

Multidisciplinary orthogeriatric care can enhance prompt ED diagnosis, optimal pre- and postoperative care, and functional recovery in older adults with bony injuries. Emergency care providers should be cognizant of prevalent geriatric syndromes including delirium and standing level falls to minimize fracture-related morbidity. Recognizing the implications of aging physiology, acute care physicians should be aware of effective alternatives to analgesia, procedural sedation, and definitive imaging to promote early surgical management and postoperative recovery.

The practice of wound care has greatly improved and evolved over the years. The emergency provider (EP) can choose from a wide variety of sutures, adhesives, strips, and surgical staples, and uses proven wound closure techniques to address this common Emergency Department (ED) patient complaint. All EPs should be comfortable and proficient in the management and care of wounds in the ED. Because wound care is responsible for a large number of malpractice claims, EPs need to be aware of practices that can limit bad outcomes and thus decrease their liability risk. EPs should follow a standard examination and ensure that there is no damage to underlying structures (ie, nerves, tendons, and vasculature), and that foreign bodies are meticulously looked for and removed if found. Discharge instructions that alert the patient on warning signs of infection, and having all patients return within 48hours for a wound check are 2 ways to optimize patients' outcomes.

Avoiding legal pitfalls of orthopedic injuries in the emergency department (ED) requires an understanding of certain high-risk injuries, their presentation, evaluation, and disposition. Various pitfalls pertaining to both upper and lower extremity injuries are discussed in detail, with recommendations regarding the history, physical examination, and radiographic techniques that minimize the risk inherent in these injuries. When approaching these injuries in the ED, a high level of suspicion coupled with appropriate evaluation and management will allow the practitioner to avoid mismanagement of these potential pitfall cases.

THE CLINICS ARE NOW AVAILABLE ONLINE!

Access your subscription at:
www.theclinics.com

GOAL STATEMENT

The goal of *Emergency Medicine Clinics of North America* is to keep practicing physicians up to date with current clinical practice in emergency medicine by providing timely articles reviewing the state of the art in patient care.

ACCREDITATION

The *Emergency Medical Clinics of North America* is planned and implemented in accordance with the Essential Areas and Policies of the Accreditation Council for Continuing Medical Education (ACCME) through the joint sponsorship of the University of Virginia School of Medicine and Elsevier. The University of Virginia School of Medicine is accredited by the ACCME to provide continuing medical education for physicians.

The University of Virginia School of Medicine designates this educational activity for a maximum of 15 *AMA PRA Category 1 Credits*™ for each issue, 60 credits per year. Physicians should only claim credit commensurate with the extent of their participation in the activity.

The American Medical Association has determined that physicians not licensed in the US who participate in this CME activity are eligible for a maximum of 15 *AMA PRA Category 1 Credits*™ for each issue, 60 credits per year.

The Emergency Medicine Clinics of North America CME program is approved by the American College of Emergency Physicians for 60 hours of ACEP Category I Credit per year.

Credit can be earned by reading the text material, taking the CME examination online at http://www.theclinics.com/home/cme, and completing the evaluation. After taking the test, you will be required to review any and all incorrect answers. Following completion of the test and evaluation, your credit will be awarded and you may print your certificate.

FACULTY DISCLOSURE/CONFLICT OF INTEREST

The University of Virginia School of Medicine, as an ACCME accredited provider, endorses and strives to comply with the Accreditation Council for Continuing Medical Education (ACCME) Standards of Commercial Support, Commonwealth of Virginia statutes, University of Virginia policies and procedures, and associated federal and private regulations and guidelines on the need for disclosure and monitoring of proprietary and financial interests that may affect the scientific integrity and balance of content delivered in continuing medical education activities under our auspices.

The University of Virginia School of Medicine requires that all CME activities accredited through this institution be developed independently and be scientifically rigorous, balanced and objective in the presentation/discussion of its content, theories and practices.

All authors/editors participating in an accredited CME activity are expected to disclose to the readers relevant financial relationships with commercial entities occurring within the past 12 months (such as grants or research support, employee, consultant, stock holder, member of speakers bureau, etc.). The University of Virginia School of Medicine will employ appropriate mechanisms to resolve potential conflicts of interest to maintain the standards of fair and balanced education to the reader. Questions about specific strategies can be directed to the Office of Continuing Medical Education, University of Virginia School of Medicine, Charlottesville, Virginia.

The faculty and staff of the University of Virginia Office of Continuing Medical Education have no financial affiliations to disclose.

The authors/editors listed below have identified no professional or financial affiliations for themselves or their spouse/partner:

Michael K. Abraham, MD, MS; Michael C. Bond, MD (Guest Editor); Jose G. Cabanas, MD; Christopher R. Carpenter, MD, MSc; Rose M. Chasm, MD; George Chiampas, DO; Lissandra Colon-Rolon, MD; Brian N. Corwell, MD; Moira Davenport, MD; Laura Diegelmann, MD; Jorge L. Falcon-Chevere, MD; Carlos F. García-Gubern, MD; Carl A. Germann, MD; Dennis P. Hanlon, MD; Eduardo Labat, MD; Heather Leonard, MD; Sanjeev Malik, MD; Patrick Manley, (Acquisitions Editor); Dana Mathew, MD; Amal Mattu, MD (Consulting Editor); Andrew D. Perron, MD; Laura Pimentel, MD; Sara Scott, MD; Michael E. Stern, MD; Sharon A. Swencki, MD; Harold Watson, MBBS, MSc, DM; Eric Williams, MBBS, MSc, DM; Jean Williams-Johnson, MBBS, MSc, DM; and Bill Woods, MD (Test Author).

Disclosure of Discussion of Non-FDA Approved Uses for Pharmaceutical Products and/or Medical Devices.
The University of Virginia School of Medicine, as an ACCME provider, requires that all faculty presenters identify and disclose any off-label uses for pharmaceutical and medical device products. The University of Virginia School of Medicine recommends that each physician fully review all the available data on new products or procedures prior to clinical use.

TO ENROLL

To enroll in the Emergency Medicine Clinics of North America Continuing Medical Education program, call customer service at 1-800-654-2452 or visit us online at www.theclinics.com/home/cme. The CME program is available to subscribers for an additional fee of $190.00.

Foreword

Orthopedic Emergencies

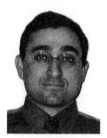

Amal Mattu, MD
Consulting Editor

In many other countries, the specialty of Emergency Medicine is referred to as "Accident and Emergency Medicine." The addition of the word "Accident" provides appropriate recognition of the fact that many patients that present for emergency care are not suffering from a medical disorder but rather are victims of accidental trauma, having sustained orthopedic injuries. It is no surprise, therefore, that management of orthopedic injuries constitutes a significant part of the practice of emergency medicine.

Orthopedic injuries certainly seem to be on the rise in emergency practice. One possible reason is that outdoor sporting activities, especially "extreme" sports, are gaining popularity worldwide. Protective equipment and safety devices are helpful but still pose no match for the high-impact nature of falls that occur during these activities. A second possible reason for the increasing incidence of orthopedic injuries is the rapid growth of the geriatric population. Elderly patients are more prone to fractures related to falls, even seemingly minor falls. Regardless of the reason for the increase in orthopedic cases in emergency practice in recent years, it is clear that emergency health care providers must have a sound knowledge in the diagnosis and management of these injuries if they are going to be effective providers.

In this issue of *Emergency Medicine Clinics of North America*, Guest Editor Dr Michael Bond brings us a comprehensive curriculum in emergency orthopedics. He has assembled an exceptional group of emergency physicians who have a particular academic interest in management of orthopedic emergencies. The "curriculum" addresses upper extremity disorders from the cervical spine down to the hand, and lower extremity disorders from the lumber spine and pelvis down to the foot. Additional articles are added which focus on special challenges in the very young and the very old. Risk management is also addressed in one article devoted to wound care and another article devoted to avoidance of the legal pitfalls.

Emerg Med Clin N Am 28 (2010) xiii–xiv
doi:10.1016/j.emc.2010.09.003
0733-8627/10/$ — see front matter © 2010 Elsevier Inc. All rights reserved.

emed.theclinics.com

This issue of *Clinics* represents an important addition to the emergency medicine literature. Experienced emergency physicians as well as emergency medicine trainees will benefit tremendously from the expertise provided in the pages that follow. Dr Bond and the authors are to be commended for providing a single resource that covers a comprehensive spectrum of orthopedic emergencies in a succinct and clinically relevant manner.

Amal Mattu, MD
Department of Emergency Medicine
University of Maryland School of Medicine
110 S. Paca Street, 6th Floor, Suite 200
Baltimore, MD 21201, USA

E-mail address:
amattu@smail.umaryland.edu

Preface

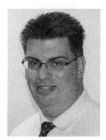

Michael C. Bond, MD
Guest Editor

This edition of *Emergency Medicine Clinics of North America* is focused on the Emergency Department (ED) management of orthopedic injuries. The treatment of orthopedic patients is a growing part of our specialty with over 42.4 million injury-related visits to the ED in 2006.[1] This fact along with the realization that immediate orthopedic consultation in the ED can often be difficult to impossible in some communities require that the emergency provider be comfortable and competent with the initial stabilization and management of orthopedic injuries. The American Association of Orthopaedic Surgeons also recognizes this and released a position statement in 2008 that acknowledges, "access to emergency orthopedic care in the United States is problematic and may get worse. At present, there is variable access to orthopedic emergency care in many communities in the United States."[2] The availability of orthopedic consultations can be an even bigger challenge when dealing with pediatric, hand, or uninsured cases.

This edition of the *Emergency Medicine Clinics of North America* provides an up-to-date, evidence-based approach to the initial management and stabilization of common and some not so common orthopedic injuries. Some notable areas to mention are the article on geriatrics where expert guidance is provided on pain control, prevention of delirium, prevention of hip fractures, and dealing with the unique pathophysiology of the elderly patient; and the article on high-risk injuries and how you can minimize your medicolegal liability while providing the highest quality of care. Other questions that are answered are: does any specific fracture predict child abuse, and what is the best maneuver to evaluate the posterolateral corner of the knee?

I hope you find this edition of the *Emergency Medicine Clinics* to be highly educational and stimulating and a useful resource as you deal with those challenging orthopedic cases. I would like to thank all the authors that spent endless hours scouring

Emerg Med Clin N Am 28 (2010) xv–xvi
doi:10.1016/j.emc.2010.09.002
0733-8627/10/$ – see front matter © 2010 Elsevier Inc. All rights reserved.

through the literature and writing their articles. I also need to thank my wife, Ginger, and family for their unwavering support, encouragement, understanding, and love.

Michael C. Bond, MD
Department of Emergency Medicine
University of Maryland School of Medicine
110 South Paca Street
Sixth Floor, Suite 200
Baltimore, MD 21201, USA

E-mail address:
mbond007@gmail.com

REFERENCES

1. Pitts SR, Niska RQ, Xu J, et al. National Hospital Ambulatory Medical Care Survey: 2006 Emergency Department Summary. National Health Statistics Reports; no. 7. Hyattsville (MD): National Center for Health Statistics; 2008.
2. Emergency Orthopaedic Care Position Statement. American Academy of Orthopaedic Surgeons and the American Association of Orthopaedic Surgeons. Available at: http://www.aaos.org/about/papers/position/1172.asp. Revised 2008. Accessed July 4, 2010.

Evaluation and Management of Acute Cervical Spine Trauma

Laura Pimentel, MD[a,b,*], Laura Diegelmann, MD[a,c]

KEYWORDS

• Cervical spine • Trauma • Fracture • Injury • Vertebrae

The evaluation and management of cervical spine injuries is a core component of the practice of emergency medicine. The incidence of serious cervical spine injuries is low but associated rates of death and disability are high; therefore, the emergency physician must have a strong knowledge base to identify these injuries as well as clinical skills that will protect the patient's spine during assessment. Cervical spine injury causes an estimated 6000 deaths and 5000 new cases of quadriplegia in the United States each year.[1] Males are affected 4 times as frequently as females.

Two to three percent of blunt trauma patients who undergo cervical spine imaging are diagnosed with a fracture. The second vertebra is most commonly injured, accounting for 24% of fractures; the sixth and seventh vertebrae together account for another 39% of fractures.[2] From a clinical perspective, it is crucial for the emergency physician to diagnose a fracture. In the NEXUS trial, 56.7% of cervical spine fractures were unstable and another 13.9% were otherwise classified as clinically significant.[2] Older age is an important risk factor for cervical spine injury: patients 65 years or older have a relative risk twice that of younger trauma victims.[3] The associated mortality rate in this age group is 24%.[4]

A disproportionate number of cervical spine injuries are associated with moderate and severe head injuries sustained in motor vehicle crashes. Head-injured patients are almost 4 times as likely to have a cervical spine injury as those without head injuries. Those at highest risk have an initial Glasgow Coma Scale (GCS) score of 8 or lower and are likely to sustain unstable injuries in the high cervical spine.[5]

[a] Department of Emergency Medicine, University of Maryland School of Medicine, 110 South Paca Street, 6th Floor, Suite 200, Baltimore, MD 21201, USA
[b] Department of Emergency Medicine, Maryland Emergency Medicine Network, 110 South Paca Street, Baltimore, MD 21201, USA
[c] Department of Emergency Medicine, University of Maryland Medical Center, 110 South Paca Street, Baltimore, MD 21201, USA
* Corresponding author. Department of Emergency Medicine, University of Maryland School of Medicine, 110 South Paca Street, 6th Floor, Suite 200, Baltimore, MD 21201.
E-mail address: lpimentel@memn.org

Emerg Med Clin N Am 28 (2010) 719–738
doi:10.1016/j.emc.2010.07.003
0733-8627/10/$ – see front matter © 2010 Elsevier Inc. All rights reserved.
emed.theclinics.com

The focus of this article is the evaluation and management of blunt cervical spine trauma by the emergency physician. The authors begin by reviewing the pertinent anatomy of the cervical spine. Specific cervical spine fractures are discussed, with an emphasis on unstable injuries and associated spinal cord pathology. The association of vertebral artery injury with cervical spine fracture is addressed, followed by a review of the most recent literature on prehospital care. The authors then review initial considerations in the emergency department, including cervical spine stabilization and airway management. The most current recommendations for cervical spine imaging with regard to indications and modalities are covered. Finally, the emergency department management and disposition of patients with spinal cord injuries are reviewed.

ANATOMY

The cervical spine consists of 7 cervical vertebrae, the spinal cord, intervertebral discs beginning at the C2-C3 interspace, a complex network of supporting ligaments, and neurovascular structures. General vertebral anatomy consists of an annular body and the vertebral arch, including the symmetric pedicles, laminae, superior and inferior articular surfaces, transverse processes, and a single posterior spinous process (**Fig. 1**A). The cervical vertebrae are smaller than their thoracic or lumbar counterparts, and each transverse process contains a foramen (foramen transversarium) (**Fig. 1**B). The first 2 and the seventh bones have exceptional anatomic features.

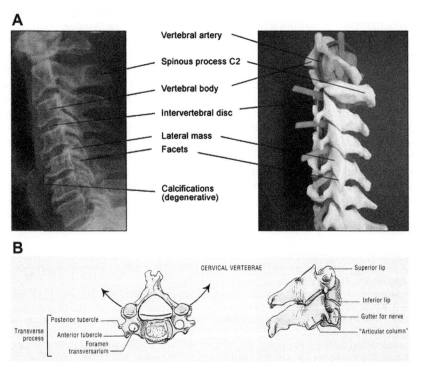

Fig. 1. (*A*) Cervical spine anatomy. (*From* EuroSpine, Patient Line, www.eurospine.org; with permission.) (*B*) Cervical vertebra. (*From* Agur AMR, Lee MJ, Anderson JE. Distinguishing features and movements. In: Grant's atlas of anatomy. 9th edition. Philadelphia: Lippincott Williams & Wilkins; 1991. p. 206; with permission.)

The first cervical vertebra is called the atlas because it supports the head. Distinct from all other vertebrae, the atlas has no body and no spinous process (**Fig. 2**); it is a ring-like structure with anterior and posterior arches separated by lateral masses on each side.[6] The superior surfaces of the lateral masses articulate with the occipital condyles of the skull, forming the atlanto-occipital joint. Functionally, this joint allows 50% of neck flexion and extension.

The second cervical vertebra, the axis, forms the surface on which the atlas pivots to allow lateral rotation of the head. The dens, also called the odontoid process, is the cranial extension of the body of the axis into the ring of the atlas; it is the most characteristic feature of C2 (see **Fig. 2**). The dens articulates with the posterior aspect of

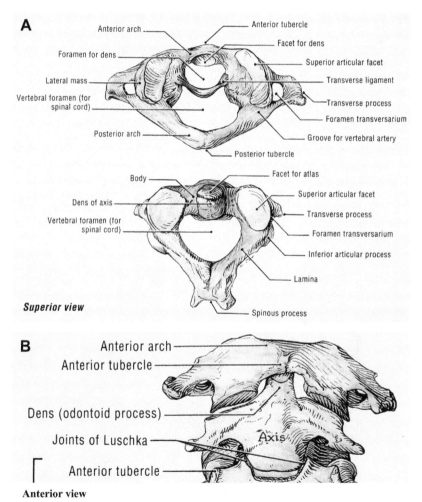

Fig. 2. (*A, B*) Cervical vertebrae 1 and 2: the atlas and axis. (*A*) Superior view. (*From* Agur AMR, Lee MJ, Anderson JE. Atlas and its transverse ligament and the axis. In: Grant's atlas of anatomy. 9th edition. Philadelphia: Lippincott Williams & Wilkins; 1991. p. 211; with permission.) (*B*) Anterior view. (*Modified from* Agur AMR, Lee MJ, Anderson JE. Articulated cervical vertebrae. In: Grant's atlas of anatomy. 9th edition. Philadelphia: Lippincott Williams & Wilkins; 1991. p. 208; with permission.)

the anterior ring of C1 and is stabilized by the transverse ligament. This articulation provides stability as the atlas pivots during rotation. Half of neck rotation occurs at this atlantoaxial joint. There is no intervertebral disc at either the atlanto-occipital or the C1-C2 joints, predisposing them to inflammatory arthritis.[7]

The distinctive feature of the seventh vertebra is its prominent spinous process. Its length extends beyond the other cervical vertebrae, rendering it palpable on physical examination. The seventh vertebra is the highest spinous process that is reliably identifiable, making it a useful landmark.[6] The length and prominence of the spinous process predispose this vertebra to fracture.

Intervertebral discs are interposed between the vertebral bodies from C2 down to the sacrum; they account for about 25% of the height of the spinal column. Structurally, discs are composed of a soft gelatinous center, the nucleus pulposus, surrounded by a cartilaginous ring of tissue (the annulus fibrosus). Functionally, discs provide support, elasticity, and cushioning to the spine. Intervertebral discs deteriorate with age; much of the gelatinous center is replaced with fibrous tissue, resulting in decreased elasticity and mobility.[8]

The cervical spine is connected and supported by a complex network of ligaments (**Fig. 3**). Three of the most important are the anterior longitudinal ligament and the posterior longitudinal ligament, which extend from the occiput to the sacrum, and the ligamentum flavum. The anterior longitudinal ligament, connecting the anterior aspects of the vertebral bodies, becomes taut and resists hyperextension. The posterior, connecting the posterior aspect of the vertebral bodies, tightens and limits hyperflexion. The posterior longitudinal ligament forms the anterior surface of the spinal canal. The ligamentum flavum connects the laminae of adjacent vertebrae and forms the posterior surface of the spinal canal. This ligament is susceptible to thickening with age and may cause spinal stenosis, resulting in cord and nerve root compression.[7] The interspinous ligaments are thin and membranous, and span the length of the spinous processes.

The blood supply to the spinal column and cord is complex. The main spinal arteries consist of a single anterior and 2 posterior vessels originating from the vertebral arteries; they run longitudinally from the medulla along the length of the cord. These arteries supply only the superior portion of the cord and are supplemented by segmental medullary arteries originating from the vertebral arteries in the cervical spine; they enter the spinal column through the intervertebral foramen. A lone vessel,

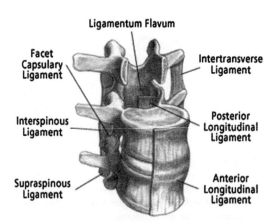

Fig. 3. Vertebral ligaments. (*Courtesy of* Goimage Media Services Inc; with permission.)

the anterior cervical artery, is particularly vulnerable to damage associated with hyperextension injuries. The result is ischemia to the anterior two-thirds of the cord, a devastating complication.[8]

When considering cervical spine anatomy in the clinical context, emergency physicians should think of the spinal column as 2 parallel entities. The vertebral bodies and associated intervertebral discs form the anterior column, which is stabilized by the anterior and posterior longitudinal ligaments. The posterior column containing the spinal cord and canal consists of the structures posterior to the anterior column: pedicles, transverse processes, superior and inferior articulating facets, laminae, and spinous process. The ligamentum flavum and the interspinous and associated ligaments stabilize the posterior column. When only one column is injured, the other provides stability, substantially lowering the risk of spinal cord injury compared with when both are compromised.[9]

The widest portion of the spinal canal is from C1 to C3, where the mid-sagittal diameter ranges from 16 to 30 mm. This diameter narrows from C4 to C7 to a range of from 14 to 23 mm. At this level, the spinal cord normally occupies 40% of the diameter of the canal in a healthy adult. Hyperextension decreases the canal diameter approximately 2 to 3 mm, which becomes clinically important in the context of hyperextension injury.[8]

The cervical spine is vulnerable to trauma; injury occurs when forces applied to the head or neck overwhelms the anatomic stabilizers of the bony and ligamentous support structures. Degenerative changes resulting in spinal stenosis increase vulnerability to cord damage, particularly with hyperextension mechanisms. Fatal injuries are most common at the craniocervical junction or atlantoaxial level.

PATHOPHYSIOLOGY

Cervical spine injuries can be considered by degree of mechanical instability. White and colleagues[10] defined the concept physiologically and radiographically. These investigators defined "stability" as limitation of displacement of the spine under applied physiologic loads, which prevents spinal cord or nerve root damage. In the adult spine, instability may be diagnosed radiographically when there is more than 3.5 mm of displacement in the sagittal plane relative to an adjacent vertebra on resting radiographs or with flexion/extension views. This work led to a complex scoring system that may be applied to injuries that are not clearly stable or unstable.

When evaluating patients in the emergency department, it is not always clear which fractures are stable. Some of the difficulty is the lack of a consistent convention for classifying cervical spine injuries. Some injuries are named, for example, the Jefferson, hangman, and clay shoveler fractures. Others are described by mechanism of injury, pathologic lesion, or combinations of the two. Another source of confusion is lack of agreement among investigators about which injuries are stable. The reality is that each cervical spine injury is unique and its relative stability depends on individual factors such as the patient's age, associated injuries, and underlying health. It is useful to consider White's strategy of combining radiologic findings with response to physiologic stress when unsure. All but the most minor cervical spine fractures in the emergency department should be treated as unstable injuries until proven otherwise.

Axial Compression Injury

The Jefferson fracture is an unstable burst fracture of the atlas caused by severe axial compression (**Fig. 4**). Diving is a common mechanism. The injury is characterized by unilateral or bilateral fractures of the anterior and posterior arches of C1. As an isolated injury, the Jefferson fracture is not usually associated with neurologic injury because of

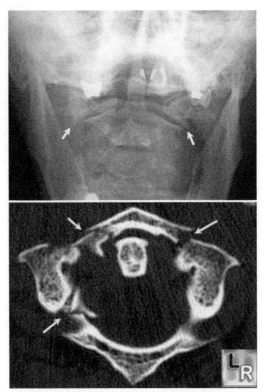

Fig. 4. Jefferson fracture: burst fracture of C1. (*Courtesy of* William Herring, MD, Philadelphia, PA and learningradiology.com. Available at: http://www.learningradiology.com/caseofweek/caseoftheweekpix2006/cow188arr.jpg.)

the width of the spinal canal at that level. However, when it is associated with rupture of the transverse ligament that stabilizes the odontoid to the anterior arch of C1, the Jefferson fracture is very unstable.[11] Associated injuries may include damage to the vertebral artery traversing the foramen transversarium and a second fracture at a lower level.[12] A Jefferson fracture may be diagnosed on an open-mouthed odontoid view by noting displacement of the lateral masses of C1 relative to C2. Overhang of C1 of 6.9 mm over the lateral mass of C2 is diagnostic of a fracture.[13] If this finding is not present but clinical suspicion remains, a computed tomography (CT) scan should be obtained.

Multiple or Complex Mechanism

Odontoid fractures may be 1 of 3 types. The mechanisms are mixed and often unclear. Flexion, extension, and rotation may contribute to the fractures. When evaluating odontoid trauma, emergency physicians should consider that the dens occupies one-third of the spinal canal, the spinal cord occupies another third, and the remaining third is empty space.

A Type I fracture is an avulsion of the tip of the dens above the transverse ligament, thought to be an avulsion fracture from the alar ligaments. In isolation, this injury is usually not associated with instability or spinal cord injury; however, Type I odontoid fractures may be seen in association with atlanto-occipital dislocation. This extremely dangerous injury must be ruled out before conservative treatment is initiated.

A Type II odontoid fracture, the most common of the 3, is localized to the base of the dens (**Fig. 5**). Ten percent of these fractures are associated with damage to the transverse ligament. This complication represents a very unstable injury associated with high mortality. Because of limited blood supply to the fractured dens, nonunion is high. Patients may be treated with halo immobilization or open surgery. Risk factors for nonunion are age older than 50 years and displacement of the fracture.[12,14] Hadley and colleagues[15] reported that displacement of 6 mm or more correlated with a 67% rate of nonunion compared with 26% when displacement was less than 6 mm.

A Type III fracture extends into the body of C2 (**Fig. 6**). It is a mechanically unstable injury because it allows the atlas and occiput to move as a unit. Nonunion is uncommon. Most patients are successfully managed with halo immobilization.

Flexion Mechanism

Among flexion injuries of the cervical spine, the 2 most unstable are the flexion teardrop fracture and the bilateral facet dislocation.[1] The flexion teardrop (**Fig. 7**) is a devastating injury in which substantial force is required to fracture the anterior inferior aspect of the vertebral body. Common mechanisms are motor vehicle crashes and diving. For the teardrop fracture to occur, there must be disruption of the ligaments of the posterior column, displacing the vertebral body posteriorly into the spinal canal. Neurologic injury is very common. The result is often the anterior cord syndrome, manifesting as quadriplegia and loss of pain and temperature sensation. The most common level for a teardrop fracture is C5.[12]

Bilateral facet dislocation is the most severe form of anterior subluxation (**Fig. 8**). At the subluxed level, the inferior facets dislocate superiorly and anteriorly to the superior articulating facets of the lower vertebra, causing complete anterior and posterior longitudinal ligamentous disruption. Subluxation of more than 50% will be seen on a lateral radiograph. Neurologic injury is common.

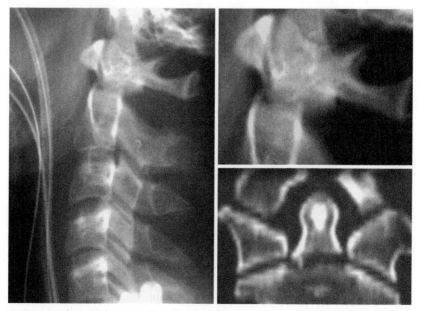

Fig. 5. Type II odontoid fracture. (*Courtesy of* Adam Flanders, MD, Department of Radiology, Thomas Jefferson University Hospital, Philadelphia, PA. Available at: www.radiologyassistant. nl/images/4911d5fd8c73bdens1.jpg.)

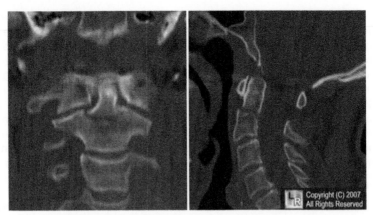

Fig. 6. Type III odontoid fracture. (*Courtesy of* William Herring, MD, Philadelphia, PA. Available at: www.mypacs.net/repos/mpv3_repo/viz/full/108,110/5,405,541.jpg.)

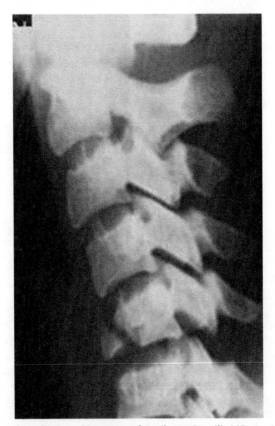

Fig. 7. Flexion teardrop flexion. (*Courtesy of* Amilcare Gentili, MD, La Jolla, CA at www.gentili.net. Available at: www.gentili.net/image.asp?ID=40&imgid=flexteardrop.jpg&Fx=Flexion+Tear+Drop+Fracture.)

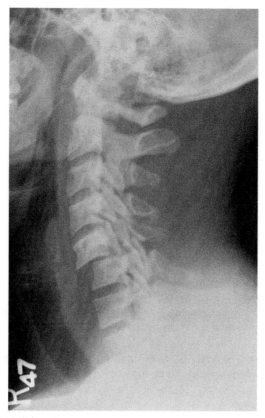

Fig. 8. Bilateral facet dislocation.

Less devastating flexion injuries of the cervical spine include wedge fractures, anterior subluxations, and clay shoveler fractures (an avulsion fracture of the spinous process of C7) (**Fig. 9**). These injuries are usually stable, without neurologic deficit. An anterior subluxation must be evaluated very carefully to rule out disruption of posterior ligaments.

Extension Mechanism

Hangman's fracture is a fracture of the pedicles of the axis or second cervical vertebra (**Fig. 10**). The usual mechanism of injury is extreme hyperextension during a diving accident or motor vehicle collision. This fracture is considered unstable because of its location, but spinal cord injury is not common because the spinal canal is widest at C2. The pedicle fracture allows decompression of the canal, preventing pressure on the spinal cord.[11]

The extension teardrop fracture is a potentially unstable injury caused by neck extension. The most common location is C2 (**Fig. 11**). This fracture is radiographically similar to the flexion teardrop fracture; however, the pathophysiology and mechanism of injury are different. In forced hyperextension, tension on the anterior longitudinal ligament causes avulsion of the anterior inferior aspect of the vertebral body. Neurologic injury is usually not severe, but it is extremely important to prevent neck extension and thus avoid injury to the anterior ligament.[12] When the extensor teardrop

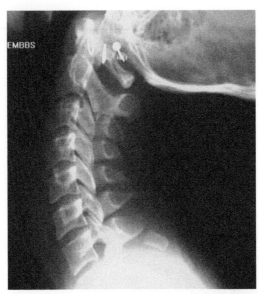

Fig. 9. Clay shoveler's fracture. (*Courtesy of* Dr Kai Ming Liau, Pulau Pinang, Malaysia. Available at: http://static.squidoo.com/resize/squidoo_images/-1/draft_lens2184941module11827967photo_1,222,874,817c7spinousfracture_clay_shovelers.jpg.)

occurs at lower levels, typically C5 to C7, central cord syndrome may be caused by buckling of the ligamentum flavum into the cord.[16]

Vertebral Artery Injury

Vertebral artery occlusion complicates 17% of cervical spine fractures.[17] The cause of occlusion is usually vasospasm or dissection. Most unilateral injuries are not

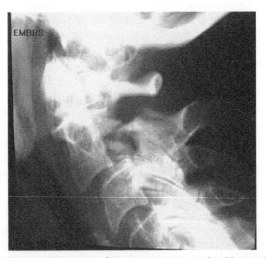

Fig. 10. Hangman's fracture. (*Courtesy of* Dr Kai Ming Liau, Pulau Pinang, Malaysia. Available at: http://static.squidoo.com/resize/squidoo_images/-1/draft_lens2184941module11827962photo_1,222,874,681c2c3subluxation.jpg.)

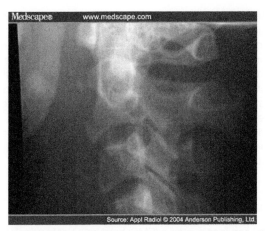

Fig. 11. Extension teardrop fracture. (*Reprinted from* Jarolimek AM, Coffey EC, Sandler CM, et al. Imaging of upper cervical spine injuries—part III: C2 below the dens. Appl Radiol 2004;33(7):9–21; with permission from Anderson Publishing Ltd.)

symptomatic because collateral blood is supplied through the Circle of Willis. When present, typical clinical findings are vertigo, unilateral facial paresthesia, cerebellar signs, lateral medullary signs, and visual field defects.[18] The clinical significance of dissection is the predisposition to thrombus formation, leading to basilar stroke. Cothren and colleagues[19] note a consistent 20% stroke rate in untreated patients. Cervical spine injuries at high risk for vertebral artery injury are fractures associated with subluxation, transverse process fractures extending into the foramen transversarium, and fractures of C1 to C3. Patients with these injuries should be screened for vertebral artery injury.[20] The gold standard test has been 4-vessel cerebrovascular angiography. The increasing availability of multislice CT scans has improved the accuracy of CT angiography for identification of vertebral artery injury.[21]

SPINAL CORD INJURY WITHOUT RADIOGRAPHIC ABNORMALITY

Most often a spinal cord injury is associated with radiographic findings such as fractures, ligamentous injuries, or subluxations. However, a spinal cord injury can occur when bony abnormalities are not present. Spinal cord injury without radiographic abnormality (SCIWORA) is defined as the presence of a spinal cord injury on magnetic resonance imaging (MRI) in the absence of a fracture or subluxation on CT or plain radiography. Most studies limit SCIWORA to injuries of the spinal cord, not just a neurologic deficit that can also represent a peripheral nerve injury or a brachial plexus injury. Once thought to be a finding primarily in children, SCIWORA has now been found to occur more often in adults. A retrospective review of the NEXUS data found that 3.3% of adult patients had SCIWORA,[22] similar to the 4.2% prevalence documented in another more recent retrospective study.[23]

SPINAL AND NEUROGENIC SHOCK

Spinal shock is the phenomenon of loss of reflexes and sensorimotor function below the level of a spinal cord injury. It manifests as flaccid paralysis, including the loss of bowel and bladder reflexes and tone. Spinal shock is a temporary physiologic response to trauma that lasts from hours to days. The degree of recovery depends on the extent of the initial insult. Even with severe injury, patients will recover spinal cord reflex arcs such as the bulbocavernosus and anal wink.[24]

Neurogenic shock refers to hemodynamic instability that occurs in high spinal cord injury, including cervical cord and T1-T4. The 3 major manifestations are hypotension, bradycardia, and hypothermia. Hypotension is the result of sympathetic denervation that causes loss of arteriolar tone and results in venous pooling. Bradycardia occurs with interruption of cardiac sympathetics, allowing unopposed vagal stimulation. A neurogenic source of shock is suggested by the combination of hypotension and bradycardia or variable heart rate response.[25,26] Loss of autonomic regulation occurs in high spinal injuries, contributing to hemodynamic instability and altered thermoregulation, typically manifesting as hypothermia.[27]

PREHOSPITAL MANAGEMENT

Emergency medical services systems (EMS) have one basic principle: deliver fast and efficient patient care for prompt transfer to a hospital. When managing cervical spine injuries, on-scene EMS personnel must rapidly triage patients and attend to the most critical injuries. When performing the initial evaluation, the ABCDEs (airway, breathing, circulation, disability, and exposure) should be monitored first. The airway must be secured before proceeding with the initial evaluation. If the airway needs immediate attention, manual in-line stabilization should be maintained at all times. The first responder must always assume that an injured patient has a spinal cold injury until proven otherwise. The initial insult causes the most damage to the cervical spine, and caution must be taken to prevent further injury. Good immobilization techniques prevent secondary injury and prevent the initial insult from progressing.

EMS personnel follow protocols when approaching a patient with a potential cervical spine injury. The first step is to survey the scene and ensure that it is safe to approach the patient. After securing the ABCs, the EMS provider can move on to the secondary survey, assessing the extent of injuries. For any trauma patient, EMS providers follow standard immobilization procedures. The physician who receives the patient in an emergency department will see various types of immobilization. The most common are the backboard, the rigid cervical collar, spider straps, and head blocks. The most important point is to secure the patient to the backboard to minimize movement in case the patient vomits and needs to be rolled onto the side to prevent aspiration. Another immobilization device is the Kendrick Extrication Device (KED),[28] which is often used to immobilize and extricate patients from vehicles.

The protocol for spinal immobilization is as follows:

1. Maintain the head in neutral in-line position with a cervical collar in place
2. Logroll the patient onto the backboard
3. Secure the torso with spider straps or buckle straps
4. Secure the head to the backboard with foam blocks or towel rolls
5. Secure the legs to the backboard.

The backboard has claimed itself as the gold standard for spine immobilization in the prehospital setting. The backboard helps maintain neutral position of the spinal column en route and helps facilitate easy transfer once at the hospital. Occipital padding achieves the most neutral position; without it 98% of the patients would be in relative extension.[29] Studies are unclear regarding how long the patient should remain on the backboard before he or she is at risk for developing complications, such as increased discomfort or pressure ulcers. Current recommendations suggest timely removal from the backboard as soon as the primary survey is complete and the patient is stable, to avoid such complications.[30]

EMERGENCY DEPARTMENT EVALUATION
Clinical Assessment

A missed cervical spine injury can have devastating consequences. When approaching the trauma patient to evaluate the cervical spine, the emergency physician should first consider whether the spine can be cleared without the use of imaging. It is best to approach the cervical spine evaluation in a structured manner. An unstructured approach to examining the cervical spine has low sensitivity compared with a more systematic approach.[31] One can apply structured clinical decision rules in alert stable patients without neurologic deficits to determine how to proceed with the workup to evaluate for a clinically significant cervical spine injury. A clinically important cervical spine injury is defined as any fracture, dislocation, or ligamentous instability demonstrated on diagnostic imaging. A clinically unimportant injury is defined as an isolated avulsion fracture of an osteophyte, an isolated fracture of a transverse process not involving a facet joint, an isolated fracture of a spinous process not involving the lamina, or a simple compression fracture involving less than 25% of the vertebral body height.

Airway Management

Patients presenting to the emergency department may require emergency airway management before a full assessment for cervical spine injuries can be performed. When approaching the trauma patient, the physician should assume that an injury to the cervical spine is present. If the patient has an associated head injury, with a GCS score of less than 9, the risk of cervical spine injury increases significantly. This patient is also the one who most likely needs an emergent airway. Lesions above C3 cause immediate need for airway management because of respiratory paralysis. Lower lesions may cause phrenic nerve paralysis or increasing respiratory distress from ascending edema. Injuries to the cervical spine may cause local swelling, edema, or hematoma formation that may obstruct the airway, necessitating intubation.

Recommendations for managing the airway of a trauma patient are[32]:

1. Rapid-sequence intubation (RSI): When managing an unconscious patient, standard drugs should be used for paralysis and induction
2. Manual in-line stabilization: An assistant firmly holds both sides of the patient's head, with the neck in the midline and the head on a firm surface throughout the procedure, to reduce cervical spine movement and minimize potential injury to the spinal cord
3. Orotracheal intubation is preferred in trauma patients requiring intubation
4. Use a tracheal tube introducer such as a Bougie or stylet
5. Have a selection of blades ready: evidence supports the use of a Macintosh blade
6. A laryngeal mask airway (LMA) can be used as a temporary device.

Manual in-line immobilization (MILI), as described by Crosby,[33] is designed to hold sufficient forces on either side of the head to prevent movement during interventions such as airway management. There are 2 approaches to MILI: (1) an assistant standing at the head of the bed grasps the patient's mastoid process with the fingertips and then cradles the occiput in the palms of the hands; or (2) an assistant standing at the side of the bed cradles the mastoids and grasps the occiput with the fingers. Once the head and neck are stabilized by one of these methods, the front of the cervical collar can be removed to increase mouth opening and visualization by direct laryngoscopy. The neck should be maintained in neutral position throughout the procedure, and the anterior aspect of the collar should be replaced promptly when it has been completed.

Ideally, MILI should prevent all movement that may worsen a spinal cord injury. In practice, this goal is not necessarily achieved. Crosby[33] found that MILI minimizes distraction and angulation at the level of injury but has no effect on subluxation at the injury site. MILI may improve laryngoscopic views compared with immobilization with a collar, sandbags, or tape. In Crosby's series, only poor views (grade 3 or 4), caused by limited mouth opening, were obtained in 64% of patients immobilized with techniques other than MILI and in 22% of the MILI group.[33] In a retrospective study, Patterson[34] evaluated neurologic outcome in patients with cervical spine injury who required emergent intubation in the emergency department. No patients in whom cervical spine injury was subsequently identified had a worsening of neurologic outcome related to immobilization. This study did not consider the specific technique used to immobilize the cervical spine, but did assume that a cervical spine injury was present in all patients presenting with trauma.

Cord-Level Findings

Neurologic deficits correlate with the level of the injury, resulting in weakness or paralysis below the lesion. There are 8 pairs of spinal nerves in the cervical spine. The dermatomal distribution for the cord at each vertebra is listed in **Fig. 12**. From C1 to C7, the nerve root exits above the level of the vertebra; from C8 and below, the nerve root exits below the level of the vertebra.

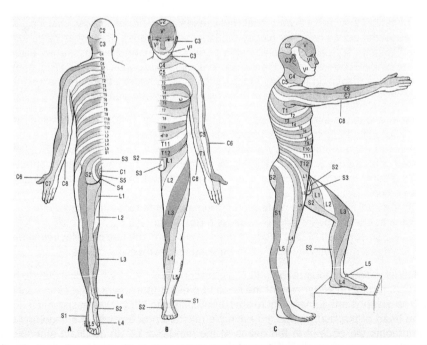

Fig. 12. Dermatome map. (*From* Agur AMR, Lee MJ, Anderson JE. Dermatomes. In: Grant's atlas of anatomy. 9th edition. Philadelphia: Lippincott Williams & Wilkins; 1991. p. 252.)

The presentation of incomplete cord injuries depends on the level and location of the lesion. The anterior column conveys motor function, pain, and temperature, and the posterior column conveys impulses related to fine touch, vibration, and proprioception. Syndromes resulting from partial injuries are described here.

Partial Cord Syndromes

Anterior cord syndrome results from compression of the anterior spinal artery, direct compression of the anterior cord, or compression induced by fragments from burst fractures. Anterior cord syndrome manifests as complete motor paralysis, with loss of pain and temperature perception distal to the lesion. Posterior cord syndrome is very rare; involvement of the posterior column is most often seen in Brown-Séquard syndrome.

Brown-Séquard syndrome is characterized by paralysis, loss of vibration sensation, and proprioception ipsilaterally, with contralateral loss of pain and temperature sensation. These signs and symptoms result from hemisection of the spinal cord, most often from penetrating trauma or compression from a lateral fracture.

Central cord syndrome, induced by damage to the corticospinal tract, is characterized by weakness in the upper extremities, more so than in the lower extremities. The weakness is more pronounced in the distal portion of the extremities. This injury is usually caused by hyperextension in a person with an underlying condition such as stenosis or spondylosis.

CERVICAL SPINE IMAGING

Two decision rules guide the use of cervical spine radiography in patients with trauma: the NEXUS Low Risk Criteria (NLC) and the Canadian C-Spine Rule (CCR). The NLC were derived from the National Emergency X-radiography Use Study (NEXUS), which was designed to identify patients who do not need diagnostic imaging to exclude a clinically significant cervical spine injury. Cervical spine radiographs are indicated for trauma patients unless they have all of the following 5 characteristics: they are alert, are not intoxicated, have no posterior midline tenderness, have no neurologic indications of the injury, and have no distracting injuries (eg, a long bone fracture, a large laceration, a crush injury, a large burn, or another injury that produces acute functional impairment). The definitions of "intoxicated" and "distracting injury" are open to interpretation, requiring physician judgment in deciding whether to obtain imaging studies.

The CCR was developed out of concern for the potentially low specificity and sensitivity of the NLC for detecting clinically significant cervical spine injuries.[35] The CCR poses 3 questions:

1. Does the patient have any high-risk factors? Patients are at higher risk if they are older than 65 years, if their mechanism of injury was "dangerous," or if they experienced paresthesia in the extremities after the injury. Examples of dangerous mechanisms of injury include fall from a height greater than 3 ft, axial load to the head, high-speed motor vehicle crash, rollover, ejection, and bicycle crash.
2. Are any low-risk factors present that would allow a safe assessment of range of motion? Low-risk criteria include simple rear-end motor vehicle crash, the ability to sit upright in the emergency department, ambulation at any point after the incident, delayed onset of neck pain, and the absence of midline cervical spine tenderness.
3. Is the patient able to actively rotate the neck 45° to the left and right? If the patient has active rotation of the neck as well as low-risk factors and the absence of

high-risk factors, then the physician can safely clear the spine without radiographic imaging.[35]

A prospective cohort study done in Canada found the CCR to be more sensitive (99.4% vs 90.7%) and specific (45.1% vs 36.8%) than the NLC for detecting injury. In addition, the CCR resulted in decreased radiography rates (55.9% vs 66.6%).[36]

Imaging Modalities

Three methods exist for imaging the cervical spine in the emergency department: plain radiographs, CT, and MRI. Each has advantages and disadvantages, and the clinical situation must be considered when deciding which method to use.

Plain radiography typically includes 3 views: anteroposterior, lateral, and odontoid. This imaging modality is falling out of favor because its false-negative rate is higher than that associated with CT. Emergency departments commonly rely on CT imaging to evaluate patients for injury. CT allows easy imaging of the cervical spine when clinically indicated. A CT scan is best for detecting bony abnormalities; it can detect 97% of osseous fractures. When ligamentous injury or spinal cord injury is suspected, MRI is indicated. Holmes and colleagues[37] reported that CT detected no spinal cord injuries and only 25% of ligamentous injuries in trauma patients. In the same series, MRI allowed discovery of all spinal cord and ligamentous injuries.

EMERGENCY DEPARTMENT MANAGEMENT

The treatment of cervical spine injuries begins after the initial clinical evaluation. After management of the airway, attention to hemodynamic support and blood pressure management is essential. Hypotension should not be attributed to neurogenic shock until blood loss or other trauma-related causes have been managed or ruled out. Regardless of etiology, it is critically important to aggressively manage hypotension in patients with cervical cord injuries. Hypotension is associated with worse outcomes and is thought to contribute to secondary injury because of reduced spinal cord perfusion.[38]

The goal for optimal spinal cord perfusion is maintenance of a mean arterial pressure of 85 to 90 mm Hg. Unstable patients require arterial lines and central venous or Swan Ganz monitoring. Initial treatment is with crystalloid. If indicated, blood transfusion should be started to correct blood loss. After volume correction, if the mean arterial pressure remains low, pressors should be initiated. A vasopressor should be chosen with the goal of treating both hypotension and bradycardia. Agents with α- and β-agonist properties, such as dopamine, norepinephrine, or epinephrine, are preferred to provide both inotropic and chronotropic support. Caution is warranted when considering the use of phenylephrine its pure stimulation of α-receptors is associated with reflex bradycardia. Bradycardia may require atropine or a pacemaker.[27,38]

In patients with a cervical spine injury and abnormal neurologic examination, the question of the efficacy and safety of methylprednisolone arises. Three multicenter, randomized, double-blind clinical trials have studied this question. Results of the National Acute Spinal Cord Injury Studies I, II, and III (NASCI I, II, and III) were published in 1984, 1990, and 1997.[39–41] The first study compared outcomes in patients treated with a 100-mg bolus of methylprednisolone and then 100 mg daily for 10 days with those of patients treated with a 1000-mg bolus and then 1000 mg per day for 10 days in 330 patients with acute spinal injury. The investigators reported no difference in neurologic recovery at 6 weeks and 6 months after injury. A control group was not used.

NASCI II used a much higher dose of methylprednisolone (a 30-mg/kg bolus followed by a 5.4-mg/kg/h infusion for 23 hours). This group was compared with patients with comparable injuries treated with a naloxone regimen or placebo. A total of 487 patients were enrolled and divided into 3 treatment arms. Patients in the methylprednisolone arm treated within 8 hours of injury had a statistically significant improvement in motor and sensory function at 6 months compared with those in the other 2 groups. The *Guidelines for the Management of Acute Cervical Spine and Spinal Cord Injuries*, published by the American Association of Neurological Surgeons (AANS), document methodological, scientific, and statistical flaws in the trial, citing numerous criticisms in follow-up publications.[38]

The NASCIS III trial compared the efficacy of methylprednisolone for 24 hours with that of a 48-hour regimen. The salient findings were that patients in all groups treated within 3 hours after injury did equally well. Among patients treated between 3 and 8 hours after injury, those receiving the 48-hour regimen were statistically significantly better at 6 weeks and 6 months than those treated for 24 hours. Unfortunately, patients treated for 48 hours also had higher rates of severe sepsis and severe pneumonia. Nevertheless, the investigators recommended 24 hours of treatment for those receiving methylprednisolone within 3 hours of injury and 48 hours of therapy for those for whom treatment started 3 to 8 hours after injury.[41] In their published guidelines, however, the AANS concludes that the available evidence does not demonstrate significant clinical benefit of treatment of patients with acute spinal cord injury with methylprednisolone for either 24 or 48 hours. The report states, "In light of the failure of clinical trials to convincingly demonstrate a significant clinical benefit of administration of methylprednisolone, in conjunction with the increased risks of medical complications associated with its use, methylprednisolone in the treatment of acute humans spinal cord injury is recommended as an option that should only be undertaken with the knowledge that the evidence suggesting harmful side effects is more consistent than the suggestion of clinical benefit."[38] The investigators suggest that emergency physicians consider the individual factors unique to each clinical case when making the decision of whether to initiate treatment. Consultation with the accepting trauma service or neurosurgeon is appropriate and encouraged.

Surprisingly little evidence exists to guide emergency physicians when treating patients with cervical strain without associated fracture or neurologic deficit. Commonly used modalities include rest, ice, analgesics, and muscle relaxants. Acetaminophen and nonsteroidal anti-inflammatory medications are the cornerstones of analgesic therapy in the United States. Turturro and colleagues[42] studied the efficacy of 800 mg ibuprofen with and without cyclobenzaprine administered to adults with acute myofascial strain. These investigators found significant pain relief at 48 hours but no incremental benefit to the use of cyclobenzaprine. Central nervous system side effects were more prevalent in the group receiving cyclobenzaprine. Cyclobenzaprine alone, however, has demonstrated efficacy in acute muscle spasm of the neck and back.[43] One study showed no difference in pain relief between patients receiving 5 mg 3 times per day and 10 mg 3 times per day. Sedation was lower in the former group. A Cochrane Review found that administration of intravenous methylprednisolone within 8 hours of injury significantly reduced pain at 1 week and decreased days lost from work at 6 months.[44] Other evidence suggests that gentle exercise and physical therapy are more efficacious than rest, soft collar, and gradual advancement of neck mobility.[45] Based on the limited evidence to date, the authors recommend gentle range of motion exercises and treatment with an analgesic such as ibuprofen. In patients with contraindications to nonsteroidal anti-inflammatory medications or palpable spasm, a muscle relaxant such as cyclobenzaprine at 5 mg 3 times per day may be substituted. All patients should follow up with a primary care physician who can arrange for physical therapy if necessary.

DISPOSITION

Early consultation with a spine or neurosurgeon is critical to optimal management of cervical spine injuries. Early intervention accomplishing closed reduction, halo traction, open reduction, or decompression of serious injuries with cord compromise provides the best patient outcomes. Critical care consultation and admission to the intensive care unit are indicated for unstable cervical spine fractures or spinal cord injury. Numerous studies document the benefits and improved neurologic outcomes of optimal hemodynamic and respiratory management. Severely injured patients frequently suffer from hypotension, cardiac instability, hypoxemia, and pulmonary dysfunction for 7 to 14 days.[38] Placement of a hard cervical collar provides protection from a secondary injury. Those with minor muscular and ligamentous strain may be treated symptomatically with analgesics or muscle relaxants and gentle range of motion exercises.

SUMMARY

Cervical spine trauma is high risk and anxiety provoking for patients and emergency physicians. A detailed understanding of the clinical approach to the patient in the field and the emergency department is essential to limit morbidity. This article has reviewed the clinical and radiographic evaluation, relevant anatomy, common fractures, and management principles. Careful study and implementation of these concepts provides the emergency physician with the necessary knowledge to safely and expertly care for this important group of injured patients.

ACKNOWLEDGMENTS

The authors thank Linda Kesselring, ELS for technical assistance in the preparation of the manuscript.

REFERENCES

1. Davenport M, Mueller J, Belaval E, et al. Fracture, cervical spine. eMedicine Specialties, Emergency Medicine, Trauma & Orthopedics; 2008 [online].
2. Goldberg W, Mueller C, Panacek E, et al. Distribution and patterns of blunt traumatic cervical spine injury. Ann Emerg Med 2001;38(1):17–21.
3. Lowery DW, Wald MM, Browne BJ, et al. Epidemiology of cervical spine injury victims. Ann Emerg Med 2001;38(1):12–6.
4. Damadi AA, Saxe AW, Fath JJ, et al. Cervical spine fractures in patients 65 years or older: a 3-year experience at a level I trauma center. J Trauma 2008;64(3): 745–8.
5. Holly LT, Kelly DF, Counelis GJ, et al. Cervical spine trauma associated with moderate and severe head injury: incidence, risk factors, and injury characteristics. J Neurosurg 2002;96(Suppl 3):285–91.
6. Gray H. Osteology. In: Goss CM, editor. Gray's anatomy. 29th edition. Philadelphia: Lea & Febiger; 1973. p. 95–286.
7. Nakano K. Neck pain. In: Ruddy S, Harris EJ, Sledge C, editors. Textbook of rheumatology. 6th edition. Philadelphia: Saunders; 2001. p. 458.
8. Devereaux MW. Anatomy and examination of the spine. Neurol Clin 2007;25(2): 331–51.

9. Maroon JC, Abla AA. Classification of acute spinal cord injury, neurological evaluation, and neurosurgical considerations. Crit Care Clin 1987;3(3):655–77.
10. White AA 3rd, Johnson RM, Panjabi MM, et al. Biomechanical analysis of clinical stability in the cervical spine. Clin Orthop Relat Res 1975;109:85–96.
11. Hockberger R, Kaji A, Newton E. Spinal injuries. In: Marx JA, Hockberger RS, Walls RM, editors. Rosen's emergency medicine: concepts and clinical practice, vol. I. 7th edition. Philadelphia: Elsevier; 2009. Chapter 40.
12. Wheeless C III. Wheeless' textbook of orthopaedics. In: Wheeless C III, Nunley J II, Urbaniak, editors. Durham (NC): Data Trace Internet Publishing, LLC; 2009.
13. Foster M. C1 Fractures. eMedicine Specialties, Orthopedic Surgery. Spine; 2009 [online].
14. Sama A, Girardi F, Cammisa F Jr. Cervical spine injuries in sports: multimedia. eMedicine Specialties, Orthopedic Surgery. Spine; 2008 [online].
15. Hadley MN, Browner C, Sonntag VK. Axis fractures: a comprehensive review of management and treatment in 107 cases. Neurosurgery 1985;17(2):281–90.
16. Guthkelch AN, Fleischer AS. Patterns of cervical spine injury and their associated lesions. West J Med 1987;147(4):428–31.
17. Taneichi H, Suda K, Kajino T, et al. Traumatically induced vertebral artery occlusion associated with cervical spine injuries: prospective study using magnetic resonance angiography. Spine (Phila Pa 1976) 2005;30(17):1955–62.
18. Saeed AB, Shuaib A, Al-Sulaiti G, et al. Vertebral artery dissection: warning symptoms, clinical features and prognosis in 26 patients. Can J Neurol Sci 2000;27(4):292–6.
19. Cothren CC, Moore EE, Ray CE Jr, et al. Screening for blunt cerebrovascular injuries is cost-effective. Am J Surg 2005;190(6):845–9.
20. Cothren CC, Moore EE, Ray CE Jr, et al. Cervical spine fracture patterns mandating screening to rule out blunt cerebrovascular injury. Surgery 2007;141(1):76–82.
21. Biffl WL, Egglin T, Benedetto B, et al. Sixteen-slice computed tomographic angiography is a reliable noninvasive screening test for clinically significant blunt cerebrovascular injuries. J Trauma 2006;60(4):745–51 [discussion: 751–2].
22. Hendey GW, Wolfson AB, Mower WR, et al. Spinal cord injury without radiographic abnormality: results of the National Emergency X-Radiography Utilization Study in blunt cervical trauma. J Trauma 2002;53(1):1–4.
23. Kasimatis GB, Panagiotopoulos E, Megas P, et al. The adult spinal cord injury without radiographic abnormalities syndrome: magnetic resonance imaging and clinical findings in adults with spinal cord injuries having normal radiographs and computed tomography studies. J Trauma 2008;65(1):86–93.
24. Atkinson PP, Atkinson JL. Spinal shock. Mayo Clin Proc 1996;71(4):384–9.
25. Bilello JF, Davis JW, Cunningham MA, et al. Cervical spinal cord injury and the need for cardiovascular intervention. Arch Surg 2003;138(10):1127–9.
26. Gondim FA, Lopes AC Jr, Oliveira GR, et al. Cardiovascular control after spinal cord injury. Curr Vasc Pharmacol 2004;2(1):71–9.
27. Wing PC. Early acute management in adults with spinal cord injury: a clinical practice guideline for health-care providers. Who should read it? J Spinal Cord Med 2008;31(4):360.
28. Howell JM, Burrow R, Dumontier C, et al. A practical radiographic comparison of short board technique and Kendrick Extrication Device. Ann Emerg Med 1989; 18(9):943–6.
29. Schriger DL, Larmon B, LeGassick T, et al. Spinal immobilization on a flat backboard: does it result in neutral position of the cervical spine? Ann Emerg Med 1991;20(8):878–81.

30. Vickery D. The use of the spinal board after the pre-hospital phase of trauma management. Emerg Med J 2001;18(1):51–4.

31. Bandiera G, Stiell IG, Wells GA, et al. The Canadian C-spine rule performs better than unstructured physician judgment. Ann Emerg Med 2003;42(3):395–402.

32. Ollerton JE, Parr MJ, Harrison K, et al. Potential cervical spine injury and difficult airway management for emergency intubation of trauma adults in the emergency department—a systematic review. Emerg Med J 2006;23(1):3–11.

33. Crosby ET. Airway management in adults after cervical spine trauma. Anesthesiology 2006;104(6):1293–318.

34. Patterson H. Emergency department intubation of trauma patients with undiagnosed cervical spine injury. Emerg Med J 2004;21(3):302–5.

35. Stiell IG, Wells GA, Vandemheen KL, et al. The Canadian C-spine rule for radiography in alert and stable trauma patients. JAMA 2001;286(15):1841–8.

36. Stiell IG, Clement CM, McKnight RD, et al. The Canadian C-spine rule versus the NEXUS low-risk criteria in patients with trauma. N Engl J Med 2003;349(26):2510–8.

37. Holmes JF, Mirvis SE, Panacek EA, et al. Variability in computed tomography and magnetic resonance imaging in patients with cervical spine injuries. J Trauma 2002;53(3):524–9 [discussion: 530].

38. Hadley M, Walters B, Grabb P, et al. Guidelines for the management of acute cervical spine and spinal cord injuries. Rolling Meadows (IL): American Association of Neurological Surgeons: Section on Disorders of the Spine and Peripheral Nervies; 2007.

39. Bracken MB, Collins WF, Freeman DF, et al. Efficacy of methylprednisolone in acute spinal cord injury. JAMA 1984;251(1):45–52.

40. Bracken MB, Shepard MJ, Collins WF, et al. A randomized, controlled trial of methylprednisolone or naloxone in the treatment of acute spinal-cord injury. Results of the Second National Acute Spinal Cord Injury Study. N Engl J Med 1990;322(20):1405–11.

41. Bracken MB, Shepard MJ, Holford TR, et al. Administration of methylprednisolone for 24 or 48 hours or tirilazad mesylate for 48 hours in the treatment of acute spinal cord injury. Results of the Third National Acute Spinal Cord Injury Randomized Controlled Trial. National Acute Spinal Cord Injury Study. JAMA 1997;277(20):1597–604.

42. Turturro MA, Frater CR, D'Amico FJ. Cyclobenzaprine with ibuprofen versus ibuprofen alone in acute myofascial strain: a randomized, double-blind clinical trial. Ann Emerg Med 2003;41(6):818–26.

43. Borenstein DG, Korn S. Efficacy of a low-dose regimen of cyclobenzaprine hydrochloride in acute skeletal muscle spasm: results of two placebo-controlled trials. Clin Ther 2003;25(4):1056–73.

44. Peloso P, Gross A, Haines T, et al. Medicinal and injection therapies for mechanical neck disorders. Cochrane Database Syst Rev 2007;3:CD000319.

45. Rosenfeld M, Gunnarsson R, Borenstein P. Early intervention in whiplash-associated disorders: a comparison of two treatment protocols. Spine (Phila Pa 1976) 2000;25(14):1782–7.

Emergent Evaluation of Injuries to the Shoulder, Clavicle, and Humerus

Sanjeev Malik, MD[a],*, George Chiampas, DO[a,b,c],
Heather Leonard, MD[a]

KEYWORDS

- Shoulder emergencies • Proximal humerus fractures
- Acromioclavicular separation • Shoulder dislocations

The shoulder is the most mobile joint in the body, serving a great many functions. In exchange for enhanced mobility, the shoulder also has inherent instability, placing it at increased risk of injury. Injuries to the shoulder girdle account for 8% to 13% of athletic injuries and are a frequent reason for seeking emergent medical attention.[1] Expertise in the acute diagnosis, stabilization, and management of these injuries is an essential part of the skill set of an emergency provider (EP).

EVALUATION

An accurate history and physical examination may be all that is required in the evaluation of the patient with shoulder pain. The EP should be careful to consider all causes of shoulder pain including infectious, bony, and soft tissue injuries, as well as referred pain from more serious pathology such as myocardial ischemia, biliary disease, and cervical injuries. Certain historical features may have prognostic value in focusing the differential for the injured patient, as shown in **Table 1**.

Physical examination of the shoulder, clavicle, and humerus involves careful inspection, palpation, passive and active range of motion testing, neurovascular assessment, strength testing, and provocative tests. As with all orthopedic examinations, evaluation of the joint proximal (cervical spine) and distal (elbow) is prudent. Whereas deformities from glenohumeral dislocations, clavicle fractures, and acromioclavicular

Disclosures: The authors have no financial interest to disclose.
a Department of Emergency Medicine, Feinberg School of Medicine, Northwestern University, 259 East Erie Street, Suite 100, Chicago, IL 60610, USA
b Bank of America Chicago Marathon, 135 South LaSalle Street, Suite 2705, Chicago, IL 60603, USA
c Northwestern University Athletics, 1501 Central Street, Evanston, IL 60208, USA
* Corresponding author.
E-mail address: s-malik@northwestern.edu

Emerg Med Clin N Am 28 (2010) 739–763
doi:10.1016/j.emc.2010.06.006
0733-8627/10/$ – see front matter © 2010 Elsevier Inc. All rights reserved.

Table 1
Suggested differential diagnosis with certain historical features

Historical Feature		Differential Diagnosis to Consider
Age	Age <40 y	Glenohumeral instability/dislocation, labral tears, acromioclavicular separations
	Age >40 y	Rotator cuff tears, proximal humerus fractures, impingement syndrome, adhesive capsulitis
Duration	Acute	Glenohumeral dislocations, acromioclavicular separations, shoulder contusions, rotator cuff tears, biceps/pectoralis rupture
	Chronic	Impingement syndrome, biceps tendinosis
Mechanism	Traumatic	Glenohumeral dislocations, acromioclavicular separations, proximal humerus fracture
	Atraumatic/repetitive microtrauma	Impingement syndrome, labral tears, glenohumeral instability, osteoarthritis
History of diabetes		Adhesive capsulitis, septic arthritis
Limitations in passive range of motion		Glenohumeral dislocations, proximal humerus fracture, adhesive capsulitis
Mechanical symptoms		Labral tear, osteoarthritis, intra-articular loose body
Muscle weakness		Rotator cuff tear, brachial plexus injury
Prior instability or dislocation		Glenohumeral instability/dislocation, impingement syndrome, labral tears, biceps tendinosis
Fever		Septic arthritis, acute cholecystitis

Data from Refs.[4,14,107]

separations are often clinically apparent, detection of effusion, ecchymosis, or erythema on visual inspection may be more subtle.

Palpation of the sternoclavicular (SC) joint, clavicle, acromioclavicular (AC) joint, and proximal humerus should be performed to assess for crepitus and tenderness. The long head of the biceps can be palpated in the intertubercular groove when the shoulder is externally rotated. In addition to palpation, accurate assessments of active and passive range of motion have diagnostic value. An individual typically can perform 170° abduction, 150° to 170° forward flexion, 90° external rotation, and internal rotation to approximately the T7 spinous level.[2,3] Active range of motion may be limited by pain or functional deficits. However, passive range of motion is preserved in most injuries. Limitations in passive range of motion should increase the suspicion for adhesive capsulitis, osteoarthritis, fracture, or dislocation.[4]

Early assessment of neurovascular structures and prompt recognition of neurovascular compromise is an essential part of the examination and a common pitfall for the EP. Electromyogram (EMG) studies suggest that neurovascular injuries occur in approximately 45% of shoulder dislocations and humeral fractures, although many are not diagnosed at the time of injury or clinically apparent.[5,6] Elderly age, inferior dislocations, fracture-dislocations, and hematoma have been associated with a higher incidence of neurovascular injury. The most commonly injured structure is the axillary nerve (37%), followed by the suprascapular (29%) and radial nerves (22%).[5] The axillary nerve provides sensation to the lateral deltoid in the distribution commonly referred to as the "policeman's badge." Although approximately 87% of neurologic injuries will recover with expectant management, the presence of neurologic or vascular compromise in the ED warrants prompt reduction of fracture fragments or dislocations and should be managed in consultation with an orthopedic surgeon.[6]

After careful neurovascular assessment, the examiner should perform strength testing of the rotator cuff (**Fig. 1**), biceps, triceps, and deltoid muscles. The supraspinatus muscle assists the deltoid muscle with abduction of the arm and is commonly assessed with the empty can test (sensitivity 0.50–0.89, specificity 0.50–0.98).[7–9] The infraspinatus and teres minor muscles are responsible for external rotation of the glenohumeral joint. Strength testing of these 2 muscles can be performed with the external rotation test (sensitivity 0.51, specificity 0.84).[9] The fourth rotator cuff muscle, the subscapularis, performs internal rotation of the glenohumeral joint and can be evaluated by the liftoff test (sensitivity 0.17–0.92, specificity 0.60–0.92).[7,9,10] For all of the above strength tests, a positive test is defined by weakness compared with the contralateral side as determined by the examiner. While individual test accuracy varies in the published literature, objective weakness has a relatively high specificity in the detection of a partial or complete rotator cuff tear.[4] The presence of pain without weakness may be suggestive of rotator cuff impingement.

In addition to the basic examination maneuvers described, there is an array of specialized provocative tests that may be indicated and have diagnostic value in the assessment of the patient with acute shoulder pain. A select few of these tests relevant to the EP are described herein. If rotator cuff impingement is suspected, the Neer[11] and Hawkins[12] tests may be performed as described in **Fig. 2**A and B. A recent pooled meta-analysis of the Neer test showed a sensitivity of 0.79 but relatively poor specificity (0.53), whereas the Hawkins test has similar sensitivity with slightly greater specificity (0.59).[7]

In patients with suspected subluxation, recent dislocation, or instability, the apprehension and relocation tests are 2 highly sensitive and specific tests that may be performed to assess for instability.[4] To perform the apprehension test, the patient should be placed in the supine position with the affected arm abducted 90° and flexed 90° at the elbow.[13] The examiner should then apply an external rotation force to the arm. If the patient develops discomfort and a sensation of impending dislocation, the test is suggestive of anterior glenohumeral instability. If the apprehension test is positive, the relocation test may also be performed with the examiner applying a posteriorly directed force to the humeral head. A decrease in patient discomfort with the relocation test further suggests anterior instability.[4,14]

The cross-arm adduction test (sensitivity 0.77) can be used to evaluate suspected acromioclavicular injuries.[15,16] With the arm forward flexed at 90°, the arm is adducted across the body toward the contralateral arm, providing a compressive force at the AC joint. Pain localized at this joint is suggestive of AC pathology. If biceps tendon pathology is suspected, the examiner may perform the Speed test (sensitivity 0.54, specificity 0.81) by resisting forward flexion with the arm extended at the elbow and the forearm supinated.[17] Palpable subluxation or pain localized in the intertubercular groove is suggestive of biceps involvement.[18]

Plain radiography is inexpensive, readily available, and adequate for the initial evaluation of most injuries to the shoulder girdle. Standard shoulder radiography should include at least 2 views: an anteroposterior (AP) view and a lateral projection, either an axillary lateral or scapular Y view. Failure to obtain a lateral projection view may result in inadequate assessment of the glenohumeral relationship. An additional AP internal or external rotation view is often performed in many hospitals but does not substitute for a true lateral projection.

An AP view and 45° cephalic tilt view is recommended for evaluation of the suspected clavicle fracture. A serendipity view (40° cephalic tilt centered on the manubrium) may be performed for better assessment of medial clavicle fractures and sternoclavicular joint injuries while a Zanca view (10°–15° cephalic tilt) may give better

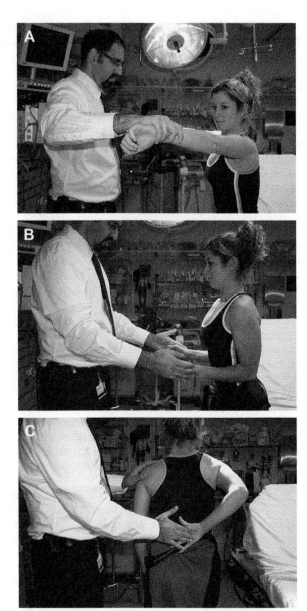

Fig. 1. Rotator cuff strength testing. (*A*) Empty can test.[8] The examiner isolates the supraspi-natus by placing the patient's arm in 90° abduction and 30° forward flexion with the elbow in full extension and the arm in internal rotation with the thumb pointed downward. The examiner then places downward pressure on the arm while the patient resists. (*B*) External rotation test. The examiner resists active external rotation by the patient with the arm adducted at the side and the elbow flexed at 90°. (*C*) Liftoff test.[10] The patient places the affected arm behind his back with the dorsum of his hand against the lumbar spine. The patient then attempts to actively lift the hand away from the spine against resistance provided by the examiner. (*Courtesy of* the Northwestern Emergency Medicine teaching file, copyright 2010; with permission.)

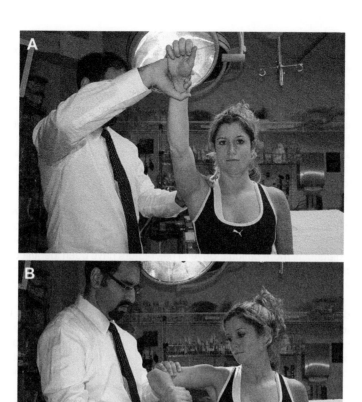

Fig. 2. Tests for impingement. (*A*) Neer[11] test. The examiner performs passive forward flexion of the arm to 180° with the arm fully pronated. Reproduction of pain above 90° suggests impingement. (*B*) Hawkins and Kennedy[12] test. The patient's arm is placed in 90° forward flexion with the elbow flexed. The examiner then forcibly internally rotates the arm. Discomfort suggests impingement.[14] (*Courtesy of* the Northwestern Emergency Medicine teaching file, copyright 2010; with permission.)

visualization of the distal clavicle and acromioclavicular joint.[19,20] Computed tomography (CT) is the test of choice in evaluating suspected sternoclavicular injuries.[21,22] Although magnetic resonance imaging (MRI) provides excellent assessment of the soft-tissue structures, it is of limited value in the acute evaluation of the patient in the ED setting.

CAUSES OF SHOULDER PAIN
Septic Arthritis

Septic arthritis is a disease that affects all age groups yet is most prevalent in children. The morbidity of associated cartilage destruction can be debilitating, and there is an 8% to 15% associated mortality rate.[23] This disease tends to affect weight-bearing joints such as the hip and knee; however, a recent case series has shown the gleno-humeral joint to be involved in 12% of cases.[24] Septic arthritis typically is a monoartic-ular process, with polyarticular presentations occurring in fewer than 20% of cases.[23]

In adults, common pathogens of monoarticular septic arthritis include *Staphylococcus aureus*, *Streptococcus pneumoniae*, and gram-negative bacilli, whereas *Haemophilus influenzae* type b (Hib) is the most common organism affecting children younger than 2 years. In young, sexually active individuals or in patients with polyar-thritic involvement, *Neisseria gonorrhoeae* is the most common offending organism.[23] Recently, septic arthritis caused by methicillin-resistant *S aureus* (MRSA) has become more prevalent and is the most common organism in some institutions.[25] Septic arthritis occurs as a result of inoculation of bacteria into the joint via either hematog-enous spread or direct injury such as recent trauma or surgery.

Children with septic arthritis often appear acutely ill with irritability, fever, tachy-cardia, and pain with any motion of the limb. Alternatively, older adults, particularly those with a prosthesis, may only have vague complaints of joint pain or swelling, making the diagnosis more difficult. Several risk factors have been identified including age older than 80 years, diabetes mellitus, rheumatoid arthritis, recent joint surgery, immunocompromised status, intravenous drug abuse, overlying skin infections, and prosthesis in conjunction with skin infections.[26]

The predominant complaint for many patients is joint pain exacerbated by move-ment, found in 85% of cases. Joint swelling is present in 78% of cases whereas fever is noted in only half of patients with septic arthritis.[23] Although there are no definitive physical examination findings of septic arthritis, certain signs may be suggestive. Identification of a potential infectious source near the shoulder such as a penetrating wound or overlying cellulitis should raise the examiner's suspicion for septic arthritis. It is also important to note any swelling and the positioning of the shoulder, as patients with septic arthritis often hold the arm in a position of comfort.

Standard laboratory evaluation should include a white blood cell count (WBC), erythrocyte sedimentation rate (ESR), and C-reactive protein (CRP) measurement in addition to blood cultures.[27] Radiographs of the shoulder are indicated to evaluate for effusion and/or bony disruption; however, the gold standard for diagnosis is syno-vial fluid analysis with cell counts, Gram stain, and culture obtained after arthrocentesis.[23,27,28]

While traditionally a WBC count greater than 50,000/mm^3 has been considered the hallmark of diagnosis, there is no absolute WBC count, ESR, or CRP value that is sensi-tive or specific enough to make the diagnosis of septic arthritis.[23,25,27,29] In fact, syno-vial WBC counts less than 50,000/mm^3 occur in 39% of cases of culture-proven septic arthritis.[28] This result may be in part due to of the increased prevalence of MRSA, which in a recent case series was found to have much lower synovial WBC counts than other organisms with an average of 15,000 WBC/mm^3.[25] A negative Gram stain also cannot exclude septic arthritis. The initial Gram stain may be negative in 55% of cases and in up to 90% of patients with gonococcal arthritis.[28] The presence of crystals on synovial analysis is highly suggestive of an alternative origin of discomfort; however, the EP must be careful to consider concurrent infection, which occurs in 1.5% of patients.[30]

There are no absolute contraindications to arthrocentesis, but relative contraindica-tions include overlying cellulitis and the presence of a prosthesis.[23] Patients with concern for septic arthritis with these conditions should be evaluated in conjunction with an orthopedic consultant.

Management includes prompt administration of antibiotics and hospital admission once the diagnosis is strongly suspected. The currently recommended choice of anti-biotics is a third generation cephalosporin or vancomycin if MRSA is a concern.[23,25]

Drainage of the affected joint is indicated, but there continues to be controversy over the optimal method. Many surgeons prefer arthroscopic debridement, permitting better visualization and irrigation, whereas others advocate serial needle aspirations, citing the advantages of the minimally invasive approach and recurrent drainage.[31] In chronic or recurrent cases, consultation with an Infectious Disease specialist may be indicated.

Bony Injuries

Glenohumeral dislocations

The shoulder is the most commonly dislocated joint in the body and accounts for 50% of large joint dislocations.[1,32] Of these, approximately 95% will be anterior dislocations with posterior and inferior dislocations occurring much less frequently.[32] Anterior glenohumeral dislocations classically occur with a traumatic, posteriorly directed force to the affected arm held in abduction and extension. Conversely, posterior dislocations occur with the arm adducted and internally rotated, as commonly seen with a seizure or lightning injury.

Patients with an anterior dislocation typically present with a squared off appearance to the shoulder due to the prominent acromium and the arm held in slight abduction. Posterior dislocations, however, result in the patient holding the arm adducted to the side of the thorax and internally rotated across his or her chest.[1] Deformity is subtle and can be easily missed clinically and radiographically. A detailed neurovascular examination with particular focus on the axillary nerve is prudent to assess for concurrent injury.[6]

Radiographs are typically performed in the ED setting to confirm the dislocation and document any concurrent fractures prereduction and postreduction. A standard shoulder radiograph series should include AP and axillary lateral or scapular Y views.[1,32,33] Obtaining an AP view alone is a common medicolegal pitfall, as 50% of posterior dislocations are missed without a lateral projection.[33,34]

In recent years, some investigators have questioned the value of both routine prereduction and postreduction radiographs in clinically obvious anterior shoulder dislocations. Delay in reduction for radiographs may result in persistent discomfort for the patient. Clinical diagnosis by an experienced EP was found to be 98% to 100% accurate when the physician listed confidence in the diagnosis as "certain."[35,36] A proposed clinical decision rule by Hendey and colleagues[37] advocates the omission of prereduction and postreduction films in the select subset of patients with recurrent dislocations and an atraumatic mechanism. The validation study of this decision rule showed a 46% reduction in radiography and a median reduction in total length of stay (LOS) of 133 minutes (46%) in the cohort that did not receive radiographs without any missed fractures or persistent dislocations found on follow-up.

Many EPs, however, advocate that either a pre- or postreduction radiograph be performed to evaluate for concurrent fracture. Approximately 17% to 25% of dislocations will have an associated clinically significant fracture.[36,38] Three factors have been found to be predictive of risk for concurrent fracture: first-time dislocation, blunt trauma, and age greater than 40. Absence of these 3 factors was found to have a sensitivity of 97% at excluding a clinically significant fracture.[36] Furthermore, the fear of iatrogenic fracture during reduction is likely overexaggerated because iatrogenic fractures are relatively rare in published case series.[37–39]

A decision regarding selective radiographs should be made with regard to the individual provider's comfort level. However, consensus exists that both pre- and postreduction films are recommended for patients with fracture-dislocations, posterior or inferior dislocations, or if the assessment of the joint status is not absolutely certain.[37]

Glenohumeral dislocations (**Fig. 3**A–D) can be safely reduced with any of several closed reduction methods, ranging from the classic techniques of Kocher and Hippocrates to newer maneuvers such as the Snowbird and Spaso techniques. Comparison studies in the literature are limited, but reported success rates are relatively similar across the spectrum of reduction techniques and do not definitively support the use of any single method.[40] A summary of these techniques is given in **Table 2**.

Glenohumeral dislocations cause tremendous discomfort for the patient, and adequate pain management is essential to the care of the patient as well as to facilitate the reduction. Classically, EPs have used either narcotic analgesia or intravenous sedation as premedication for the reduction. These methods provide excellent analgesia for patients and have a high rate of success.[41] However, risks of complications including respiratory depression and aspiration must be considered. As such, alternative methods including intra-articular anesthetics, regional anesthesia with ultrasound guided interscalene blocks, and nitrous oxide are currently being researched.[40,42–44]

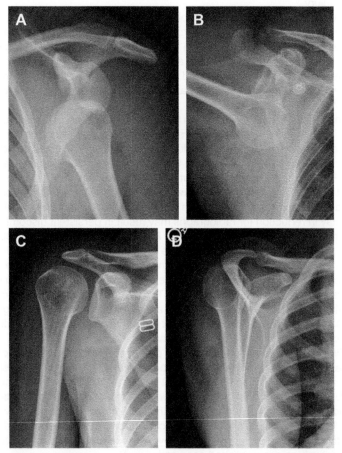

Fig. 3. Glenohumeral dislocations. (*A*) AP view of an anterior glenohumeral dislocation. (*B*) AP view of luxatio erecta dislocation. (*C*) AP view of posterior glenohumeral dislocation. Note that radiographic signs are subtle and easily missed. (*D*) Scapular Y view showing humeral head migration posteriorly in the same patient as in *C*. (*Courtesy of* the Northwestern Emergency Medicine teaching file, copyright 2010; with permission.)

Table 2
Comparison of common glenohumeral reduction techniques

Technique	No. of Operators	Position	Description	Disadvantages	Success Rate
Modified Hippocratic (traction–countertraction)	Two	Supine	One operator provides a longitudinal traction force with the arm slightly abducted. Second operator provides countertraction (typically with a bed sheet wrapped around the thorax in the axilla)	Requires significant force	86%
Kocher[127,128]	One	Seated	Starting position: arm should be adducted at the side with elbow flexed. Gently adduct the arm further and externally rotate the arm. When resistance is felt, the arm is forward flexed upwards and then internally rotated	Higher incidence of fracture	72%–100%
Milch[127,129,130]	One	Supine	Starting position: arm fully abducted above the head with extended elbow. Apply longitudinal traction and external rotation of arm	None	70%–89%
Scapular manipulation[131]	Two	Prone	One operator provides downward traction to arm forward flexed 90°. Second operator attempts to adduct and medially rotate inferior border of scapula	Difficult to monitor sedation, operator dependent	79%–90%
External rotation[132,133]	One	Supine/ seated	Starting position: arm fully adducted at side with elbow flexed. Perform slow passive external rotation of arm	None	80%–90%
Stimson[42,134]	One	Prone	Arm hangs off stretcher in 90° forward flexion and 5–10 pound weights attached to affected arm (can combine with scapular)	Equipment; difficult to monitor sedation	91%–96%
Snowbird[135]	Two	Seated	Starting position: patient seated in chair with arm adducted and flexed at elbow. Operator applies downward traction by placing foot in a loop of stockinette wrapped around the patient's forearm	None	97%
Spaso[126,136]	One	Supine	Starting position: arm forward flexed 90° toward the ceiling. Apply longitudinal traction toward ceiling and passive external rotation	Operator back discomfort (rare)	67%–91%

Data from Ufberg JW, Vilke GM, Chan TC, et al. Anterior shoulder dislocations: beyond traction-countertraction. J Emerg Med 2004;27(3):301–6.

Studies over the last 15 years have shown that the use of intra-articular lidocaine (IAL) provides equivalent success rates in reduction and patient comfort with a significantly lower rate of complications—0.8% for IAL versus 16.8% for intravenous sedation with benzodiazepines and narcotics.[40,41] Fear of iatrogenic infection has thus far been unfounded with no cases of iatrogenic septic joint in more than 280 patients published in the literature.[40,45] In addition, reductions performed with IAL result in a significant decrease in total ED LOS of 51 to 110 minutes and an overall decrease in cost.[42,45] Newer methods of intravenous sedation with etomidate and propofol may have lower complication rates and shorter recovery times than the classic medications used in these studies, but further studies to compare these newer agents with IAL have yet to be performed.[46] Intra-articular lidocaine is an excellent alternative to intravenous sedation and is the preferred method of the authors.

Patients should be referred to an orthopedic surgeon for follow-up. Counseling patients on the risk of recurrent dislocation is advised. Patients younger than 30 years have a 50% to 64% risk of recurrent dislocation with decreasing incidence of recurrence with age.[47] Surprisingly, patients with associated greater tuberosity fractures are at significantly lower risk of recurrence than patients without fracture.[48] In those without fracture, the high rate of recurrence is attributed to disruption of the inferior glenohumeral ligament-labrum complex, commonly referred to as the bankart lesion. This lesion occurs in 97% of first-time glenohumeral dislocations.[47]

Stabilization of the bankart lesion is hypothesized to be a key factor in reducing the risk of recurrence. Although usual treatment uses an internal rotation sling, MRI studies have shown better anatomic reduction of the bankart lesion with the shoulder in external rotation.[49,50] A prospective clinical trial of 198 patients in Japan showed a 38.2% relative risk reduction for recurrent dislocation at 2 years in patients immobilized in an external rotation sling for 3 weeks compared with the conventional internal rotation sling.[51] Albeit promising, the optimal degree of external rotation has yet to be determined, and a validation study in Israel was unable to produce similar success.[52]

The duration of immobilization has unclear effects on recurrence rates in the published literature. Increased length of immobilization from 1 to 4 weeks in a standard internal rotation sling has not been shown to reduce recurrence rates, and some studies suggest that no immobilization is necessary.[47,53] Other studies suggest that longer immobilization may be beneficial at reducing recurrence rates for the patients younger than age 30.[54,55]

The duration of immobilization in an external rotation sling has also been studied without clear consensus; however, a recent MRI based study showed improved anatomic alignment of the bankart lesion with prolonged immobilization (5 weeks vs 3 weeks) in external rotation.[50] Follow-up studies are needed to determine if this results in a clinically significant decrease in recurrence rates.

While further research is needed to determine both the optimal technique and duration of immobilization, the existing literature suggests an external rotation sling may be more effective at reducing recurrence rates and is surprisingly well tolerated by patients.[47,51,52] There is insufficient data thus far to recommend any particular duration of immobilization.[53]

Proximal humerus fractures

Proximal humeral fractures account for up to 5% of all fractures that present to the ED and are the third most common fracture in the elderly.[56] Most patients who suffer this injury are elderly, with greater than 70% of these fractures occurring in females older than 60 years.[56–58] Although most risk factors for proximal humeral factors are ultimately related to advanced age, other related risk factors include poor balance, previous falls, limitations in ambulation, insulin-dependent diabetes, and maternal history of a hip fracture.[59,60] As the general population ages, these fractures are likely to become even more prevalent. Studies in Finland and the United States have demonstrated a threefold increase in the number of proximal humerus fractures from 1970 through 2002.[58,61]

The most common mechanism of injury in the elderly is a fall at an oblique angle onto an outstretched hand, with between 75% and 87% of these occurring secondary to a fall from standing height or less.[56,62,63] Proximal humerus fractures in younger populations tend to result from high mechanism trauma with a direct blow to the lateral shoulder.[56]

These patients frequently hold their arm in adduction and complain of increased pain with movement.[1] It may be difficult to assess for a step-off or obvious deformity in these patients because of the surrounding musculature. However, most patients will have distinct point tenderness over the proximal humerus. Given the location of the axillary nerve and the brachial plexus, it is imperative to check for neurologic deficits, as an estimated 36% of proximal humerus fractures are associated with some type of neurovascular injury.[64] The course of the axillary nerve makes these injuries more common in patients who also have a dislocation or displaced fracture.[65] Fractures of the anatomic neck of the humerus place vascular structures including the axillary artery and its branches, the anterior and posterior circumflex arteries, at greater risk of injury.[64,65]

The primary classification system for proximal humerus fractures is the Neer[66] classification system, which is based on anatomic relationships and relative displacement. This system involves separating the proximal humerus into 4 anatomic parts: the humeral head, humeral shaft, and the greater and lesser tuberosities. Based on this anatomic relationship, the system further classifies these fractures based on the displacement of one or more parts. Displacement must be greater than 1 cm or angulation greater than 45° from normal position. Unfortunately, the Neer system has been demonstrated to have poor intra- and interobserver reliability.[67–69]

Treatment of most proximal humeral fractures in the ED can be managed conservatively with pain control and orthopedic referral. More than 80% of all fractures of the proximal humerus are nondisplaced or minimally displaced.[70,71] Conservative management for these patients consists of ice and a traditional sling. Prolonged immobilization for up to 3 weeks has historically been recommended on discharge, but recent data suggest that earlier range of motion and physical therapy after 1 week may actually result in decreased pain and improved functional outcomes.[72–74] Simple range of motion exercises such as pendulum swings and wall walk-ups should be encouraged and can be quickly demonstrated in the ED setting.

Clavicle fractures

Fractures of the clavicle occur in 30 to 64 per 100,000 people per year, accounting for approximately 2.6% to 5% of all fractures and up to 44% of all fractures of the shoulder joint.[1,21] The majority of patients with clavicle fractures are male, commonly between the ages of 15 and 30 years. A second peak in incidence occurs in women older than 80 years.[75,76] Clavicular fractures are also the most common fractures in children.[1]

Clavicular fractures can be classified by the Allman system, which is based on the anatomic location of the fracture.[77] The middle one-third of the clavicle (Type I) is the most common location for a fracture, encompassing between 69% and 80% of all clavicular fractures. Fractures in the distal (or lateral, Type II) one-third of the clavicle account for 21% to 28% of all fractures, whereas proximal (or medial, Type III) one-third fractures are relatively uncommon, occurring in only 2% of all clavicular fractures.[21,75] Both distal and proximal clavicular fractures are seen more commonly in the elderly, presumably due to the weaker trabecular bone at the ends of the clavicle secondary to aging.[21,76]

Fractures of the clavicle in young persons frequently require a high-impact mechanism such as those experienced during collision sports or a motor vehicle collision. Unlike adolescents and young adults, the older population tends to fracture after a low-energy trip and fall.[21,75]

Injured patients usually guard and hold the affected arm close to the body. The subcutaneous location of the clavicle allows for appreciation of tenting, palpation of step-offs or deformities, and ecchymosis. It is critically important to complete a full neurovascular examination in addition to the standard musculoskeletal examination because of the proximity of the brachial plexus and subclavian vessels. Although rare, cases of resultant pneumothoraces have been reported with displaced clavicular fractures.[78]

Clavicular fractures traditionally have been managed with conservative care including ice, anti-inflammatories, short-term immobilization, and physical therapy. Immobilization may be performed with a traditional sling or a figure-of-8 brace.[21] It was originally theorized that the figure-of-8 brace, which pulls the patient's shoulders up and back, would have been more beneficial, but recent research has demonstrated that this type of splint has been associated with more brachial plexus injuries, nonunion, and patient discomfort.[79] As a result, patients should be placed in a traditional sling or a sling and swathe.[79,80] Use of the sling may be discontinued when pain allows.[21] Gentle range of motion exercises should be encouraged early to improve functional recovery and prevent complications such as adhesive capsulitis and muscle atrophy. Overhead activity is typically restricted until comfort allows and radiographic healing is evident.[81]

Conservative care remains the consensus for management of nondisplaced fractures.[21,82] Recent evidence, however, suggests that the rates of nonunion for certain types of clavicular fractures are greater than previously believed; and some of these patients may have better outcomes with surgical management. In an analysis of 2144 patients across 22 studies, the overall rate of nonunion for conservatively managed clavicular fractures is 5.9% compared with 2.5% for patients managed operatively.[83] Increased age, female gender, and displacement and comminution of the fracture have been found to be independent predictors of nonunion.[84] In particular, displaced mid-shaft clavicular fractures have an alarming 15.1% rate of nonunion, but surgical fixation has been shown to decrease nonunion rates to 2.2%.[83] In addition, fractures with greater than 1.5 cm shortening are associated with increased risk of nonunion, decreased shoulder strength, and patient dissatisfaction.[82,85] As such, the current literature supports the consideration of surgical management for acute, displaced, and/or shortened, mid-shaft clavicular fractures.

For lateral clavicular fractures, the large majority are nondisplaced and managed conservatively. Similar to mid-shaft fractures, displacement of lateral clavicular fractures is associated with an approximately 11% rate of nonunion.[84] Many surgeons advocate operative repair of these fractures; but recent studies suggest higher rates of complications than previously believed and nonunion of these fractures may be relatively asymptomatic, particularly in the elderly.[21,86] Medial clavicular fractures are rare and typically managed nonoperatively. While acute management in the ED remains conservative for all clavicular fractures, orthopedic referral for operative consideration is advised for acute displaced mid-shaft and distal clavicular fractures.

Acromioclavicular separations

Injuries to the AC joint are a frequent cause of shoulder pain, particularly in the young athlete. AC injuries are the most common shoulder injury associated with contact sports, and occur 5 times more frequently in men than in women.[87] This joint serves as the roof of the shoulder and consists of 2 groups of ligaments: the acromioclavicular ligaments and the coracoclavicular ligaments. A fall directly on the adducted shoulder places these structures at risk of injury.[1,88]

All patients with pain to the superior aspect of the shoulder and traumatic mechanism should be suspected to have an AC injury. Tenderness to palpation at the AC joint and pain with cross-arm adduction further supports the diagnosis.[15,16] However, the examiner should note that pain should localize at the AC joint to be suggestive of injury, as similar discomfort may be noted with other conditions such as impingement.

Standard shoulder radiographs are indicated to evaluate the injury. An axillary lateral view is recommended to help detect AP displacement, while a 15° cephalic tilt view (Zanca view) may be beneficial as well.[87,88] Radiographic findings of AC separations include widening of the AC joint greater than 3 mm and an increase in the coracoclavicular distance (CCD) greater than 13 mm.[88,89] Stress views with a weight attached to the affected arm are of limited clinical utility and no longer recommended.[88]

Injuries to the AC joint should be classified according to severity using the Rockwood classification ranging from milder Type I and II injuries to the more severe Type III to VI injuries (**Fig. 4**).[90] The Rockwood classification and its findings are described in detail in **Table 3**.

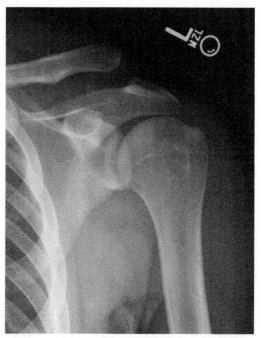

Fig. 4. Type III acromioclavicular separation Note widening of the AC joint and increased coracoclavicular distance. (*Courtesy of* the Northwestern Emergency Medicine teaching file, copyright 2010; with permission.)

Table 3
Rockwood classification of acromioclavicular injuries and associated findings

Type	Pathology	Clinical Findings	Radiographic Findings	ED Management	Definitive Management
Type I	AC sprain, CC intact	AC tenderness	Normal	Sling 7–10 days, pain control	Conservative
Type II	AC torn, CC sprain	AC tenderness	AC >3 mm	Sling 2–3 weeks, pain control	Conservative
Type III	AC torn, CC torn, D and T torn	AC tenderness, deformity	AC >3 mm, CCD >13 mm, 25%–100% displacement	Sling, pain control	Controversial, nonoperative[a]
Type IV	AC torn, CC torn, D and T torn, posterior displacement of clavicle through trapezius	Prominent acromium	AC >3 mm, CCD >13 mm, Posterior displacement of clavicle on axillary lateral	Sling, pain control, neurovascular assessment	Surgical
Type V	AC torn, CC torn, D and T torn, severe superior displacement of clavicle	Deformity	AC >3 mm, CCD >13 mm, 100%–300% displacement	Sling, pain control	Surgical
Type VI	AC torn, CC intact, inferior displacement of clavicle subcoracoid	Associated trauma	AC >3 mm, CCD decreased	Sling, pain control, neurovascular assessment	Surgical

Abbreviations: AC, acromioclavicular; CC, coracoclavicular; CCD, coracoclavicular distance; D, deltoid attachment at clavicle; T, trapezius attachment at clavicle.
[a] Management of Type III injuries is controversial. Nonoperative management is most common but surgical management may be considered in select populations.

Data from Simovitch R, Sanders B, Ozbaydar M, et al. Acromioclavicular joint injuries: diagnosis and management. J Am Acad Orthop Surg 2009;17(4):207–19; and Williams GR, Nguyen VD, Rockwood CR. Classification and radiographic analysis of acromioclavicular dislocations. Appl Radiol 1989;18:29–34.

Whereas definitive management of AC injuries depends on classification of injury, initial management of all AC injuries in the ED focuses on diagnosis, pain management, and appropriate referral to an orthopedic specialist. Although various braces have been developed, a traditional sling can be used for immobilization and comfort for most individuals.[88,91] Cryotherapy and nonsteroidal anti-inflammatories (NSAIDs) are likely adequate for pain management.[91]

Patients with Type I and II injuries can be managed conservatively with a sling for comfort until acute pain resides, at which time a gentle range of motion exercise program and strengthening program can be initiated. In more severe injuries (Types IV–VI), surgical repair is the treatment of choice.[88,89,91] Definitive management of Type III injuries, however, has changed over the years and remains controversial. Operative repair had commonly been performed but is now falling out of favor amongst orthopedists. A review of the literature suggests that patients managed non-operatively have equivalent rates of satisfactory outcome and pain control with earlier return to work, fewer complications, and better range of motion than patients managed operatively.[87,92,93] A select subset of patients including noncontact athletes, overhead workers, and laborers may still be considered for operative repair, although the literature supporting this is limited.[93]

Sternoclavicular dislocations

Although SC dislocations are the least common accounting for less than 1% of all dislocations, they can be quite serious.[1] Most of these injuries occur because of direct or indirect force to the shoulder secondary to high-speed motor vehicle collisions or contact sports.[94,95] Patients younger than 25 years commonly suffer physeal fractures rather than a true dislocation, as the growth plates remain open until this age.[19]

There are 2 different types of SC dislocations, anterior and posterior. Anterior dislocations are up to 9 times more common, with posterior dislocations being rare.[95] Complications from anterior dislocations are usually benign; however, complications from posterior dislocations may occur in up to 30% of patients and can be lethal due to the close proximity of the trachea, esophagus, and great vessels.[94,96]

Anterior dislocations result from an anterolateral force, which results in the shoulder being pulled posteriorly and the clavicle being compressed toward the sternum. Posterior dislocations can result from either a posterolateral force to the shoulder or a direct hit to the medial clavicle.[1,94]

Patients with SC dislocations present with shoulder or anterior chest pain. Such patients resist all movement of the shoulder joint, and hold the affected shoulder flexed at the elbow and adducted at the side.[1] Some patients may also complain of shortness of breath, paresthesias, or dysphagia. A thorough physical examination is indicated, beginning with stabilization of the airway, breathing, and circulation. On inspection, the affected shoulder is often shortened. The medial aspect of the clavicle may be more prominent in anterior dislocations, whereas in posterior dislocations the examination is more nonspecific, with localized tenderness at the SC joint being the only finding.[19,94]

Although often performed initially in the evaluation of SC injuries, plain radiographs are of limited utility secondary to shadowing of nearby structures.[19] A serendipity view may give additional information, but CT is the imaging modality of choice. In addition, CT angiography is often indicated to assess for concurrent vascular injury.[19,96]

Anterior SC dislocations are unstable and often continue to be unstable after treatment.[1,19,94] These dislocations can be reduced via closed reduction in the ED. The most common technique involves placing the patient supine with a rolled towel between his or her shoulder blades. The affected shoulder is then abducted and traction is applied while an assistant applies posterior pressure to the medial clavicle.[95,97,98] This technique can be performed with procedural sedation or local anesthesia. After reduction, these patients are immobilized in a figure-of-8 sling or a clavicle harness for up to 4 to 6 weeks. Orthopedic follow-up is appropriate. Although many of these dislocations ultimately remain unstable after treatment, they rarely cause functional impairment.[1,19] Operative treatment is only indicated after continued failed conservative treatment and loss of function.[97]

Unlike anterior dislocations, posterior dislocations are optimally treated in the operating room. Because of the location of vital mediastinal structures, all reduction techniques, whether open or closed, should be performed in consultation with an orthopedic surgeon and cardiothoracic surgeon.[98] Closed reduction was successful in a French case series of athletes in approximately half of patients when performed within 48 hours.[99]

Closed reduction may be attempted with traction to the abducted and extended arm. If this is unsuccessful, a sterile towel clip may be used to pull the medial clavicle out from behind the sternum.[1] An alternative technique involves caudal traction to the adducted arm with posterior pressure on both shoulders.[100] If closed reduction fails or if there is delayed presentation longer than 48 hours or an associated disruption to the medial clavicular physis, open reduction is indicated.[99] Unlike anterior dislocations, posterior dislocations are usually stable post reduction.[98] Patients should be placed in a figure-of-8 strap for 6 to 8 weeks with the appropriate orthopedic follow-up.[19,97]

Soft-Tissue Injuries

Adhesive capsulitis

Adhesive capsulitis, commonly referred to as a frozen shoulder, is a significant cause of shoulder discomfort in patients. Patients typically will have insidious onset of progressive pain, stiffness, and loss of motion.[101] The exact mechanism of the disease is not well understood. It most frequently affects women between the ages of 40 and 70 years, and is more common in patients with endocrine disorders such as diabetes and thyroid disease.[102] Approximately 20% of diabetic patients will suffer from adhesive capsulitis compared with 2% to 5% of the general population.[102,103] A recent prospective study of patients with adhesive capsulitis without known diabetes showed that 51.9% would meet criteria for having prediabetes.[103]

Diagnosis is made on clinical examination and exclusion of alternative diagnoses including rotator cuff impingement. Patients typically will have profound limitations in range of motion, with forward flexion less than 100° and a greater than 50% loss in external rotation.[102] Adhesive capsulitis often can be differentiated from other conditions by its limitation in passive range of motion, which is typically preserved in rotator cuff conditions.[101]

ED management should be directed at pain control and appropriate referral to an orthopedic specialist. Initiation of pain medication with NSAIDs or oral steroids is recommended.[102] A recent meta-analysis showed that patients with adhesive capsulitis may have short-term improvement in pain and range of motion with use of oral steroids compared with placebo, but this benefit may not be maintained beyond 6 weeks.[104] The mainstay of outpatient treatment is physical therapy, but may include adjunctive treatments including corticosteroid injections and operative manipulations.[102] In addition, patients suspected of having adhesive capsulitis should be referred for diabetic screening.[102,103]

Rotator cuff injuries

Injuries to the rotator cuff are a very common cause of shoulder pain, particularly in patients older than 40 years.[105,106] These injuries include a spectrum of illness ranging from inflammatory and degenerative conditions referred to as impingement syndrome to acute tears in the tendons of the rotator cuff.

Impingement syndrome, which incorporates rotator cuff strains, tendonitis, and subacromial bursitis, occurs as a result of mechanical irritation of the rotator cuff tendons on the anteroinferior portion of the acromium.[107] It is likely to occur in patients with a hooked acromium, present in approximately 40% of patients.[108] Rotator cuff tears are very common, affecting 7% to 30% of the elderly, and may occur because of an acute traumatic injury or from progression of impingement.[109–111]

Injuries to the rotator cuff are diagnosed with history and physical examination findings. Patients with rotator cuff pathology often localize pain to the lateral deltoid, and frequently complain of increased pain with overhead activity and "night pain."[32] In addition, patients will have limitations in active range of motion due to discomfort but preserved passive range of motion. Neer and Hawkins tests for impingement (see **Fig. 2**A,B) may be positive.[11,12] True weakness in the affected extremity is suggestive of a rotator cuff tear but may be clinically difficult to distinguish from weakness secondary to pain. A diagnostic injection of 10 mL of 1% lidocaine into the subacromial space may be performed to assist in the diagnosis of impingement syndrome. Improvement in discomfort after injection is suggestive of rotator cuff impingement. Persistent weakness increases suspicion for rotator cuff tear.[11,107]

Radiographs should be performed to exclude alternative diagnoses, but are usually nondiagnostic. Superior migration of the humeral head toward the acromium (acromiohumeral distance <7 mm) can be suggestive of a cuff tear, while the presence of a hooked type acromium increases the likelihood of impingement.[112,113]

Definitive diagnosis of rotator cuff tears can be difficult in the ED setting. The EP must have a high index of suspicion, particularly in elderly patients with a traumatic mechanism or dislocation. A recent Danish study found that 50% of patients aged 50 to 69 who present to the ED with shoulder pain after an acute traumatic injury have a rotator cuff tear if radiographs are normal and the patient is unable to abduct to 90°.[114] In addition, 35% to 84% of patients older than 40 years with a first-time dislocation suffer a concurrent rotator cuff tear.[115]

Treatment of rotator cuff pathology in the ED includes ice, analgesia typically with NSAIDs, a sling for comfort, and a referral to an appropriate specialist. A subacromial corticosteroid injection may improve short-term symptoms of impingement, although efficacy has not been validated in the published literature.[116] Caution is advised to avoid injection into the tendon itself, which may cause weakening and theoretical increased risk of rupture.[116,117] Impingement and partial thickness rotator cuff tears often improve with conservative management, including physical therapy. Full thickness tears should be considered for operative repair.[107]

Pectoralis rupture

Acute ruptures of the pectoralis major tendon are an important, albeit rare, cause of shoulder pain. While intuitively thought of as a chest muscle, the pectoralis major provides significant strength for adduction and internal rotation of the shoulder, and patients often complain of shoulder weakness as the initial presenting complaint.[118] Injuries to the pectoralis typically occur in young athletes, almost exclusively in males. The most frequently described activity precipitating this injury is weight training, particularly the bench press.[119,120]

Diagnosis in the ED should be suspected on the basis of history and physical examination, as radiographs are rarely diagnostic. Patients may describe an acute onset of pain or an audible pop, followed by weakness in the affected arm. Ecchymoses in the upper arm or axilla and weakness in adduction and internal rotation may be noted on physical examination. Abduction and external rotation of the arms may demonstrate an asymmetry in the axilla.[118]

Operative repair is the treatment of choice when possible, as 90% of patients have an "excellent "or "good" outcome compared with only 17% for those treated conservatively.[119,120] Early diagnosis by the EP and appropriate referral is imperative, as a delay in operative treatment has been associated with poorer outcomes.[119]

Bicipital tendinosis/biceps tendon rupture

Another common cause of discomfort in the patient with shoulder pain is bicipital tendinosis. The long head of the biceps tendon sits in the intertubercular groove of the proximal humerus and attaches to the glenoid labrum proximally. The biceps brachii is responsible for elbow flexion and supination of the forearm. Bicipital tendinosis occurs in isolation in only 5% of cases and is often associated with injuries to the rotator cuff, particularly the subscapularis tendon.[121,122]

This condition usually occurs in older individuals aged 40 to 60 years but sometimes occurs in the young athlete with repetitive overhead activity. Patients complain of a dull throbbing pain anteriorly, worse with overhead motion. Tenderness in the intertubercular groove with the arm in 10° internal rotation and discomfort with the Speed test is suggestive of the diagnosis.[122,123]

Acute tendon rupture is an unfortunate complication of bicipital tendinosis, often lending to presentation to the ED. Isolated tears of the long head of the biceps tendon account for 97% of biceps tendon ruptures.[124] Patients describe an acute onset of pain in the anterior shoulder and weakness with flexion. The classic "Popeye" deformity may be present on examination as the biceps muscle belly retracts distally. In addition, patients may demonstrate weakness in supination and have pain with the Speed test.[122]

Treatment of bicipital tendinosis in the ED is also conservative, using ice, NSAIDs, and physical therapy.[123] For acute biceps tendon ruptures, early diagnosis in the ED and appropriate referral to an orthopedic specialist aid in ideal patient outcomes. No consensus exists on the optimal treatment course for these patients. Whereas some investigators have advocated similar strength outcomes in patients managed conservatively, others have demonstrated a 21% residual loss in supination strength and 8% loss in elbow flexion in those managed conservatively, with no appreciable strength loss in those who underwent surgical repair.[124,125] Patients do, however, have an earlier recovery and return to work if managed nonoperatively.[124]

SUMMARY

Injuries to the shoulder girdle account for a large number of visits to the ED and cause significant morbidity for patients. While by no means a comprehensive review of all injuries to the shoulder girdle, this article provides a focused, up-to-date review of the literature on emergent conditions of the shoulder seen in the ED and their optimal management, with an emphasis on dangerous medicolegal pitfalls.

REFERENCES

1. Daya M. Shoulder. In: Marx JA, Hockberger RS, Walls RM, editors. Rosen's emergency medicine. 5th edition. Philadelphia: Mosby; 2002. p. 576–606.

2. Boone DC, Azen SP. Normal range of motion of joints in male subjects. J Bone Joint Surg Am 1979;61(5):756–9.
3. AAOS. Joint motion. Method of measuring and recording. Chicago: AAOS; 1965.
4. Burbank KM, Stevenson JH, Czarnecki GR, et al. Chronic shoulder pain: part I. Evaluation and diagnosis. Am Fam Physician 2008;77(4):453–60.
5. de Laat EA, Visser CP, Coene LN, et al. Nerve lesions in primary shoulder dislocations and humeral neck fractures. A prospective clinical and EMG study. J Bone Joint Surg Br 1994;76(3):381–3.
6. Visser CP, Coene LN, Brand R, et al. The Incidence of nerve injury in anterior dislocation of the shoulder and its influence on functional recovery. A prospective clinical and EMG study. J Bone Joint Surg Br 1999;81(4):679–85.
7. Hegedus EJ, Goode A, Campbell S, et al. Physical examination tests of the shoulder: a systematic review with meta-analysis of individual tests. Br J Sports Med 2008;42(2):80–92.
8. Jobe FW, Moynes DR. Delineation of diagnostic criteria and a rehabilitation program for rotator cuff injuries. Am J Sports Med 1982;10:336–9.
9. Park HB, Yakota A, Gill HS, et al. Diagnostic accuracy of tests for the different degrees of subacromial impingement syndrome. J Bone Joint Surg Am 2005; 87(7):1446–55.
10. Gerber C, Krushell RJ. Isolated rupture of the tendon of the subscapularis muscle. Clinical features in 16 cases. J Bone Joint Surg Br 1991;73(3): 389–94.
11. Neer CS 2nd. Impingement lesions. Clin Orthop Relat Res 1983;173:70–7.
12. Hawkins RJ, Kennedy JC. Impingement syndrome in athletes. Am J Sports Med 1980;8:151–7.
13. Harryman DT, Sidles JA, Clark JM, et al. Translation of the humeral head on the glenoid with passive glenohumeral motion. J Bone Joint Surg Am 1990;72: 1334–43.
14. Woodward TW, Best TM. The painful shoulder, part I. Clinical evaluation. Am Fam Physician 2000;61(10):3079–88.
15. McLaughlin HL. On the frozen shoulder. Bull Hosp Joint Dis 1951;12:383–90.
16. Chronopoulos E, Kim TK, Park HB, et al. Diagnostic value of physical tests for isolated chronic acromioclavicular lesions. Am J Sports Med 2004;32(3): 655–61.
17. Kibler BW, Sciascia AD, Hester P, et al. Clinical utility of traditional and new tests in the diagnosis of biceps tendon injuries and superior labrum anterior and posterior lesions in the shoulder. Am J Sports Med 2009;37(9):1840–7.
18. Bennett WF. Specificity of the Speed's test: arthroscopic technique for evaluating the biceps tendon at the level of the bicipital groove. Arthroscopy 1998; 14(8):789–96.
19. MacDonald PB, Lapionte P. Acromioclavicular and sternoclavicular joint injuries. Orthop Clin North Am 2008;39:535–45.
20. Rockwood CA, Wirth MA. Injuries to the sternoclavicular joint. In: Rockwood CA, Green DP, Bucholz RW, et al, editors. Rockwood and green's fractures in adults. 4th edition. Philadelphia: Lippincott Raven; 1996. p. 1415–71.
21. Khan LA, Bradnock TJ, Robinson CM, et al. Fractures of the clavicle: current concepts review. J Bone Joint Surg Am 2009;91:447–60.
22. Hanby CK, Pasque CB, Sullivan JA. Medial clavicle physis fracture with posterior displacement and vascular compromise: the value of three dimensional computed tomography and duplex ultrasound. Orthopedics 2003;26:81–4.

23. Margaretten ME, Kohlwes J, Moore D, et al. Does this adult patient have septic arthritis? JAMA 2007;297(13):1478–88.
24. Lossos IS, Yossepowitch O, Kandel L, et al. Septic arthritis of the glenohumeral joint. A report of 11 cases and review of the literature. Medicine (Baltimore) 1998;77(3):177–87.
25. Frazee B, Fee C, Lambert L. How common is MRSA in septic arthritis. Ann Emerg Med 2009;54(5):695–700.
26. Kaandorp CJ, Van Schaardenburg D, Krijnen P, et al. Risk factors for septic arthritis in patients with joint disease: a prospective study. Arthritis Rheum 1995;38:1819–25.
27. Li SF, Henderson J, Dickman E, et al. Laboratory tests in adults with monoarticular arthritis: can they rule out a septic joint? Acad Emerg Med 2004;11(3): 276–80.
28. McGillicuddy DC, Shah KH, Friedberg RP, et al. How sensitive is the synovial fluid white blood cell count in diagnosing septic arthritis? Am J Emerg Med 2007;25(7):749–52.
29. Li SF, Cassidy C, Chang C, et al. Diagnostic utility of laboratory tests in septic arthritis. Emerg Med J 2007;24(2):75–7.
30. Shah K, Spear J, Nathanson LA, et al. Does the presence of crystal arthritis rule out septic arthritis? J Emerg Med 2007;32(1):23–6.
31. Manadan AM, Block JA. Daily needle aspiration versus surgical lavage for the treatment of bacterial septic arthritis in adults. Am J Ther 2004;11(5):412–5.
32. Blake R, Hoffman J. Emergency Department evaluation and treatment of the shoulder and humerus. Emerg Med Clin North Am 1999;17(4):859–76.
33. Hawkins RJ, Neer CS II, Pianta RM, et al. Locked posterior dislocation of the shoulder. J Bone Joint Surg Am 1987;69:9–18.
34. Clough TM, Bale RS. Bilateral posterior shoulder dislocation: the importance of the axillary radiographic view. Eur J Emerg Med 2001;8(2):161–3.
35. Hendey GW. Necessity of radiographs in the emergency department management of shoulder dislocations. Ann Emerg Med 2000;36(2):108–13.
36. Shuster M, Abu-Laban R, Boyd J. Prereduction radiographs in clinically evident anterior shoulder dislocation. Am J Emerg Med 1999;17:653–8.
37. Hendey GW, Chally MK, Stewart VB. Selective radiography in 100 patients with suspected shoulder dislocation. J Emerg Med 2006;31(1):23–8.
38. Emond M, Le Sage N, Lavoie A, et al. Clinical factors predicting fractures associated with an anterior shoulder dislocation. Acad Emerg Med 2004;11(8): 853–8.
39. Kahn JH, Mehta SD. The role of post-reduction radiographs after shoulder dislocation. J Emerg Med 2007;33(2):169–73.
40. Kuhn JE. Treating the initial anterior shoulder dislocation—an evidence-based medicine approach. Sports Med Arthrosc 2006;14(4):192–8.
41. Fitch RW, Kuhn JE. Intraarticular lidocaine versus intravenous procedural sedation with narcotics and benzodiazepines for reduction of the dislocated shoulder: a systematic review. Acad Emerg Med 2008;15(8):703–8.
42. Miller SL, Cleeman E, Auerbach J, et al. Comparison of intra-articular lidocaine and intravenous sedation for reduction of shoulder dislocations: a randomized, prospective study. J Bone Joint Surg Am 2002;84(12):2135–9.
43. Underhill TJ, Wan A, Morrice M. Interscalene brachial plexus blocks in the management of shoulder dislocations. Arch Emerg Med 1989;6:199–204.
44. Gleeson AP, Graham CA, Meyer AD. Intra-articular lidocaine versus Entonox for reduction of acute anterior shoulder dislocation. Injury 1999;30(6):403–5.

45. Ng VK, Hames H, Millard WM. Use of intra-articular lidocaine as analgesia in anterior shoulder dislocation: a review and meta-analysis of the literature. Can J Rural Med 2009;14(4):145–9.
46. Miner JR, Burton JH. Clinical practice advisory: emergency department procedural sedation with propofol. Ann Emerg Med 2007;50:182–7.
47. McNeil NJ. Postreduction management of first-time traumatic anterior shoulder dislocations. Ann Emerg Med 2009;53(6):811–3.
48. Hovelius L, Olofsson A, Sandström B, et al. Nonoperative treatment of primary anterior shoulder dislocation in patients forty years of age and younger. a prospective twenty-five-year follow-up. J Bone Joint Surg Am 2008;90(5): 945–52.
49. Itoi E, Sashi R, Minagawa H, et al. Position of immobilization after dislocation of the glenohumeral joint. A study with use of magnetic resonance imaging. J Bone Joint Surg Am 2001;83(5):661–7.
50. Scheibel M, Kuke A, Nikulka C, et al. How long should acute anterior dislocations of the shoulder be immobilized in external rotation? Am J Sports Med 2009;37(7):1309–16.
51. Itoi E, Hatakeyama Y, Sato T, et al. Immobilization in external rotation after shoulder dislocation reduces the risk of recurrence. A randomized controlled trial. J Bone Joint Surg Am 2007;89(10):2124–31.
52. Finestone A, Milgrom C, Radeva-Petrova DR, et al. Bracing in external rotation for traumatic anterior dislocation of the shoulder. J Bone Joint Surg Br 2009; 91(7):918–21.
53. Smith TO. Immobilisation following traumatic anterior glenohumeral joint dislocation: a literature review. Injury 2006;37(3):228–37.
54. Maeda A, Yoneda M, Horibe S, et al. Longer immobilization extends the "symptom-free" period following primary shoulder dislocation in young rugby players. J Orthop Sci 2002;7:43–7.
55. Kiviluoto O, Pasila M, Jaroma H, et al. Immobilisation after primary dislocation of the shoulder. Acta Orthop Scand 1980;51:915–9.
56. Court-Brown CM, Garf A, McQeen MM. The epidemiology of proximal humeral fractures. Acta Orthop Scand 2001;72:365.
57. Lauritzen JB, Schwarz P, Lund B, et al. Changing incidence and residual lifetime risk of common osteoporosis-related fractures. Osteoporos Int 1993;3: 127–32.
58. Nordqvist A, Petersson CJ. Incidence and causes of shoulder girdle injuries in an urban population. J Shoulder Elbow Surg 1995;4:107.
59. Lee SH, Dargent-Molina P, Breart G. Risk factors for fractures of the proximal humerus: results from the EPIDOS prospective study. J Bone Miner Res 2002; 17:817–25.
60. Nguyen TV, Center JR, Sambrook PN, et al. Risk factors for proximal humerus, forearm and wrist fractures in elderly men and women: the Dubbo Osteoporosis Epidemiology Study. Am J Epidemiol 2001;153:587–95.
61. Palvanen M, Kannus P, Niemi S, et al. Update in the epidemiology of proximal humeral fractures. Clin Orthop Relat Res 2006;442:87–92.
62. Kelsey JL, Browner WS, Seeley DG, et al. Risk factors for fractures of the distal forearm and proximal humerus. The Study of Osteoporotic Fractures Research Group. Am J Epidemiol 1992;135:477–89.
63. Palvanen M, Kannus P, Parkkari J, et al. The injury mechanisms of osteoporotic upper extremity fractures among older adults: a controlled study of 287 consecutive patients and their 108 controls. Osteoporos Int 2000;11:822–31.

64. Bahrs C, Rolauffs B, Dietz K, et al. Clinical and radiological evaluation of minimally displaced proximal humeral fractures. Arch Orthop Trauma Surg 2009; 130(5):673–9.
65. Visser CP, Coene LN, Brand R, et al. Nerve lesions in proximal humeral fractures. J Shoulder Elbow Surg 2001;10:421.
66. Neer CS 2nd. Displaced proximal humerus fractures. I. Classification and evaluation. J Bone Joint Surg Am 1970;52(6):1077–89.
67. Siebenrock KA, Gerber C. The reproducibility of classification of fractures of the proximal end of the humerus. J Bone Joint Surg Am 1993;75:1751–5.
68. Sidor ML, Zuckerman JD, Lyon T, et al. The Neer classification system for proximal humeral fractures: an assessment of interobserver reliability and intraobserver reproducibility. J Bone Joint Surg Am 1993;75:1745–50.
69. Bernstein J, Adler LM, Blank JE, et al. Evaluation of the Neer System of classification of proximal humeral fractures with computerized tomographic scans and plain radiographs. J Bone Joint Surg Am 1996;78:1371–5.
70. Eiff P, Hatch R, Calmbach W. Fracture management for primary care. Philadelphia: Saunders; 2003.
71. Handoll HH, Gibson JN, Madhok R, et al. Interventions for treating proximal humeral fractures in adults. Cochrane Database Syst Rev 2003;4:CD000434.
72. Lefevre-Colau MM, Babinet A, Fayad F, et al. Immediate mobilization compared with conventional immobilization for the impacted nonoperatively treated proximal humeral fracture: a randomized controlled trial. J Bone Joint Surg Am 2007;89(12):2582–90.
73. Kristiansen B, Angermann P, Larsen TK, et al. Functional results following fractures of the proximal humerus: a controlled clinical study comparing two periods of immobilization. Arch Orthop Trauma Surg 1989;108:339.
74. Hodgson S, Stanley S, Mawson S. Timing of physiotherapy in management of fractured proximal humerus: randomised controlled trial. Physiotherapy 2002; 88(12):763.
75. Postacchini F, Stefano G, De Santis P, et al. Epidemiology of clavicle fractures. J Shoulder Elbow Surg 2002;11(5):452–6.
76. Robinson CM. Fractures of the clavicle in the adult: epidemiology and classification. J Bone Joint Surg Br 1998;80:476–84.
77. Allman FI. Fractures and ligamentous injuries of the clavicle and its articulation. J Bone Joint Surg Am 1967;49:774–84.
78. Geraci G, Pisello F, Sciume C, et al. [Clavicle fracture complicated by pneumothorax. Case report and literature review]. G Chir 2007;28(8–9):330–3 [in Italian].
79. Anderson K, Jenson PO, Lauritzen J. Treatment of clavicular fractures: figure of eight bandages versus a simple sling. Acta Orthop Scand 1987;58:71–4.
80. Nordqvist A, Redlund-Johnell I, von Scheele A, et al. Shortening of the clavicle after fracture: incidence and clinical significance- a five year follow-up of 85 patients. Acta Orthop Scand 1997;68:349.
81. Jeroy KJ. Acute midshaft clavicle fractures. J Am Acad Orthop Surg 2007;15(4): 239–48.
82. Smekal V, Oberladstaetter J, Struve P, et al. Shaft fractures of the clavicle: current concepts. Arch Orthop Trauma Surg 2009;129(6):807–15.
83. Zlowodzki M, Zelle BA, Cole PA, et al. Evidence-Based Orthopaedic Trauma Working Group. Treatment of acute midshaft clavicle fractures: systematic review of 2144 fractures: on behalf of the Evidence-Based Orthopaedic Trauma Working Group. J Orthop Trauma 2005;19:504–7.

84. Robinson CM, Court-Brown CM, McQueen MM, et al. Estimating the risk of nonunion following nonoperative treatment of a clavicular fracture. J Bone Joint Surg Am 2004;86(7):1359–65.
85. McKee MD, Pedersen EM, Jones C, et al. Deficits following nonoperative treatment of displaced midshaft clavicle fractures. J Bone Joint Surg Am 2006;88(1):35–40.
86. Kona J, Bosse MJ, Staeheli JW, et al. Type II distal clavicle fractures; a retrospective review of surgical treatment. J Orthop Trauma 1990;4:115–20.
87. Bishop JY, Kaeding C. Treatment of the acute traumatic acromioclavicular separation. Sports Med Arthrosc 2006;14(4):237–45.
88. Simovitch R, Sanders B, Ozbaydar M, et al. Acromioclavicular joint injuries: diagnosis and management. J Am Acad Orthop Surg 2009;17(4):207–19.
89. Rios CG, Mazzocca AD. Acromioclavicular joint problems in athletes and new methods of management. Clin Sports Med 2008;27(4):763–88.
90. Williams GR, Nguyen VD, Rockwood CR. Classification and radiographic analysis of acromioclavicular dislocations. Appl Radiol 1989;18:29–34.
91. Nuber GW, Bowen MK. Acromioclavicular joint injuries and distal clavicle fractures. J Am Acad Orthop Surg 1997;5(1):11–8.
92. Phillips AM, Smart C, Groom AF. Acromioclavicular dislocation: conservative or surgical therapy. Clin Orthop 1998;353:10–7.
93. Spencer EE Jr. Treatment of Grade III acromioclavicular joint injuries: a systematic review. Clin Orthop Relat Res 2007;455:38–44.
94. Ferrera PC, Wheeling HM. Sternoclavicular joint injuries. Am J Emerg Med 2000;18:58.
95. Yeh GL, Williams GR. Conservative management of sternoclavicular injuries. Orthop Clin North Am 2000;31:189.
96. Ono K, Inagawa H, Kiyota K, et al. Posterior dislocation of the sternoclavicular joint with obstruction of the innominate vein: a case report. J Trauma 1998;44:381.
97. Bicos J, Nicholson G. Treatment and results of sternoclavicular joint injuries. Clin Sports Med 2003;22:359–70.
98. Robinson CM, Jenkins PJ, Markham PE, et al. Disorders of the sternoclavicular joint. J Bone Joint Surg Br 2008;90(6):685–96.
99. Laffosse JM, Espie A, Bonnevialle N, et al. Posterior dislocation of the sternoclavicular joint and epiphyseal disruption of the medial clavicle with posterior displacement in sports participants. J Bone Joint Surg Br 2010;92(1):103–9.
100. Buckerfield CT, Castle ME. Acute traumatic retrosternal dislocation of the clavicle. J Bone Joint Surg Am 1984;66:379–85.
101. Kelley MJ, McClure PW, Leggin BG. Frozen shoulder: evidence and a proposed model guiding rehabilitation. J Orthop Sports Phys Ther 2009;39(2):135–48.
102. Brue S, Valentin A, Forssblad M, et al. Idiopathic adhesive capsulitis of the shoulder: a review. Knee Surg Sports Traumatol Arthrosc 2007;15(8):1048–54.
103. Tighe CB, Oakley WS Jr. The prevalence of a diabetic condition and adhesive capsulitis of the shoulder. South Med J 2008;101(6):591–5.
104. Buchbinder R, Green S, Youd JM, et al. Oral steroids for adhesive capsulitis. Cochrane Database Syst Rev 2006;4:CD006189.
105. Jobe FW, Kvitne RS, Giangarra CE. Shoulder pain in the overhand or throwing athlete. The relationship of anterior instability and rotator cuff impingement. Orthop Rev 1989;18:963–75.
106. Bigliani LU, Levine WN. Subacromial impingement syndrome. J Bone Joint Surg Am 1997;79(12):1854–68.

107. Ahmad CS, Yamaguchi K, Wolfe I, et al. The shoulder. In: Scuderi GR, McCann PD, editors. Sports medicine a comprehensive approach. 2nd edition. Philadelphia: Elsevier Mosby; 2005. p. 227–48.
108. Bigliani LU, Morrison DS, April EW. The morphology of the acromion and rotator cuff: importance. Orthop Trans 1986;10:228.
109. SooHoo NF, Rosen P. Diagnosis and treatment of rotator cuff tears in the emergency department. J Emerg Med 1996;14(3):309–17.
110. Moosmayer S, Smith HJ, Tariq R, et al. Prevalence and characteristics of asymptomatic tears of the rotator cuff: an ultrasonographic and clinical study. J Bone Joint Surg Br 2009;91(2):196–200.
111. Yamamoto A, Takagishi K, Osawa T, et al. Prevalence and risk factors of a rotator cuff tear in the general population. J Shoulder Elbow Surg 2009; 19(1):116–20.
112. Kotzen LM. Roentgen diagnosis of rotator cuff tear: a report of 48 surgically proven cases. Am J Roentgenol Radium Ther Nucl Med 1971;112:507–11.
113. Moosikasuwan JB, Miller TT, Burke BJ. Rotator cuff tears: clinical, radiographic, and US findings. Radiographics 2005;25(6):1591–607.
114. Sørensen AK, Bak K, Krarup AL, et al. Acute rotator cuff tear: do we miss the early diagnosis? A prospective study showing a high incidence of rotator cuff tears after shoulder trauma. J Shoulder Elbow Surg 2007;16(2):174–80.
115. Stayner LR, Cummings J, Andersen J, et al. Shoulder dislocations in patients over 40 years of age. Orthop Clin North Am 2000;31(2):231–9.
116. Gruson KI, RUchelsman DE, Zuckerman JD. Subacromial corticosteroid injections. J Shoulder Elbow Surg 2008;17(1 Suppl):118S–130S.
117. Soslowsky LJ, Thomopoulos S, Esmail A, et al. Rotator cuff tendinosis in the animal model: role of extrinsic and overuse factors. Ann Biomed Eng 2002;30: 1057–63.
118. Ryan SA, Bernard AW. Pectoralis major rupture. J Emerg Med 2008. [Online]. DOI:10.1016/j.jemermed.2008.05.002.
119. Bak K, Cameron EA, Henderson IJ. Rupture of the pectoralis major: a meta-analysis of 112 cases. Knee Surg Sports Traumatol Arthrosc 2000;8:113–9.
120. Pochini Ade C, Einisman B, Andreoli CV, et al. Pectoralis major muscle rupture in athletes: a prospective study. Am J Sports Med 2010;38(1):92–8.
121. Post D, Benca P. Primary tendinitis of the long head of the biceps. Clin Orthop 1989;246:117–25.
122. Patton WC, McCluskey GM 3rd. Biceps tendinitis and subluxation. Clin Sports Med 2001;20(3):505–29.
123. Churgay CA. Diagnosis and treatment of biceps tendinitis and tendinosis. Am Fam Physician 2009;80(5):470–6.
124. Mariani EM, Cofield RH, Askew LJ, et al. Rupture of the tendon of the long head of the biceps brachii: surgical versus nonsurgical treatment. Clin Orthop 1988; 228:223–9.
125. Carroll RE, Hamilton LR. Rupture of biceps brachii—a conservative method of treatment. J Bone Joint Surg Am 1968;49:1016.
126. Yuen MC, Yap PG, Chan YT, et al. An easy method to reduce anterior shoulder dislocation: the Spaso technique. Emerg Med J 2001;18(5):370–2.
127. Beattie TF, Steedman DJ, McGowan A, et al. A comparison of the Milch and Kocher techniques for acute anterior dislocation of the shoulder. Injury 1986; 17(5):349–52.
128. Kocher T. Eine neue Reductionsmethode fur Schuiterverrenkung. Berl Klin Wochenschr 1870;7:101–5 [in German].

129. Johnson G, Hulse W, McGowan A. The Milch technique for reduction of anterior shoulder dislocations in an accident and emergency department. Arch Emerg Med 1992;9(1):40–3.
130. Milch H. Treatment of dislocation of the shoulder. Surgery 1938;3:732–40.
131. Baykal B, Sener S, Turkan H. Scapular manipulation technique for reduction of traumatic anterior shoulder dislocations: experiences of an academic emergency department. Emerg Med J 2005;22(5):336–8.
132. Marinelli M, de Palma L. The external rotation method for reduction of acute anterior shoulder dislocations. J Orthop Trauma 2009;10(1):17–20.
133. Eachempati KK, Dua A, Malhotra R, et al. The external rotation method for reduction of acute anterior dislocations and fracture-dislocations of the shoulder. J Bone Joint Surg Am 2004;86(11):2431–4.
134. Stimson LA. An easy method of reduction dislocation of the shoulder and hip. Med Rec 1900;57:356.
135. Westin CD, Gill EA, Noyes ME, et al. Anterior shoulder dislocation. A simple and rapid method for reduction. Am J Sports Med 1995;23(3):369–71.
136. Fernández-Valencia JA, Cuñe J, Casulleres JM, et al. The Spaso technique: a prospective study of 34 dislocations. Am J Emerg Med 2009;27(4):466–9.

Management and Treatment of Elbow and Forearm Injuries

Jorge L. Falcon-Chevere, MD[a,*], Dana Mathew, MD[b,c],
Jose G. Cabanas, MD[c,d], Eduardo Labat, MD[e]

KEYWORDS

- Elbow injury • Forearm injury • Nightstick • Galeazzi
- Monteggia • Essex-Lopresti • Supracondylar fractures
- Elbow dislocation

Orthopedic injuries to the upper extremity are frequently seen in the emergency department (ED). The emergency medicine practitioner (EP) must be proficient in recognizing these injuries and their associated complications, and be able to provide appropriate orthopedic management. This article highlights the most frequent forearm and elbow injuries seen in the ED.

FOREARM ANATOMY

Two bones form the forearm, the radius (lateral) and ulna (medial). The elbow capsule holds both bones together proximally while the anterior and posterior radioulnar ligaments carry out the same task in the distal radioulnar joint (DRUJ). The forearm muscles, pronator quadratus, pronator teres, and supinator also help maintain the unified movement of bones. The interosseous membrane further stabilizes both bones, while dividing the forearm into the flexor and extensor muscle compartments.

The median nerve or its anterior interosseous branch innervates all the flexor muscles except for the flexor carpi ulnaris and the ulnar aspect of the flexor digitorum profundus, which are innervated by the ulnar nerve. The anterior interosseous nerve

[a] Department of Emergency Medicine, University of Puerto Rico School of Medicine, Hospital UPR Dr Federico Trilla, 65th Infantry Avenue Km 3.8, Carolina, PR 00985, USA
[b] WakeMed Health & Hospitals, Emergency Services Institute, 3000 New Bern Avenue, Raleigh, NC 27610, USA
[c] Department of Emergency Medicine, University of North Carolina at Chapel Hill, 170 Manning Drive, CB# 7594, Chapel Hill, NC 27599-7594, USA
[d] WakeMed Health & Hospitals, Clinical Research Unit, Emergency Services Institute, 3000 New Bern Avenue, Raleigh, NC 27610, USA
[e] Department of Diagnostic Radiology, University of Puerto Rico School of Medicine, Rio Piedras, PR 00926, USA
* Corresponding author. Department of Emergency Medicine, University of North Carolina at Chapel Hill, Chapel Hill, NC.
E-mail address: jfalconc@gmail.com

Emerg Med Clin N Am 28 (2010) 765–787
doi:10.1016/j.emc.2010.07.005
0733-8627/10/$ – see front matter © 2010 Elsevier Inc. All rights reserved.

commences from the posterior aspect of the median nerve. As discussed later, any lesion to this nerve will be translated to weakness or loss of interphalangeal joint flexion of the thumb and index finger. The radial nerve and its terminal muscle ramification, the posterior interosseous nerve, innervate the muscles from the extensor compartment.[1]

The radial and ulnar arteries arise from the brachial artery. The radial artery runs along the radial bone to the wrist. Distally it forms the deep palmar arch. A superficial branch arises at the level of the wrist and contributes to the superficial palmar arch. The ulnar artery runs along the ulnar bone to the wrist. One of its branches is the common interosseous artery, which divides into anterior and posterior interosseous arteries. The anterior interosseous artery accompanies the median nerve over the anterior aspect of the interosseous membrane. The posterior interosseous artery passes through the interosseous membrane reaching the extensor compartment.[1]

FOREARM FRACTURES

The nightstick fracture is an isolated fracture of the midshaft of the ulnar. The mechanism of injury is direct trauma (ie, a blow from a nightstick) to the distal forearm. Associated with the defensive move in raising the arm to protect the head and face against a blow, it is considered a simple injury, given that it is not associated with ligamentous disruption of the boney structures (**Fig. 1**). Nightstick fractures are considered a stable fracture when the displacement is less than 50% of cortical width and there is no injury to the interosseous membrane.[1] This fracture should be immobilized in a long arm splint; it is not a surgical fracture unless angulation is less than 15° with more than 50% to 75% fracture displacement.[2] Fractures involving the middle and proximal third of the ulnar shaft are at an increased risk for malunion or other complications. These fractures often require both surgical correction and longer periods of immobilization in a long arm cast.[2] If the fracture is displaced as explained, open reduction and internal fixation is needed to preclude angulation, rotation, and shortening of the ulnar length.[3]

Fractures of the radius and ulna (both-bone fractures) are complex injuries that typically require surgical correction, as they are inherently unstable and difficult to treat successfully.[4–6] The evaluation and management in the ED includes a focused physical examination, neurovascular assessment, analgesia, splint immobilization, and early orthopedic consultation. Radiographic evaluation should include forearm, wrist, and elbow radiographs.

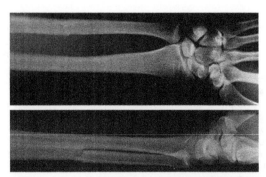

Fig. 1. Anteroposterior and lateral views of a minimally displaced isolated fracture of the ulnar bone. (*From* Eiff MP, Calmbach WL, Hatch RL. Radius and ulnar injuries. In: Fracture management for primary care. 2nd edition. Philadelphia: Saunders; 2002. p. 116–47; with permission.)

An EP must be proficient in the identification of forearm fractures such as the Galeazzi, Monteggia, and Essex-Lopresti fractures, and be aware of the potential complications of these fractures. Undiagnosed fractures or missed dislocations can result in complications such as extremity weakness, chronic pain, or decreased range of motion.

Galeazzi Fracture-Dislocation

In 1934, fractures of the middle and distal third of the radius associated with instability of the DRUJ were described by Galeazzi.[7] This rare fracture accounts for 3% to 7% of all forearm fractures.[8,9] The Galeazzi fracture-dislocation mechanism of injury is usually a fall on an outstretched hand in forced pronation.[9-11] The patient presents with distal forearm swelling, pain, radial deformity, and ulnar head prominence.

Radiographs confirm the diagnosis and at least 2 views (anteroposterior [AP] and lateral) should be evaluated. In the lateral view, a dorsal angulation of the distal radial fracture is seen as well as dorsal displacement of the ulnar head (**Fig. 2**). The AP view illustrates radioulnar space widening and radial length shortening (**Fig. 3**).

Galeazzi's fracture-dislocations are unstable injuries. Definitive treatment for this injury should be operative. It has been reported that up to 90% of adult patients treated conservatively could suffer poor outcomes.[12] Occasionally, if the radial fracture is distal, a closed reduction of both radius and the DRUJ can be accomplished under conscious sedation or a hematoma block. The arm is placed in a long arm splint and urgent orthopedic consultation is obtained.[13] Immobilization should be done with a long arm cast in supination.

Common complications associated with the unrecognized or untreated DRUJ disruption are chronic pain and weakness with associated diminished supination and pronation.

Monteggia Fracture-Dislocation

A Monteggia fracture-dislocation consists of a fracture to the proximal third of the ulna with a concomitant dislocation of the radial head.[6] Its mechanism of injury has been described as forced pronation of the forearm on an outstretch hand, or direct trauma to the dorsal aspect of the ulna.

Monteggia fracture-dislocations have been categorized into 4 types by the Bado classification.[14] Each type is described depending on the location of the ulnar fracture and the direction of the radial head dislocation (**Table 1**).

Physical examination shows a swollen forearm and elbow, with associated pain in the area of the fracture, decreased range of motion, and shortening of the forearm.

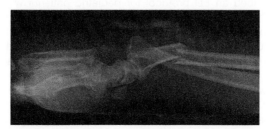

Fig. 2. Galeazzi fracture-dislocation, lateral view. Distal third radial fracture and associated distal radioulnar joint (DRUJ) dislocation. (*Courtesy of* E. Labat, MD, University of Puerto Rico Diagnostic Radiology Program.)

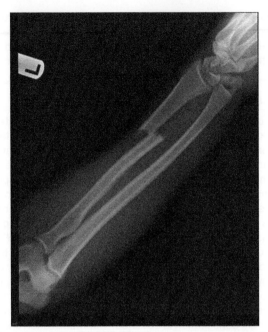

Fig. 3. Galeazzi fracture-dislocation, AP view. Fracture of distal radial fracture. Notice the DRUJ separation and radial bone shortening. (*Courtesy of* E. Labat, MD, University of Puerto Rico Diagnostic Radiology Program.)

Clinically, tenderness to palpation at the DRUJ in the presence of an ulnar fracture should raise suspicion for a Monteggia lesion.[13] It is necessary to complete a thorough neurovascular evaluation, as it can be associated with a radial nerve injury. Injury to this nerve manifests as weakness or paralysis of extension in the fingers or thumb. The sensory branch is not typically involved.[15]

Radiographs confirm the diagnosis. In the forearm AP view, a proximal ulna fracture will be evident. It is important for an adequate evaluation of this lesion to include elbow radiographs to avoid missing the radial head dislocation. In 20% to 50% of patients, the diagnosis is not made at initial evaluation.[9,16] One simple technique the EP can use to avoid missing a proximal dislocation is to draw a line through the long axis of the radius at the elbow in the lateral radiography. This line should intersect the capitellum regardless of the degree of elbow flexion or extension.[9,16] In 2004 David-West and colleagues[17] described an ED protocol for pediatric patients with painful swollen elbow to reduce the incidence of missed cases. This protocol recommended orthopedic consultation if the ulna was bent in association with a displaced radial head or if there was a classic Monteggia pattern. It also recommended repeating radiographs 1 week after the accident if unsure about radial head displacement, because early treatment of this injury improves the outcome.

As with the Galeazzi fracture-dislocation, definitive treatment of the Monteggia fracture-dislocation is surgical. ED management consists of immobilization with a long arm splint, analgesics, and urgent orthopedic consult.[13]

Complications of this rare orthopedic fracture-dislocation are malunion or nonunion (>2%, especially if Monteggia type IV) of the ulnar fracture, a missed radial head dislocation (60%) that could produce chronic elbow pain along with reduced supination

Type	Definition	Film/Diagram
1	Fracture of the ulnar diaphysis at any level with anterior displacement of the radial head	
2	Fracture of the ulnar diaphysis at any level with posterior displacement of the radial head	
3	Fracture of the ulnar diaphysis at any level with lateral displacement of the radial head	
4	Fracture of the proximal third of the radius and ulna at the same level with an anterior dislocation of the radial head	

Table 1
Bado classification

Photos Courtesy of E. Labat, MD, University of Puerto Rico Diagnostic Radiology Porgram.

and pronation, and posterior interosseous nerve injuries that range between 3% and 63%, as shown in several studies.[14,18–23]

Essex-Lopresti Injury

Essex-Lopresti injury is a rare complex injury of the forearm consisting of a fracture of the head of the radius, rupture of the interosseous membrane, and disruption of the DRUJ (**Fig. 4**).[24] The mechanism of injury is longitudinal force to the outstretched hand that causes impaction of the capitellum and radial head, with subsequent rupture of the interosseous membrane and radial shortening greater than 2 mm. The diagnosis is often missed in the ED and can be a challenge if the initial evaluation is focused solely on the radial head fracture, causing one to overlook the more serious

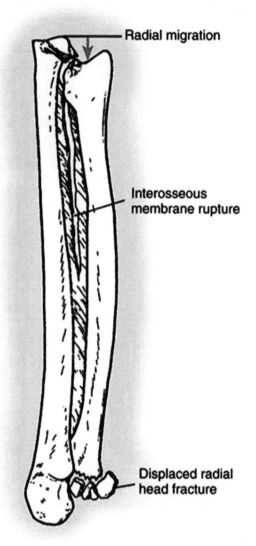

Radial migration

Interosseous membrane rupture

Displaced radial head fracture

Fig. 4. Essex-Lopresti fracture-dislocation. (*From* Edwards GS, Jupiter JB. Radial head fractures with acute distal radioulnar dislocation: Essex-Lopresti revisited. Clin Orthop Relat Res 1988;234:61; with permission.)

interosseous membrane (IOM) injury.[25,26] To avoid missing the IOM injury the EP can use bedside sonography. The medical literature cites several studies wherein sonography has been shown to be useful in the detection of rupture of the IOM, with up to 96% accuracy.[26–30] Wallace[28] described that the transducer should be placed over the dorsal aspect of the forearm oriented transversely. Failla and colleagues[27] described the IOM as a very hyperechoic structure (**Fig. 5**), with the central third of the IOM seen as a thick, continuous white line. Any disruptions of the IOM show a break in this continuity of the white line, representing the IOM.

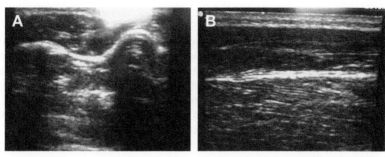

Fig. 5. (*A, B*) Radio-ulnar Interosseous membrane. (*A*) Transverse forearm view. (*B*) Longitudinal forearm view. Any discontinuity of this hyperechoic structure suggest IOM disruption. (*Courtesy of* Jorge L. Falcon-Chevere, MD, Faculty at University of Puerto Rico Emergency Medicine Residency Program, Carolina, PR.)

The patient should be initially immobilized in a well-padded and well-molded long posterior splint that extends to the distal palmar crease to immobilize the wrist.[26] The EP must provide adequate analgesia and an emergent orthopedic consult. The definitive treatment is an open reduction and internal fixation (ORIF), or radial head implant if ORIF is not possible.

A complete neurovascular evaluation and documentation is needed. The nerve most commonly affected is the posterior interosseous nerve. Physical examination will show pain on evaluation, inability to extend thumb or other digits at metacarpophalangeal (MCP) joints, and if in complete palsy, the patient will continue to have wrist extension but will be unable to extend the wrist at neutral or in ulnar deviation, and will be able to extend the digits at the interphalangeal joints but not at MCP joints.[31] Evaluation of the flexor and extensor muscle compartment is imperative, as a compartment syndrome may ensue. With time this complex orthopedic injury can cause chronic wrist pain, elbow stiffness, and arthritis requiring operative reconstructive procedure if not properly treated.

ELBOW INJURIES

The elbow is a complex joint, and a good knowledge of its anatomy is crucial to properly assess and treat traumatic injuries in the ED. Some describe the elbow as a trochleogingylomoid joint, in reference to its flexion and extension movement (ginglymoid), and its supination and pronation movement (trochoid) at the ulnohumeral and radioulnar articulations, respectively.[32] Bony stability is provided primarily by the ulnotrochlear joint and secondarily by the radiocapitellar articulation. The distal humerus provides the proximal articular bony surface involving the capitellum and the trochlea.

The elbow is anatomically stabilized by a group of ligaments and muscles. The main ligaments are the medial collateral ligament (MCL) and the lateral collateral ligament (LCL). The MCL originates at the medial epicondyle and is further divided into the anterior, posterior, and transverse ligaments. The anterior MCL inserts on the coronoid process of the ulna and provides primary stability for valgus stress movements. The LCL divides into the radial collateral ligament, lateral ulnar collateral ligament, annular ligament, and the accessory collateral ligament. The LCL originates from the lateral epicondyle, and segments are attached at different regions of the annular ligament and the crista supinatoris. The lateral ulnar collateral ligament provides varus stability to the elbow. The radial collateral ligament stabilizes the radial head. All these ligaments account for 50% of elbow stability.[33,34]

Muscles that cross the elbow offer a significant amount of protection as well as functional stability to the joint. Specifically, 4 groups of muscles allow for flexion and extension of the elbow, wrist, and digits. In addition, they allow for forearm supination and pronation. The biceps brachii, the brachioradialis, and the brachialis are contained in the anterior compartment and are responsible for elbow flexion. The posterior compartment contains the triceps brachii and the anconeus, which provides extension of the joint. A general anatomic rule is that the flexor-pronator muscles originate at the medial epicondyle while the extensor-supinator muscles originate from the lateral epicondyle.[34–36]

From the neurologic standpoint, there are 4 main nerves in the forearm that EPs must evaluate at the time of an injury: the median, ulnar, musculocutaneous, and radial nerves. Damage to any one nerve can cause a different set of clinical manifestations. Neurologic damage will depend on the type of fracture as it relates to the anatomic path of the nerve. For instance, the median nerve is most commonly injured in supracondylar humerus fractures. This nerve innervates the flexor pronators, finger flexors, and thenar muscles within the anterior compartment of the forearm. The median nerve passes anteriorly to and runs medially and parallel to the brachial artery. By contrast, the ulnar nerve passes posterior to the medial epicondyle of the humerus. This nerve can be damaged with a fracture of the medial epicondyle. If damaged, it can cause radial hand deviation with wrist flexion due to paralysis of the flexor carpi ulnaris muscle, loss of flexion of the ring and little fingers at the distal interphalangeal (DIP) joint and the metacarpophalangeal (MP) joint due to paralysis of the flexor digitorum profundus muscle, loss of extension of the ring and little finger at the DIP and proximal interphalangeal (PIP) joints, and loss of adduction and abduction of the fingers due to paralysis of the interosseous muscles.[34–36]

The radial nerve supplies all the extensor muscles of the posterior compartments of the upper arm. This nerve crosses anterior to the lateral epicondyle of the humerus. Damage is most commonly caused by a midshaft fracture of the humerus. If damaged, extension of the wrist and digits are lost and supination is compromised. There is sensory loss of the posterior arm, posterior forearm, and lateral dorsum of the hand. A wrist drop can be seen on clinical examination. The musculocutaneous nerve travels in the lateral antecubital fossa and innervates elbow flexor muscles. Physical examination findings and pertinent abnormalities are summarized in **Table 2**.

After any extremity trauma, radiographs are necessary to evaluate for fractures and dislocations. A series of imaging studies are necessary to guide initial management. AP, lateral, and oblique views are usually sufficient for the initial evaluation. On lateral view, a distended anterior fat pad also known as the "sail sign" is suggestive of an occult fracture and should be treated accordingly.[37] A posterior fat pad is always considered pathologic and is highly suggestive of a fracture. Evaluation of alignment is equally important. Several lines are used to evaluate alignment on the radiographs, including the anterior humeral line, radiocapitellar line, and the Baumann angle.[38,39] These angles may be difficult to evaluate in some patients, especially in the pediatric population, because of continued development of ossification centers that appear at different ages in childhood. EPs may choose to order a comparative radiograph if unable to differentiate an ossification center from an acute fracture. However, it should be treated as a fracture if clinically suspected.

Distal humeral fractures are usually seen in children between the ages of 3 and 11 or in adults older than 50 years. Up to 60% of all elbow fractures are classified as supracondylar.[40] In children, they generally are caused by a fall on outstretched hand

Table 2
Physical examination findings and pertinent abnormalities of elbow injuries

Nerve	Innervations	Fracture	Strength Loss	Sensory Deficits	Physical Examination
Median	Flexors of the forearm	Supracondylar	Flex of index, middle fingers at DIP, PIP, and MP. Abduction/opposition and flexion of the thumb	Palmar and dorsal portions of the index, middle, and half of the ring finger. Palmar portion of the thumb	Ulnar deviation during flexion. Thenar eminence atrophy. When trying to make a fist the index and middle finger will remain straight
Ulnar	Flexor carpi ulnaris, flexor digitorum profundus, interosseus	Medial epicondyle fracture	DIP/MP ring and little finger flexion. Extension of the ring and little finger at DIP/PIP. Adduction/abduction of fingers	Palmar and dorsal half of ring and little finger	Loss of thumb adduction, radial deviation with wrist flexion, no flexion or extension of ring and little finger at DIP
Radial	Wrist extensor and supinator muscles	Midshaft humerus fracture, badly fitted crutch	Extensor compartment	Posterior arm, forearm and lateral dorsum of hand	Wrist drop, supination difficulty
Musculocutaneous	Elbow flexors	Axilla injury	Elbow flexion and supination	Lateral surface of the forearm	"Waiter's tip" position

(FOOSH) injury, or by a direct blow to the elbow. These injuries are classified as extension or flexion supracondylar fractures, respectively. The classification is based on the mechanism of injury and the distal fragment displacement.[34] Extension fractures account for 95% to 98% of all supracondylar fractures.[37,41]

Radiographically, a fat pad or anterior humeral line abnormality may be the only indication of a supracondylar injury (**Fig. 6**A).[42,43] Another radiographic technique that can highlight a supracondylar injury is evaluation of the Baumann angle, described as the angle between the physeal line of the lateral condyle of the humerus and a line perpendicular to the long axis of the humeral shaft. A normal angle is defined to be between 8° and 28°. A very small Baumann angle (<8°) is a warning to the orthopedic surgeon that

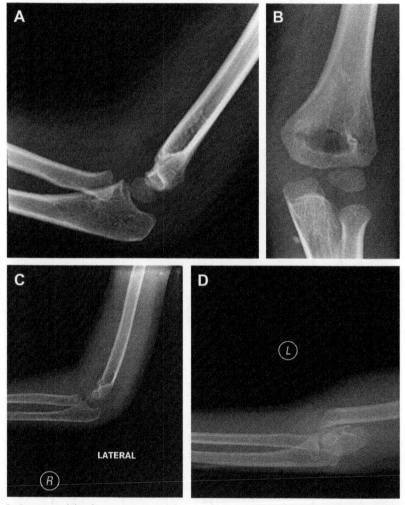

Fig. 6. Supracondylar fracture type I. (*A*) Lateral view. Notice the anterior and posterior fat pad signs (*B*) AP view. (*C*) Supracondylar fracture type II with displacement of the distal humerus, lateral view. Notice the anterior and posterior fat pad signs with displacement of distal humerus. (*D*) Supracondylar fracture type III, lateral view. Notice deformity and unstable joint. (*Courtesy of* E. Labat, MD, University of Puerto Rico Diagnostic Radiology Program.)

a varus deformity exists.[37] Supracondylar fractures are divided into 3 types (I, II, and III) and is known as the Gartland classification, first described in 1959.[34,44–46] These types describe the associated amount of displacement, with type I having no displacement and type III having complete displacement and full cortex disruption.[44]

Clinical evaluation is important because it can provide information on the type of injury and ultimate disposition. EPs must identify neurovascular complications such as prolonged capillary refill, loss of radial pulse, and possible anterior interosseous nerve palsy.[37] Common clinical findings include pain out of proportion to the amount of swelling at the elbow. Nondisplaced supracondylar fractures (type I) (see **Fig. 6**A, B) are commonly managed conservatively with a long arm splint with 90° flexion at the elbow and the forearm in a neutral position, or a double sugar-tong splint, then discharge with rest, ice, compression, and elevation (RICE), pain control, and follow-up in 1 to 2 days. Ideally, this should be done in consultation with an orthopedic surgeon.[37]

Type II distal humerus injuries (see **Fig. 6**C) have minimal displacement (2 mm) with the posterior periosteum intact[47]; up to 25% of these fractures may not be visible on plain radiographs.[40] In a type III distal humerus injury (see **Fig. 6**D), the patient may present to the ED holding the extremity in an abduction-extension position with swelling and tenderness at the elbow. Type II is an intrinsically unstable fracture.[48] Type II and III distal humerus injuries are commonly treated by closed reduction with percutaneous pinning.[47] ORIF is usually required if a rotational deformity exists, the brachial artery is trapped (ie, vascular compromise), or reduction cannot be maintained. If a type II distal humerus fracture has subtle displacement or a complete reduction can be obtained it may be treated with a posterior splint or percutaneous pinning, but ORIF is also used given the possibility of complications.[45]

All supracondylar fractures need to be treated aggressively, given the high risk of malunion and potential for neurovascular injury.[49] Vascular compromise secondary to supracondylar fractures ranges from 5% to 12%.[45] The most common complications are malunion, a loss of the carrying angle resulting in a cosmetic disruption, and neuropraxia (a stretch of the nerve) that usually fully recovers within 1 year. Splinting and orthopedic follow-up should be initiated for any child with focal tenderness at the distal humerus after a trauma, even with negative radiographs. All type III supracondylar fractures and any type II with displacement or angulation require emergent orthopedic consultation. Any supracondylar fracture that requires manipulation needs admission because of the increased risk of compartment syndrome.

Rarely, supracondylar fractures can be classified as flexion injuries, which account for only 2% of supracondylar fractures.[37] The patient typically presents holding the elbow in a flexed position. There are similar subgroups as with extension fractures, types I, II, and III. It is important that Garland classification be used only for extension supracondylar fractures. Differences from the extension fractures include that type I can be minimally displaced, type II is a fracture through the posterior cortex with the anterior cortex remaining intact, and the distal fragment in type III is displaced anterior and proximal. Type I may be splinted in a long arm posterior splint with the elbow flexed at 90°. Types II and III require emergent orthopedic consultation, with type III commonly requiring ORIF.

In contrast to supracondylar fractures, transcondylar fractures occur frequently in the elderly. The mechanism of injury tends to be similar to supracondylar fractures, but the fracture line transverses both condyles just proximal to the articular surface of the elbow and within the joint capsule. These fractures are classified as flexion and extension, with the distal humeral portion anterior or posterior to the proximal segment, respectively. The fractures can develop a callus between the olecranon and the coronoid fossa, obstructing the range of motion within the joint space.[34] Given that most patients are elderly and commonly osteopenic, improved outcome has been found with emergent orthopedic consult and ORIF.[50]

Olecranon Injuries

The integrity of the olecranon is essential for normal function of the elbow. These injuries account for 10% of fractures within the elbow[51] and are frequently comminuted, occurring more frequently in adults than children after direct trauma to the elbow.[19] Rarely, a forceful contraction of the triceps muscle secondary to a fall can cause a transverse or oblique fracture through the olecranon.[52]

Patients with olecranon injuries will present with pain and tenderness to palpation over the olecranon area. The inability to extend the elbow against force after a traumatic event is considered highly suggestive of an olecranon injury.[51] Special attention should be made to the ulnar nerve when performing the neurovascular examination; this is accomplished by examining for motor weakness and sensorial abnormalities along the palmar aspect of the fifth digit and hypothenar eminence.

Radiographic studies must include a lateral view, which should be evaluated for bone disruption, the degree of comminution, and the degree of displacement. Several classification systems have been created to describe theses injuries.[53–55] The Mayo Clinic classification is commonly used and describes fractures on the basis of displacement, stability, and comminution. Type I fractures are stable and nondisplaced, type II are displaced and unstable but with joint stability (ie, not dislocated), and type III (**Fig. 7**) have an unstable joint. Types II and III are subdivided into A (noncomminuted) and B (comminuted).[55] Mayo type III injuries are associated with poor functional outcomes.[51] No fracture displacement in a 90° position suggests the triceps aponeurosis is likely intact and the injury is stable. If there is a greater than 2 mm displacement, the patient may need an orthopedic consult for possible ORIF.[52] However, there have been reports of cases with good functional outcomes in elderly patients despite significant displacement. In a case series of 13 patients treated nonoperatively with a mean age 81.8 years and greater than 5 mm displacement, only 1 had a poor functional outcome.[53] Occasionally, olecranon fracture will be associated with an elbow dislocation noted by posterior displacement of the ulna.[52]

The majority of patients with nondisplaced injuries can be managed conservatively as outpatients with standard treatment including RICE, a long arm posterior splint with adequate padding for 3 to 4 weeks, and pain control. The joint should be immobilized in 45° to 90° of flexion. Patients should be provided with detailed instructions regarding outpatient follow-up within 5 to 7 days for a repeat radiograph. Limited range of motion exercises should be started within 3 weeks as instructed by an orthopedic specialist. Patients should return to the ED in the event of increased swelling, worsening pain, paresthesia, or numbness. Common complications include nonunion, which has been reported in up to 1% of patients, with typical symptoms of pain, instability, or loss of joint motion.[56]

Displaced fractures or fractures with elbow dislocations need immediate orthopedic consult for ORIF, especially in young patients. These patients should be observed for any clinical signs of limb deterioration. All patients who present with clinical signs of neurologic injury require orthopedic consultation for disposition. The majority of olecranon injuries will have good functional outcomes.[56–58]

Elbow Dislocation

The elbow is the second most common large joint dislocated in the adult patient, preceded only by shoulder dislocation.[32] Typically the result of a fall, dislocation predominantly affects the nondominant arm, as the dominant arm is used to shield

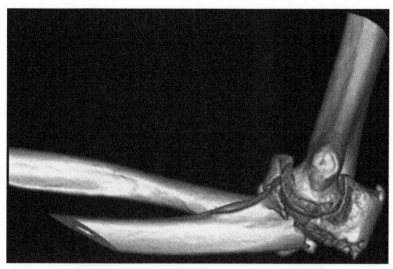

Fig. 7. Computed tomography (CT) reconstruction of displaced olecranon fracture type III. (*Courtesy of* E. Labat, MD, University of Puerto Rico Diagnostic Radiology Program.)

the body from the fall. These injuries occur twice as much in males as in females. Almost 50% of elbow dislocations are associated with sport activities.[59] Elbow dislocations are classified according to the displaced direction of the ulna relative to the distal humerus. This classification divides elbow dislocations into posterior, anterior, and divergent. Posterior dislocations are subdivided based on the final relationship between the humerus and the olecranon, and include posterior, posterolateral, posteromedial, and pure lateral dislocations.[32]

Anterior dislocations are especially rare, accounting for only 1% to 2% of all elbow dislocations.[59] Two mechanisms of injury are related to anterior elbow dislocation: a blow to the posterior portion of a flexed elbow or a forceful forearm extension to an extended elbow. Clinically, the patient has a swollen elbow, pain, and decreased range of motion. The elbow is fully extended with the forearm supinated. The diagnosis can be made clinically, and confirmed with plain radiographs (AP and lateral) of the elbow (**Fig. 8**).

A thorough neurovascular examination should be done on initial assessment. This lesion can be associated with a vascular injury to the brachial artery. The patient should be provided analgesics, and if no neurovascular injury is suspected the arm should be splinted in its current position to avoid potential injuries until radiographs can be obtained. Initial radiologic studies can be portable to avoid a delay in reduction.

Anterior dislocation reduction is performed with distal traction on the wrist and backward pressure on the forearm. An assistant provides countertraction by grasping the humerus with both hands.[60] It is important to reassess the neurovascular function after the procedure. Immediate orthopedic referral is recommended.

The posterior elbow dislocation is the most common type, accounting for 80% to 90% of dislocations.[59] Its mechanism of injury has been well studied,[61,62] consisting of a fall on an outstretched hand with an extended elbow. It is known that valgus stress plays an important role in this injury.[59,63] The final disruption occurs to the medial structures, damaging the lateral ulnar collateral ligament, the joint capsule, and medial ulnar collateral ligament. With a slightly flexed elbow, a tear in the MCL complex occurs and the elbow dislocates.[32]

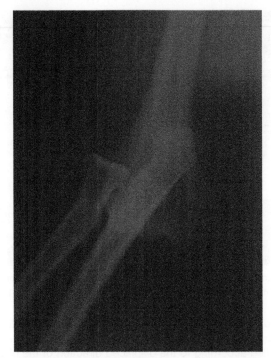

Fig. 8. Anterior elbow dislocation. (*Courtesy of* Wanda L. Rivera-Bou, MD, Faculty at University of Puerto Rico Emergency Medicine Residency Program, Carolina, PR.)

The patient arrives at the ED with the elbow flexed at 45° with pain, decreased range of motion, shortening of the forearm, and absence of the normal relation of the epicondyles to the tip of the olecranon.[64] The diagnosis can be made clinically, and confirmed with radiographs of the elbow (**Fig. 9**). Special attention should be paid to exclude fractures of the radial head, coronoid process, or distal ulna. Treatment and the risk of brachial artery injury (5%–13%) is the same as with anterior elbow dislocations; however, the median nerve can also be damaged.[65,66]

Closed reduction should be performed under conscious sedation. There are several methods to reduce a posterior elbow dislocation. When using the traction method (**Fig. 10**), one operator flexes the elbow 90° and supinates the forearm while applying

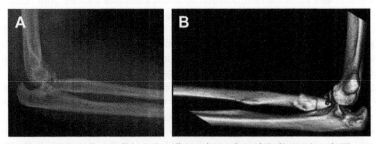

Fig. 9. (*A, B*) Posterior elbow dislocation (lateral view) and 3-dimensional CT scan reconstruction. Note the posterior elbow dislocation and associated radial head fracture. (*Courtesy of* E. Labat, MD, University of Puerto Rico Diagnostic Radiology Program.)

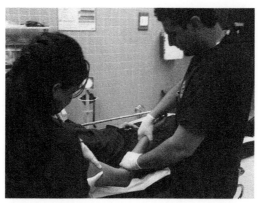

Fig. 10. Traction method. (*Courtesy of* Jorge L. Falcon-Chevere, MD, Faculty at University of Puerto Rico Emergency Medicine Residency Program, Carolina, PR.)

posterior pressure to the humerus, while a second operator applies downward pressure on the proximal forearm.[67]

Another technique to reduce a posterior elbow dislocation is the Mayo technique (**Fig. 11**), the performance of which requires only one person. The patient is positioned supine on the stretcher with the arm held overhead. Holding the patient's arm above his or her head, a valgus force is applied and the forearm supinated. When the elbow joint unlocks, an axial force can be applied to reduce the elbow.

The Parvin method (**Fig. 12**) requires placing the patient to lie prone with the humerus resting on the table and the forearm hanging perpendicular to the table.[68] The table, proximal to the elbow joint, should support the humerus. The EP pulls down at the wrist or applies 10 lb (4.5 kg) of weight to the wrist. Reduction should occur over a period of minutes. The EP may guide the olecranon into place if needed.

The Meyn and Quigley method (**Fig. 13**) is done with the patient in the prone position. The forearm is allowed to hang over the edge of the stretcher, then gentle downward traction is applied to the wrist with one hand, using the other hand to guide reduction of the olecranon.[69]

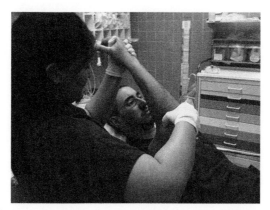

Fig. 11. Mayo technique. (*Courtesy of* Jorge L. Falcon-Chevere, MD, Faculty at University of Puerto Rico Emergency Medicine Residency Program, Carolina, PR.)

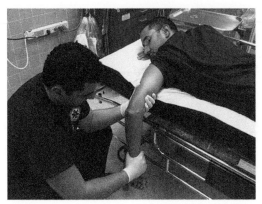

Fig. 12. Parvin method. (*Courtesy of* Jorge L. Falcon-Chevere, MD, Faculty at University of Puerto Rico Emergency Medicine Residency Program, Carolina, PR.)

The Puller technique is done with the patient supine. The operator holds the patient's wrist with one hand and applies traction to the supinated forearm with the elbow flexed. With the other hand the operator applies downward pressure on the patient's proximal forearm to release the coronoid process.[70]

After the procedure the neurovascular function of the arm is reassessed and documented.[59,63] In particular, the status of the median nerve, the ulnar nerve, and the brachial artery is determined, as these are most frequently affected, and can be injured through the manipulation during the examination.[63,71] The wrist and shoulder are evaluated to rule out concomitant injuries, which occur in 10% to 15% of cases.[59]

The arm is immobilized with a long arm posterior splint and an arm sling. Patients may be discharged home if there are no neurovascular complications, fractures, and joint instability, and a successful reduction; otherwise orthopedic referral is warranted. Instability, pain, or recurrent dislocations may complicate posterior elbow dislocation.

Medial and lateral elbow dislocations are rare injuries with a poorer prognosis as compared with the true posterior dislocation. The mechanism of injury is similar to a posterior dislocation, but with medial or lateral forces that displace both bones as a whole in the medial or lateral direction.[64]

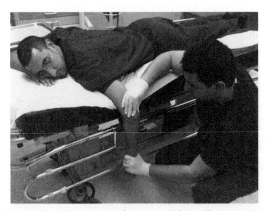

Fig. 13. Mein-Quigley method. (*Courtesy of* Jorge L. Falcon-Chevere, MD, Faculty at University of Puerto Rico Emergency Medicine Residency Program, Carolina, PR.)

On plain radiographs of a medial dislocation, the trochlear notch articulates with the medial epicondyle and the radial head articulates with the trochlea (**Fig. 14**). In the lateral dislocation, the trochlear notch articulates with the capitellum. These dislocations are reduced with the same technique as for the posterior elbow dislocation.[64]

The divergent elbow dislocation is a rare type of dislocation that predominates in the pediatric population, secondary to joint laxity.[71,72] These injuries commonly occur between the ages of 4 and 10 years.[73] There is dislocation of the elbow and dissociation of the radius and ulna, secondary to rupture of the annular ligament and the IOM.[74] The injury involves disruption of all 3 joints comprising the elbow: the radiocapitellar, ulnotrochlear, and proximal radioulnar joints.[75] There are 2 types of divergent elbow dislocations, anteroposterior and medial-lateral (transverse).[76]

Treatment can be achieved through closed reduction and immobilization in a long plaster splint with 90° elbow flexion in full supination for 5 weeks,[75] or through ORIF.

Divergent elbow dislocations may be associated with recurrent subluxation of the radial head or coronoid process fractures.[74] Other known complications of this lesion are compartment syndrome, ulnar or median neuropraxia, elbow instability, and residual disability.[71]

In general terms the indications for emergent surgical repair of an elbow dislocation are open elbow dislocation, nonreducible dislocation, neurovascular impairment, acute compartment syndrome, postreduction instability, and elbow dislocations with unstable fractures.[59,63]

Radial Head Fractures

Radial head fractures are common orthopedic injuries in the adult and pediatric population.[77] These injuries are responsible for up to 5.4% of all adult fractures,[78] and account for 20% to 33% of elbow fractures.[79,80] The mechanism of injury is described as a fall on an outstretched hand with a pronated forearm or with the elbow in slight flexion, or a direct blow to the lateral elbow.[80] The patient presents to the ED with

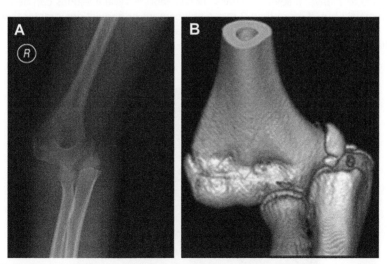

Fig. 14. (A, B) Medial Elbow dislocation AP view and 3-dimensional CT scan reconstruction. In medial dislocation the trochlear notch articulates with the medial epicondyle and the radial head articulates with the trochlea. Note the medial elbow dislocation and associated medial epicondyle fracture. (Courtesy of E. Labat, MD, University of Puerto Rico Diagnostic Radiology Program.)

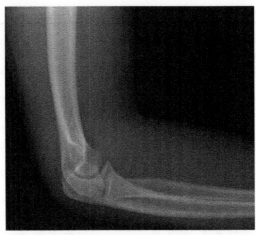

Fig. 15. Radial head fracture (Mason type 1). (*Courtesy of* E. Labat, MD, University of Puerto Rico Diagnostic Radiology Program.)

tenderness over the radial head distal to the lateral epicondyle. Movement exacerbates the pain in the forearm.[80]

Radial head fractures are classified according to the Mason classification system.[81] Type I (62%) are fractures without displacement (**Fig. 15**). Type II (20%) are fractures with displacement (**Fig. 16**), and type III (18%) are comminuted fractures involving the whole head (**Fig. 17**).

The management of these injuries is guided by the Mason classification. Type I radial head fractures are treated conservatively: the elbow is placed in a posterior splint for 5 to 7 days, followed by early mobilization.[82] Type II injuries can be treated conservatively but, if more than 2 mm displacement or angulations greater than 30° occur, they are repaired with ORIF.[80,82] Type III radial head fractures require ORIF or radial head replacement.[83]

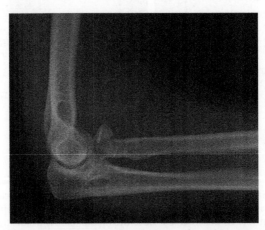

Fig. 16. Radial head fracture (Mason type II). (*Courtesy of* E. Labat, MD, University of Puerto Rico Diagnostic Radiology Program.)

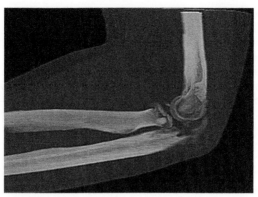

Fig. 17. Radial head fracture (Mason type III). (*Courtesy of* E. Labat, MD, University of Puerto Rico Diagnostic Radiology Program.)

Orthopedic consultation is warranted for Mason types II and III in the ED. Early management includes analgesia and placing the elbow in an arm sling for comfort. Radiographs must include elbow, distal humerus, and forearm views.

Complications of radial head fractures include chronic pain, inability to fully extend the elbow, and loss of motion.

SUMMARY

EPs must be proficient in the acute management of forearm and elbow injuries. Most forearm and elbow orthopedic injuries are initially evaluated in the ED and require imaging studies, adequate limb immobilization, rest, ice and analgesia. Most nondisplaced fractures without neurovascular involvement can be treated nonoperatively in consultation with an orthopedic specialist. However, a subset of injuries such as elbow dislocations, complex forearm fracture-dislocations, and displaced supracondylar fractures are potentially limb-threatening injuries that require immediate identification and timely intervention in the ED to avoid neurovascular complications and functional impairment. Early recognition of neurovascular complications improves the outcome in many of these injuries.

REFERENCES

1. Perry CR, Elstrom JA. Handbook of fractures. 2nd edition. St Louis (MO): McGraw Hill; 2000. p. 132.
2. Villarin LA Jr, Belk KE, Freid R. Emergency department evaluation and treatment of elbow and forearm injuries. Emerg Med Clin North Am 1999;17(4):843–58, vi.
3. Woolfrey KGH, Woolfrey MR, Eisenhauer MA. Wrist and forearm. In: Marx, Hockberger, Walls, editors. Rosen's emergency medicine concepts and clinical practice. 7th edition. Philadelphia: Mosby; 2007. p. 541.
4. Scott Black W, Becker JA. Common forearm fractures in adults. Am Fam Physician 2009;80(10):1096–102.
5. Eiff MP, Hatch R, Calmbach WL. Radius and ulna fractures. In: Fracture management for primary care. 2nd edition. Philadelphia: Saunders; 2003. p. 116–47.
6. Freeland AE, Kregor PJ. Treatment of isolated fractures of the ulnar shaft. Orthopedics 1997;20(11):1081–2.

7. Giannoulis FS, Sotereanos DG. Galeazzi fractures and dislocations. Hand Clin 2007 May;23(2):153–63.
8. Faierman E, Jupiter JB. The management of acute fractures involving the distal radio-ulnar joint and distal ulna. Hand Clin 1998;14:213–29.
9. Perron AD, Hersh RE, Brady WJ, et al. Orthopedic pitfalls in the ED: Galeazzi and Monteggia fracture dislocation. Am J Emerg Med 2001;19:225–8.
10. Kraus B, Horne G. Galeazzi fractures. J Trauma 1985;25:1093–5.
11. Morgan WJ, Breen TF. Complex fractures of the forearm. Hand Clin 1994;10: 375–90.
12. Hughston JC. Fracture of the distal radial shaft: mistakes in management. J Bone Joint Surg Am 1957;39:249–64.
13. Newton EJ, Love J. Emergency department management of selected orthopedic injuries. Emerg Med Clin North Am 2007;25:763–93.
14. Bado JL. The Monteggia lesion. Clin Orthop Relat Res 1967;50:71–86.
15. Perron AD, Brady WJ. Evaluation and management of the high-risk orthopedic emergency. Emerg Med Clin North Am 2003;21:159–204.
16. Storen G. Traumatic dislocation of the radial head as an isolated lesion in children. Acta Clin Scand 1969;116:144.
17. David-West KS, Wilson NI, Sherlock DA, et al. Missed Monteggia injuries. Injury 2005;36:1206–9.
18. Eathiraju S, Mudgal CS, Jupiter JB, et al. Monteggia fracture-dislocations. Hand Clin 2007;23:165–77.
19. Boyd HB, Boals JC. The Monteggia lesion: a review of 159 cases. Clin Orthop 1969;66:94–100.
20. Lloyd-Roberts GC, Buckhill TM. Anterior dislocation of the radial head in children aetiology, natural history and management. J Bone Joint Surg Br 1977;59(4): 402–7.
21. Smith FM. Monteggia fracture: an analysis of twenty-five consecutive fresh injuries. Surg Gynecol Obstet 1947;85:630–40.
22. Bruce HE, Harvey JP Jr, Wilson JC Jr. Monteggia fractures. J Bone Joint Surg Am 1974;56(8):1563–76.
23. Stein F, Grabias SL, Deffer PA. Nerve injuries complicating Monteggia lesions. J Bone Joint Surg Am 1971;53(7):1432–6.
24. Jungbluth P, Frangen TM, Arens S, et al. The undiagnosed Essex-Lopresti injury. J Bone Joint Surg Br 2006;88(12):1629–33.
25. Edwards GS, Jupiter JB. Radial head fractures with acute distal radioulnar dislocation: Essex-Lopresti revisited. Clin Orthop 1998;234:61–9.
26. Dodds SD, Yeh PC, Slade JF 3rd, et al. Essex-Lopresti injuries. Hand Clin 2008; 24(1):125–37.
27. Failla JM, Jacobson J, van Holsbeeck M. Ultrasound diagnosis and surgical pathology of the torn interosseous membrane in forearm fractures/dislocations. J Hand Surg Am 1999;24(2):257–66.
28. Wallace AL. Magnetic resonance imaging or ultrasound in assessment of the interosseous membrane of the forearm. J Bone Joint Surg Am 2002;84(3):496–7.
29. Jaakkola JI, Riggans DH, Lourie GM, et al. Ultrasonography for the evaluation of forearm interosseous membrane disruption in a cadaver model. J Hand Surg Am 2001;26(6):1053–7.
30. Matsuoka J, Beppu M, Nakajima H, et al. Ultrasonography for the interosseous membrane of the forearm. Hand Surg 2003;8(2):227–35.
31. Posterior Interosseous Nerve Compression Syndrome. Wheeles atlas of orthopedia online. Original Text by Clifford R. Wheeless, III, MD. Last updated by Clifford

R. Wheeless, III, MD, December 13, 2008. Available at: http://www. wheelessonline.com/ortho/posterior_interosseous_nerve_compression_syndrome. Accessed August 30, 2010.

32. Bryce CD, Armstrong AD. Anatomy and biomechanics of the elbow. Orthop Clin North Am 2008;39:141–54.

33. Sellards R, Kuebrich C. The elbow: diagnosis and treatment of common injuries. Prim Care 2005;32:1–16.

34. Geiderman JM. Humerus and elbow. In: Marx J, Hockberger R, editors. Emergency medicine: concepts and clinical practice. 6th edition. Philadelphia: Mosby; 2006. p. 647–69.

35. Plancher KD, Lucas TS. Fracture dislocations of the elbow in athletes. Clin Sports Med 2001;20(1):59–76.

36. Moore KL, Agur AMR. Upper limb. In: Moore K, Agur A, editors. Essential of clinical anatomy. 2nd edition. Baltimore (MD): Lippincott Williams & Wilkins; 2002. p. 435–42.

37. Shrader MW. Pediatric supracondylar fractures and pediatric physeal elbow fractures. Orthop Clin North Am 2008;39:163–71.

38. Chuirazzi DM, Riviello RJ. The elbow and distal humerus. In: Schwartz D, Reisdorff E, editors. Emergency radiology. St Louis (MO): McGraw-Hill; 2000. p. 77–100.

39. Lins RE, Simovitch RW, Waters PM. Pediatric elbow trauma. Orthop Clin North Am 1999;30(1):119–32.

40. Simon RR, Koenigsknecht SJ. Fractures of the distal humerus. In: Medina M, Noujaim S, Holton B, editors. Emergency orthopedics—the extremities. 4th edition. St Louis (MO): McGraw-Hill; 2001. p. 234.

41. Mangwani J, Nadarajah R, Paterson JM. Supracondylar humeral fractures in children: ten years experience in a teaching hospital. J Bone Joint Surg Br 2006;88:362–5.

42. Corbett RH. Displaced fat pads in trauma to the elbow. Injury 1978;9:297–8.

43. Skaggs DL, Mirzayan R. The posterior fat pad sign in association with occult fracture of the elbow in children. J Bone Joint Surg Am 1999;81:1429–33.

44. Crowther M. Elbow pain in pediatrics. Curr Rev Musculoskelet Med 2009;2:83–7.

45. Brubacher JW, Dodds SD. Pediatric supracondylar fractures of the distal humerus. Curr Rev Musculoskelet Med 2008;1:190–6.

46. Gartland J. Management of supracondylar fractures of the humerus in children. Surg Gynecol Obstet 1959;109:145–54.

47. Omid R, Choi PD, Skaggs DL. Supracondylar humeral fractures in children. J Bone Joint Surg Am 2008;90(5):1121–32.

48. Queally JM, Paramanathan N, Walsh JC, et al. Dorgan's lateral cross-wiring of supracondylar fractures of the humerus in children: a retrospective review. Injury 2010;41:568–71.

49. Ryan LM. Evaluation and management of supracondylar fractures in children. In: Bachur RG, editor. UpToDate. Waltham (MA): UpToDate; 2009.

50. Kuntz DG Jr, Baratz ME. Fractures of the elbow. Orthop Clin North Am 1999 Jan; 30(1):37–61.

51. Rommens PM, Kuchle R, Schneider RU, et al. Olecranon fractures in adults: factors influencing outcome. Injury 2004;35:1149–57.

52. Newman SDS, Mauffrey C, Krikler S. Olecranon fractures. Injury 2009;40(6): 575–81.

53. Browner BD, Jupiter JB, Levine AM, et al. Skeletal trauma. Philadelphia: Saunders; 1992.

54. Colton CL. Fractures of the olecranon in adults: classification and management. Injury 1973;5(2):121–9.
55. Morrey BF, Adams RA. Fractures of the proximal ulna and olecranon. In: Morrey BF, editor. The elbow and its disorders. Philadelphia: WB Saunders; 1993. p. 405–28.
56. Papagelopoulos PJ, Morrey BF. Treatment of nonunion of olecranon fractures. J Bone Joint Surg Br 1994;76(4):627–35.
57. Karlsson MK, Hasserius R, Karlsson C, et al. Fractures of the olecranon: a 15- to 25-year followup of 73 patients. Clin Orthop Relat Res 2002;403:205–12.
58. Bailey CS, MacDermid J, Patterson SD, et al. Outcome of plate fixation of olecranon fractures. J Orthop Trauma 2001;15(8):542–8.
59. Kuhn MA. Acute elbow dislocations. Orthop Clin North Am 2008;39(2):155–61, v.
60. McNamara R. Management of common dislocations. In: Roberts JR, Hedges JR, editors. Clinical procedures in emergency medicine. 3rd edition. Philadelphia: W.B. Saunders; 1998. p. 834.
61. Morrey BF, An KN, Stormont TJ. Force transmission through the radial head. J Bone Joint Surg Am 1988;70:250–6.
62. Kalicke T, Westhoff J, Wingenfeld C, et al. Fracture dislocation of the elbow involving the coronoid process. Unfallchirurg 2003;106:300–5.
63. Jungbluth P, Hakimi M, Linhart W, et al. Current concepts: simple and complex elbow dislocations—acute and definitive treatment. Eur J Trauma Emerg Surg 2008;34:120–30.
64. Geiderman JM, Torbati SS. Humerus and elbow. In: Marx J, Hockberger R, editors. Emergency medicine: concepts and clinical practice. 7th edition. Philadelphia: Mosby; 2009. p. 545–66.
65. Platz A, Heinzelmann M, Ertel W, et al. Posterior elbow dislocation with associated vascular injury after blunt trauma. J Trauma 1999;46:948.
66. Rao SB, Crawford AH. Median nerve entrapment after dislocation of the elbow in children: a report of two cases and review of literature. Clin Orthop 1995; 312:232.
67. Lavine LS. A simple method of reducing dislocations of the elbow joint. J Bone Joint Surg Am 1953;35:785.
68. Parvin RW. Closed reduction of common shoulder and elbow dislocations without anesthesia. Arch Surg 1957;75:972.
69. Meyn MA, Quigley TB. Reduction of posterior dislocation of the elbow by traction on the dangling arm. Clin Orthop 1974;103:106.
70. Kumar A, Ahmed M. Closed reduction of posterior dislocation of the elbow: a simple technique. J Orthop Trauma 1999;13(1):58–9.
71. Afshar A. Divergent dislocation of the elbow in an 11-year-old child. Arch Iran Med 2007;10(3):413–6.
72. Altuntas AO, Balakumar J, Howells RJ, et al. Posterior divergent dislocation of the elbow in children and adolescents: a report of three cases and review of the literature. J Pediatr Orthop 2005;25:317–21.
73. Vicente P, Orduna M. Transverse divergent dislocation of the elbow in a child. A case report. Clin Orthop 1993;294:312–3.
74. Andersen K, Mortensen AC, Gron P. Transverse divergent dislocation of the elbow. A report of two cases. Acta Orthop Scand 1985;56:442–3.
75. Basanagoudar P, Pace A. Unusual dislocation of the elbow in a child-review of literature. J Trauma 2008;65:E18–20.
76. Sovio OM, Tredwell SJ. Divergent dislocation of the elbow in a child. J Pediatr Orthop 1986;6:96–7.

77. Laugharnea E, Porter KM. Fractures of the radial head and neck. Trauma 2009; 11:249–58.
78. Morrey BF. Radial head fracture. In: Morrey BF, editor. The elbow and its disorders. 3rd edition. Philadelphia: Saunders; 2000. p. 341–64.
79. McKee MD, Jupiter JB. Trauma to the adult elbow and fractures of the distal humerus. Part 1: trauma to the adult elbow. In: Browner BD, Jupiter JB, Levine AM, et al, editors, Skeletal trauma: fractures, dislocations, ligamentous injuries, vol. 2. 2nd edition. Philadelphia: W.B. Saunders; 1998. p. 1455–83.
80. Black WS, Becker JA. Common forearm fractures in adults. Am Fam Physician 2009;80(10):1096–102.
81. Mason ML. Some observations on fractures of the head of the radius with a review of one hundred cases. Br J Surg 1954;42:123–32.
82. Madsen JE, Flugsrud G. Radial head fractures: indications and technique for primary arthroplasty. Eur J Trauma Emerg Surg 2008;34:105–12.
83. Ikeda M, Sugiyama K, Kang C, et al. Comminuted fractures of the radial head. Comparison of resection and internal fixation. J Bone Joint Surg Am 2005; 87(1):76–84.

The Emergent Evaluation and Treatment of Hand and Wrist Injuries

Michael K. Abraham, MD, MS[a,b,]*, Sara Scott, MD[a,c]

KEYWORDS

- Hand and wrist injuries • Emergency physician
- Emergent evaluation • Treatment

Injuries to the hand and wrist can pose a challenge for the emergency physician. These injuries are not life threatening, however, the complexity of the area can pose many diagnostic and treatment dilemmas. The anatomy of the hand is complex, which allows for the dexterity, strength, and adaptability of the most functional aspect of the musculoskeletal system. The evaluation and management of injuries to this area can be time consuming and pose a significant medicolegal risk to the emergency physician. Improperly diagnosed and managed injuries can lead to chronic pain, inability to perform activities of daily living, and even seemingly minor injuries can lead to missed work causing a significant cost to the individual and society.[1] The purpose of this article is to review injuries to the hand and wrist and discuss diagnostic studies and treatment plans that the emergency physician can use to treat patients effectively and minimize their exposure to risk.

ANATOMY

The wrist is comprised of 8 carpal bones arranged in 2 transverse rows. The proximal row is important in that it connects the radius and the ulna to the distal row of carpal bones. The proximal row of carpal bones, listed ulnar to radial, consist of the triquetrum, lunate, and scaphoid. The distal carpal row, listed ulnar to radial, is composed of the hamate, capitate, trapezoid, and trapezium. The eighth carpal bone, the pisiform, is actually a sesamoid bone enclosed in the sheath of the flexor carpi ulnaris tendon and is located

[a] Department of Emergency Medicine, University of Maryland School of Medicine, 110 South Paca Street, 6th Floor Suite 200, Baltimore, MD 21201, USA
[b] Department of Emergency Medicine, Upper Chesapeake Medical Health, 500 Upper Chesapeake Drive, Bel Air, MD 21014, USA
[c] Department of Emergency Medicine, Mercy Medical Center, 301 St Paul Place, Baltimore, MD 21202, USA
* Corresponding author. Department of Emergency Medicine, University of Maryland School of Medicine, 110 South Paca Street, 6th Floor Suite 200, Baltimore, MD 21201.
E-mail address: mabra003@umaryland.edu

Emerg Med Clin N Am 28 (2010) 789–809
doi:10.1016/j.emc.2010.06.004
0733-8627/10/$ – see front matter © 2010 Elsevier Inc. All rights reserved.

emed.theclinics.com

in an anterior plane to the other carpal bones (**Fig. 1**A). Radiographically, the carpal bones form 3 arcs, commonly referred to as Gilula's carpal arcs. Arc I forms the proximal artic-ulating surfaces of the triquetrum, lunate, and scaphoid. Arc II forms the distal articulating surface of the same 3 bones. Arc III outlines the proximal articulating surface of the capi-tate and hamate. In a normal wrist, these 3 arcs should form smooth curves and there should be no overlap between lines (see **Fig. 1**B). The anatomic snuff box is clinically significant in that it encompasses the scaphoid bone and a branch of the radial artery. The medial border of the box is the tendon of the extensor pollicis longus (EPL) and the lateral border is the tendon of the abductor pollicis longus (APL).

Moving distally from the carpal bones is a row of metacarpals. Distal to the metacarpals are 3 rows of phalanges, with the exception of the thumb, which has only 2 phalanges.

The 3 main nerves that control the hand and wrist are the median, ulnar, and radial nerves and their branches. Understanding of their course and areas of inner-vation are crucial to performing regional anesthesia and blocks. If there is signif-icant injury to the hand or wrist patients may not tolerate a digital or hematoma block. In these cases, the use of ultrasound guidance can be helpful in localizing the nerve and reducing complications when performing regional blocks.

FRACTURES OF THE HAND

It is estimated that half of all hand injuries are fractures and that phalanx and meta-carpal fractures account for more than 40% of all upper extremity fractures.[2]

First Metacarpal

The dexterity of the human hand relies on the thumb and its functionality depends on its extensive mobility. The thumb is estimated to account for approximately 1 million emergency department (ED) visits per year.[3] The wide range of motion of the

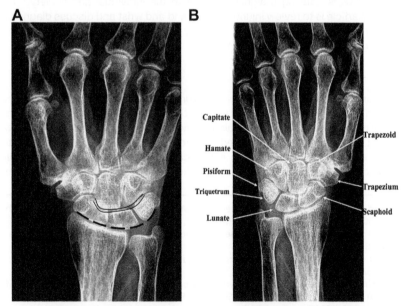

Fig. 1. (*A*) Normal PA film of the hand with carpal bones identified. The articulation between the proximal row of carpal bones and the distal forearm should have a smooth curvature. (*B*) The lines between the distal and proximal carpal bones should also form an arc. Note the distance between the scaphoid and lunate is less than 3 mm.

carpometacarpal (CMC) joint allows for the first metacarpal to withstand a wide variety of forces without injury. However, when the thumb is injured it can lead to significant changes in patients' quality of life.

On physical examination one should attempt to evaluate the pinching strength of the thumb. This is known as Froment's sign. A change in strength is usually attributed to a ligamentous injury or fracture of the first metacarpal that produces an ulnar neuropathy. Plain films with specific attention to the thumb are usually sufficient to diagnose a fracture or dislocation. The most common fracture of the first metacarpal is a Bennett fracture that was first described in 1882 (**Fig. 2**). This fracture is defined as an intraarticular fracture at the base of the CMC joint of the thumb.[4] The fractured fragment is often a triangular piece of bone. Because of the ligamentous forces applied by the APL there is dorsal displacement of the first metacarpal. This injury is a result of an axial load on a partially flexed metacarpal, for example a closed-fist injury. A similar fracture is the Rolando fracture first described in 1910. This fracture is also an intraarticular fracture of the CMC joint, but in this case the fracture has a *T* or *Y* shape. Because of the pull of the APL there is once again dorsal displacement of the first metacarpal.[4]

These fractures are inherently unstable and will require placement of a splint in the ED and discussion with a hand specialist. In addition to the instability of the fractures, closed reduction in the ED can be difficult because of the dual innervation of the thumb. Both the median and radial nerves contribute to the innervation making a regional block difficult. Hematoma blocks are not recommended for these fractures as most are intraarticular, which will increase the rate of complications. The placement of a thumb spica or modified thumb spica splint is usually sufficient in the ED.[3] The long-term management of these fractures frequently requires an operative procedure,

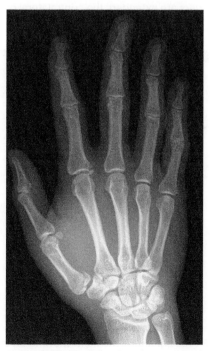

Fig. 2. An example of a Bennett fracture of the thumb metacarpal. Notice the intraarticular component of the fracture and the triangular shape of the bone fragment.

whether open reduction with internal fixation or transcutaneous pinning. There is extensive debate over what the best definitive treatment is, which is beyond the scope of this article. These fractures should be discussed with your local hand surgeon to optimize the patients' treatment plan and follow-up.

Digital Metacarpals

The metacarpals account for approximately one-third of all hand fractures. They usually result from a direct axial load on the metacarpal row. Logically, for this to occur the proximal phalanges must be flexed as in a closed-fist injury. Fractures of the metacarpals can, however, also occur with blunt trauma directly to the metacarpals as in a crush injury.

The diagnosis of these injuries is based on obtaining plain radiographs of the hand in the posteroanterior (PA), lateral, and oblique views. The key to the management of these fractures is based on the amount of angulation and rotational deformity that is present. Fracture of the neck of the fifth metacarpal is known as a boxer's fracture and is the most common metacarpal fracture (**Fig. 3**). Reduction should be attempted if there is more than 35° to 40° of volar angulation. The second and third metacarpals, however, are allowed less angular deformity and as such need to be reduced if there is more than 5° to 10° of angulation, respectively. One simplified view is to allow 5°, 10°, 20°, and 30° of angulation for the index, middle, ring, and small fingers, respectively.[5]

Although angulation is determined by radiologic studies, the rotational deformity is usually based on the physical examination and is important in these fractures. There are 3 relevant examination findings based on the presence of rotational deformity. When the hand is uninjured all of the phalanges should point to the scaphoid when the fist is closed, there should be no finger overlap, and the nails should all lie in the same plane when the fingers are extended; the contralateral or injured hand can serve

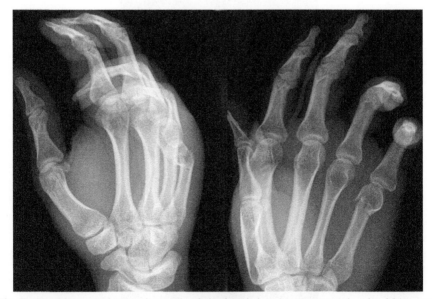

Fig. 3. An oblique and PA radiograph of the hand showing an example of a fifth metacarpal, or Boxer fracture. Notice the angulation of the head of the metacarpal. This injury would necessitate reduction in the emergency department.

as a reference.[4] Rotational deformities may also be seen on radiologic studies. The width of the cortex of the bone on opposite sides of the fracture line should be the same size. A difference in width is usually caused by the distal fragment being rotated so that the bone is not in the same plane as the proximal portion.

Immediate reduction in the ED is warranted if there is any evidence of rotational deformity. However, rotation deformities are inherently unstable and it may be difficult to maintain any reduction obtained in the ED. Reduction of metacarpal shaft or neck fractures can be accomplished with local hematoma or wrist block anesthesia using 1% lidocaine with epinephrine. The fracture is then reduced using a maneuver described by Jahss[6] in 1938. In the Jahss' maneuver, the metacarpophalangeal (MCP) and proximal interphalangeal (PIP) joints of the affected metacarpal are flexed to 90°. The fracture is then reduced by pressing up on the proximal phalanx and pushing the proximal metacarpal dorsally. Patients should then be placed in an ulnar gutter splint with the wrist flexed at 30° and the MCP joint flexed at 90°. Fracture of the second (**Fig. 4**) and third metacarpals should be reduced as needed and placed in a volar or radial gutter splint. If there is a rotational deformity, the fingers should be buddy taped to prevent misalignment before placing the splint. It should be noted that all of these injuries ultimately require an evaluation by a hand specialist. The patients' occupation, age, and the details of the injury will dictate the timeliness of the follow-up.

Phalangeal Fractures

The proximal, middle, or distal phalanges are easily injured and fractures are common. Unlike most other bones in the body, the digits are unprotected from a force in almost any direction, which can result in fractures that are displaced, angulated, rotated, or any combination of these. There may also be an intraarticular component to the

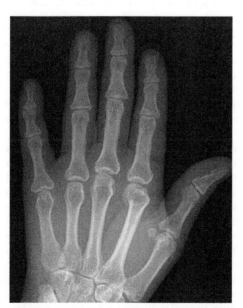

Fig. 4. Fracture of the second metacarpal. Notice how the articular surface is angulated in the ulnar direction. This injury will be difficult to reduce in the emergency department. Proper treatment will require placement in a radial gutter splint and referral for open reduction and fixation.

fractures, making for a difficult and often impossible reduction in the ED. Despite proper treatment, the most commonly cited long-term complaint is joint stiffness.[7] The diagnosis of these injuries is made with conventional radiographs. All 3 views (PA, lateral, and oblique) must be obtained with specific instruction to the radiologist to focus on the affected digit.

Although patients may be in pain, and thus significantly limit the examination, examination of both flexor tendon and the extensor tendon mechanisms is crucial. In addition, a good neurologic and vascular examination should be completed before any digital or hematoma block. After patients are given proper analgesia, the examination of the tendons can be revisited, usually with more success. Previously, the teachings were that digital blocks should be done with 1% or 2% lidocaine without epinephrine. This practice has been challenged recently and the use of lidocaine with epinephrine is not only safe but preferred in the management of digital injuries.[8]

Damage to the proximal or middle phalanx, especially the dorsal aspect, is important because improper treatment can lead to a Boutonniere deformity. This deformity is described as a flexion at the PIP with hyperextension at the distal interphalangeal (DIP) joint. The difficulty for the emergency physician lies in the fact that this injury may not be immediately present on physical examination. A boutonniere deformity usually develops weeks after the patients' initial injury. The mechanisms that control the movement of the PIP joint are complex. The extension of the digit is not controlled by a singular tendon but by a combination of tendons and sheaths that attach to the dorsal surface of both the distal and middle phalanx. Flexion is controlled by the flexor digitorum profundus (FDP), which inserts on the distal phalanx, and the flexor digitorum superficialis (FDS), which inserts on the middle phalanx. The delicate balance between the extensor mechanism over the dorsal PIP joint and the flexors is altered because of the injury. As the healing progresses, the now-dominant FDS creates constant flexion at the PIP joint. Because the extensor tendon mechanism has slipped down toward the volar surface of the phalanx, the pull of the extensor tendon causes extension of the DIP joint, thus giving the characteristic presentation.[9]

Fractures of the proximal and middle phalanges should be treated with a gutter splint, either radial or ulnar, depending on the location of the injury. These splints should leave the wrist extended at 30° and the MCP flexed to 90°. This position will allow for the remainder of the uninjured digits to maintain mobility. Once again if there is rotational deformity the digits can be buddy taped before splinting. This procedure must be done with caution, however, because a rotational deformity can be exacerbated with splinting.

Fractures of the distal phalanx provide additional treatment challenges. These fractures, similar to the middle and proximal phalanx, have tendinous attachments that can result in deformities and functional disability. They also have a unique anatomic characteristic: the nail. Fractures of the distal phalanx are classified, from distal to proximal, as a tuft, shaft, or articular surface fracture. Diagnosis of these injuries requires 3 dedicated plain radiographs of the affected digit. Distal tuft injuries are common and can be time consuming for the emergency physician to manage. These injuries usually result from a crushing force to the digit, such as a hammer or car door. Along with the fracture, there is usually some injury to the nail and the nail bed. If the fracture is open patients should undergo intense irrigation, intravenous antibiotics, and tetanus prophylaxis. If the nail is intact and there is a subungual hematoma, the nail should be left in place and the hematoma drained. If, however, the nail is damaged, the nail should be removed and the nail bed repaired with absorbable sutures. After the repair of the nail bed, the nail should be replaced and used as a physiologic splint. This procedure can be achieved by placing a horizontal mattress suture at the base of the nail, with careful attention to avoid the nail matrix. In the event that the nail is not damaged, but the fracture is open, the soft tissue must be repaired with attention paid to maintaining the anatomy as normal as possible.

Fractures of the shaft and articular surface of a phalanx can also pose problems. The most concerning of these is an avulsion fracture at the base of the distal phalanx. This fracture can be associated with a mallet deformity, in which patients cannot extend the distal phalanx. If this fracture is mismanaged, a swan neck deformity may occur. Just like the Boutonniere deformity develops weeks after injury, the swan neck deformity may take weeks to be recognized clinically (**Fig. 5**). The swan neck deformity is characterized by extension at the PIP with flexion of the DIP, caused by the unopposed action of the FDP.

Treatment of distal phalanx fractures includes splinting to ensure immobilization of the DIP joint. Every attempt should be made to leave full mobility of the PIP joint. Thus, unless there is also an injury of the more proximal bones, a gutter splint should be avoided. If there is concern for an avulsion injury on the dorsal aspect of the distal phalanx, the splint must keep the joint in full extension for 8 to 10 weeks.[10] Any joint mobility during this time could exacerbate the injury and render any healing useless.

Any open fracture of the finger requires emergent evaluation by a hand specialist, especially if amputation, either partial or full, is a component. Otherwise most injuries can be splinted and patients referred to a hand specialist. The patients' demographics (eg, age, occupation) can necessitate an orthopedic or plastic surgery consult even for a minor injury.

DISLOCATIONS

Just as with any joint in the body, dislocations in the hand are possible. Dislocations of the DIP and PIP are more common than others, and in fact the PIP is the most dislocated joint in the body.[11] Most dislocations are evident on physical examination.

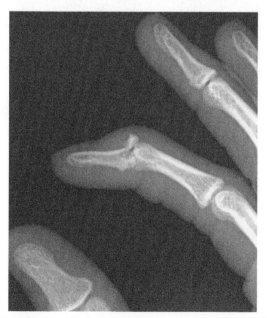

Fig. 5. Lateral radiograph of a distal phalanx fracture. Although a seemingly minor injury, failure to properly treat this fracture can lead to a boutonniere deformity. Proper treatment is splinting the joint in full extension for 8 to 10 weeks.

A plain radiograph should be obtained to ensure that there are no associated fractures. After a neurologic examination, the affected area can be anesthetized with a regional or digital block. MCP joints are rarely dislocated as an isolated injury. These dislocations commonly occur with a fracture. MCP dislocations are difficult to reduce and will need operative repair the majority of the time (**Fig. 6**).

PIP dislocations are common, especially during sporting events, making this a common injury among young, active individuals. Often the reduction is performed before evaluation in the ED. The dislocation can occur in the dorsal, volar, or lateral directions. Dorsal dislocations are usually easily reduced and treated with splinting in 20° to 30° of flexion. Volar dislocations are also easily reduced; however, their treatment is different. A volar dislocation can cause damage to the central extensor slip, which as discussed previously, predisposes patients to developing a boutonnière deformity. If a volar dislocation is treated the same as a dorsal dislocation, and splinted in flexion, the treatment will exacerbate the development of the boutonniere deformity. Therefore, volar dislocations must be splinted in full extension and necessitate follow-up with a specialist. Lateral dislocations can be reduced and buddy taped or splinted in slight flexion after reduction. The most common long-term complication of PIP dislocations is persistent swelling and stiffness.

LIGAMENT AND TENDON INJURIES

Ligament and tendon injuries can be challenging to correctly diagnosis in the ED. Aside from a laceration, where you can see damage to the tendon, the diagnosis often

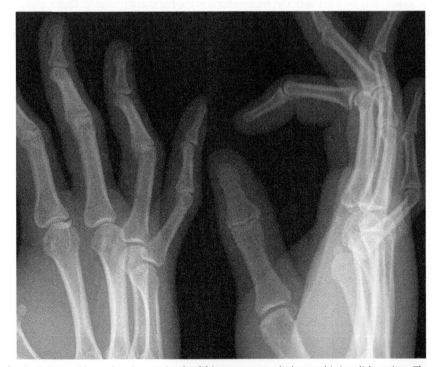

Fig. 6. A PA and lateral radiograph of a fifth metacarpophalangeal joint dislocation. These injuries can be difficult to reduce secondary to interposed soft tissue and will often need operative management.

cannot be made by inspection alone. Further complicating the diagnosis is the fact that patients often do not present to the ED at the time of injury and conventional radiography is often normal. Diagnosis can be made by high-resolution ultrasound with fairly good accuracy.[12] This modality, however, is either not available or underutilized at many centers, decreasing its usefulness. Another modality that can be used in diagnosis and for operative planning is MRI.[13] Although becoming more practical, the use of MRI for non–life-threatening emergencies in the ED is controversial and usually not warranted. Unfortunately, improper treatment of these injuries may lead to boutonniere and swan neck deformities of the digits so early diagnosis is important to prevent these complications.

A commonly encountered sports-related injury is damage to the FDP. This injury is caused by a forced extension of the partially flexed DIP joint. This injury is usually seen in football and rugby players when the finger gets caught in the opponents jersey while trying to make a tackle, and is commonly referred to as a jersey finger.[14] Because of the physics and anatomy of the digits, the ring finger is most susceptible to this injury.[15] The key to this injury lies in the diagnosis. Because the limited range of motion caused by the injury to the FDP is attributed to pain and swelling, the injury is missed. The finger is placed in a splint in slight flexion for comfort, but this does not treat the injury. Treatment is usually operative, because the flexor tendon tends to retract and can retract as proximally as the palm.

Injury to the ulnar collateral ligament of the thumb, called game-keepers thumb, secondary to forced abduction is commonly seen in ski-pole injuries.[16] This injury is associated with damage to the ulnar collateral ligament and is associated with a metacarpal avulsion fracture. An injury with this mechanism is usually treated conservatively. Plain films should be obtained to assess for fractures. In the acute setting, an examination of the first CMC joint for laxity can be limited by pain and swelling. These patients should, without exception, be placed in a thumb spica splint and arranged for prompt follow-up with a hand specialist. The hand specialist can evaluate patients after the swelling has subsided and possibly determine the need for an MRI or ultrasound. Most cases will need operative management, although conservative treatment with casting can produce good outcomes.[17]

INJURIES PERTAINING TO THE WRIST

The complex motions of the wrist are supported by an intricate framework of bones and their soft-tissue connections. Injuries to the wrist can have devastating functional results because of the small passages for the neurovascular bundles to traverse. Carpal bone fractures account for approximately 20% of all the fractures of the hand and wrist.[18]

Scaphoid Injuries

The scaphoid bone is located on the radial side of the proximal row of carpal bones. It is the most commonly fractured carpal bone and a delay in fracture diagnosis of 1 to 2 weeks can increase the chances of a poor outcome.[19] The mechanism of most injuries is an axial load to a hyperextended wrist as in a fall on an outstretched hand (FOOSH).[20] The issue with scaphoid fractures lies in the high incidence of avascular necrosis (AVN) and nonunion that results from its tenuous blood supply. The blood supply of the scaphoid enters from the dorsal side in the middle of the bone. The proximal surface of the scaphoid, the most important because of its articular surface, is supplied by nutrient arteries. Approximately 15% of fractures of the scaphoid waist result in malunion or nonunion. AVN will occur approximately 30%

of the time with more proximal fractures having a higher than 80% incidence of AVN.[19–21]

Diagnosis of these fractures (**Fig. 7**) can be difficult and, because of the risk for complications, there is a significant cost to the health care system from overtreatment of these injuries.[22] Diagnosis of scaphoid injuries should begin with a thorough physical examination and diagnostic imaging. Radiographs are required in all cases. The practitioner can obtain plain radiographs of the wrist with a dedicated scaphoid view, although these miss the diagnosis in almost 10% of fractures.[23] There is a significant debate as to whether the use of either CT or MRI is cost effective in the diagnosis of scaphoid injury. Studies have shown that the specificity and sensitivity of CT scans are approximately 90%, with a negative predictive value of 0.99 in one study, thus CT scans are unlikely to miss a fracture.[24,25] MRI has good specificity, sensitivity, and low interobserver variability; the issue with MRI lies in the limited availability and prohibitive cost.[26–28] The final modality that can be used in the diagnosis of a scaphoid fractures is a bone scan. This testing modality, however, is of limited utility in the emergent setting.

In a suspected fracture, with no definite evidence of fracture on imaging, placement of a thumb spica splint and referral to a hand specialist for follow-up in 7 to 10 days with repeat films is a commonly accepted practice. If there is a documented fracture, a placement of a long-arm thumb spica splint and immediate consultation with a hand specialist is necessary because of the long-term complications of these fractures.[29]

Hamate Injuries

The hamate is located on the ulnar side in the distal row of carpal bones. Hamate fractures are rare and account for only 1.7% of all carpal bone fractures.[30] Fractures can occur in either the body of the hamate or the hook, with the latter being more

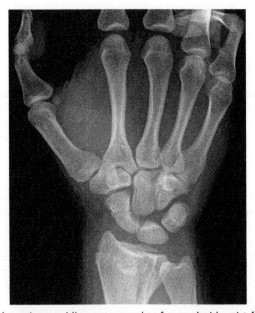

Fig. 7. PA view of the wrist providing an example of a scaphoid waist fracture and a distal radius fracture.

common.[31] Hook of the hamate fractures typically occurs in sports involving racquets, clubs, or bats. During a swing, the base of the club, bat, or racquet forcefully impacts the hook of the hamate causing a fracture. Other mechanisms of injury of the hamate include a FOOSH or the impact of power tools or machinery into the ulnar aspect of palm.

Patients with a fracture of the hook of the hamate will typically complain of ulnar-sided wrist pain and will have pain with palpation in the hypothenar area. Paresthesias in the ulnar distribution may also be found. Forcing patients to actively grasp with the affected hand will cause pain on the ulnar side of the palm.[32]

Although rare, hook of the hamate fractures should be suspected in patients with the appropriate antecedent history and any of the previously mentioned physical examination findings. Diagnostic imaging may include standard wrist films, specialized views, or CT. In standard radiography, a hook of the hamate fracture can be identified on the PA view of the wrist by the loss of the oval, dense cortical ring shadow over the hamate (**Fig. 8A**).[30] This finding can be missed if the radiograph is not done properly or if the fracture is at the base. Therefore, if a hook of the hamate fracture is suspected clinically and standard plain films do not show any abnormalities, special radiographic studies should be ordered. These studies may include a carpal tunnel view (see **Fig. 8B**), a supinated oblique view with the wrist dorsiflexed, or a lateral view projected through the first web space with the thumb abducted.[33] These views can sometimes be difficult to obtain in acutely injured patients when wrist mobility is limited by pain and swelling.

Recent literature has shown the sensitivity of plain radiography to be as low as 40% for detection of hamate fractures.[18] CT is superior to plain radiography in the detection of fractures of the hamate.[18,34,35] Because of the limitations and lack of sensitivity of plain films, CT should be considered in patients with clinically suspected fractures of the hook of the hamate and negative radiographs.

Early diagnosis of hamate fractures is important because missed fractures can lead to significant disability and serious complications, including tendon rupture.[36] Treatment in the acute setting involves immobilization with the wrist in slight flexion and

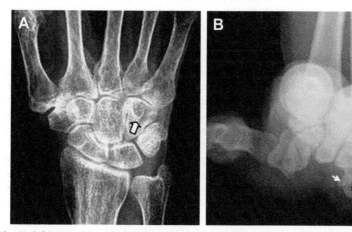

Fig. 8. (A) Normal PA view of wrist demonstrating the eye sign (*white arrow*). The eye sign is produced by an intact hook of the hamate bone. (B) Normal carpal tunnel view of the wrist. Arrow indicates the hook of the hamate. Asterisk denotes the pisiform. This view is used to more clearly demonstrate pisiform and hamate fractures.

the fourth and fifth MCP joints in maximum flexion. Immobilizing the thumb is also recommended to minimize the pull of the thenar muscles on the hook by the transverse carpal ligament.[37] Follow-up hand evaluation is recommended within 1 week.

Fractures through the body of the hamate are less common than fractures through the hook of the hamate and often occur as the result of an axial load to the clenched fist. These fractures are usually associated with concurrent injuries to the fourth and fifth CMC joints and metacarpal bases. Unlike fractures through the hook of the hamate, fractures through the body of the hamate can usually be identified by plain radiography. Early immobilization in a volar short-arm splint, with the hand in position of function, and hand follow-up is recommended for these fractures.

Triquetral Injuries

The triquetrum is located on the ulnar side of the wrist in the proximal row of carpal bones. Triquetral fractures account for 18.3% of all carpal bone fractures, making the triquetral bone the second most commonly fractured carpal bone.[30] Triquetral fractures are classified as either chip fractures, which involve just the dorsal ridge, or triquetral body fractures.

Triquetral chip fractures are the more common of the two and occur with a fall onto an ulnarly deviated wrist in dorsiflexion. Triquetral body fractures are typically caused by direct force to the bone as the result of a high-energy impact. On examination, there may be swelling noted and limitation of wrist flexion and extension.

Imaging should include standard radiographs. The chip fracture is usually best identified on the lateral or oblique view as a bone fragment. The body fracture is most easily identified on the PA view.[31] Because fractures of the body of the triquetrum are often associated with perilunate fracture dislocations, care should be taken to carefully inspect the triquetrum in patients with greater arc injuries to prevent missing a triquetral body fracture. Likewise, identification of a triquetral body fracture should prompt a search for a perilunate ligamentous injury. If suspicion remains high for a triquetral fracture despite normal plain radiographs, a repeat radiograph with the hand in slight pronation or a CT scan should be considered.

Treatment of dorsal chip fractures consists of immobilization in an ulnar gutter splint and rarely requires more than 4 weeks of immobilization.[37] Treatment of the triquetral body fracture also involves immobilization but may require more immediate orthopedic follow-up if there is a suspicion for concurrent greater arc injuries.

Pisiform Injuries

The pisiform bone is a sesamoid bone that lies on the volar surface of the wrist. It articulates only with the triquetrum. The pisiform is rarely fractured and accounts for only 1.3% of all carpal bone fractures.[30] Pisiform fractures are most often caused by a direct blow, such as might occur during a fall on an outstretched hand. Less commonly the pisiform can be avulsed by the flexor carpi ulnaris during forced wrist hyperflexion or from the strain of lifting a heavy object.

Patients with fractures of the pisiform complain of ulnar-sided wrist pain that is accentuated by resisted wrist flexion. Physical examination demonstrates pain over the pisiform. Occasionally, ulnar nerve palsy may result from a pisiform fracture because the pisiform serves as the ulnar wall of the Guyon's canal, which houses the ulnar nerve.[38]

Diagnosis of a pisiform fracture is difficult on standard radiographs because adjacent and overlying bones prevent an unobstructed view of the pisiform. If a pisiform fracture is suspected special views, such as a carpal tunnel view (see **Fig. 8**B) or a reverse oblique view with the wrist in 30° of supination, can be helpful in imaging the pisiform. In children, diagnosis of pisiform fractures is made more complicated by the fact that the pisiform is the last carpal bone to ossify, and the multiple ossification centers may give this bone a fragmented appearance until 12 years of age.[38] CT can be used if clinical suspicion of pisiform fracture persists despite normal or nondiagnostic plain radiographs.

Treatment of a pisiform fracture is immobilization in an ulnar gutter splint for 3 to 4 weeks. If ulnar nerve palsy is present, hand-specialist consultation should be obtained for possible surgical decompression.[39] However, most ulnar nerve palsies that are present at initial presentation will resolve in 8 to 12 weeks and require only close observation.[33]

Capitate Injuries

The capitate is the largest carpal bone and is located centrally in the distal row of carpal bones. Capitate fractures are uncommon, accounting for only 1.9% of all carpal bone fractures, and generally occur in association with other carpal bone injuries, namely scaphoid fractures and perilunate dislocations. Isolated fractures of the capitate are rare, and in fact account for only 0.3% of all carpal injuries.[30,40] Because they are rare, capitate fractures should prompt a search for an associated perilunate ligamentous injury.

The mechanism of injury of the capitate is generally a direct blow to the dorsum of the hand or a fall on an outstretched hand. Capitate fractures can also occur as part of a greater arc injury in association with a perilunate dislocation. Patients with a fracture of the capitate will present with pain and swelling located in the dorsum of the wrist. Direct palpation of the capitate will accentuate the pain.

Standard radiographs of the wrist will most likely reveal the fracture on the PA view. However, isolated, nondisplaced fractures of the capitate can be subtle on plain radiographs. In one study, plain radiography had a sensitivity of 0% and failed to identify any capitate fractures, compared with CT, which had a diagnostic sensitivity of 100%.[18]

Early identification and diagnosis of capitate fracture is essential because the capitate, like the scaphoid, is at risk for AVN and nonunion. Nondisplaced fractures can be immobilized with a short-arm thumb spica cast,[41] whereas displaced fractures or those associated with carpal dislocations require immediate hand-specialist consultation.

Lunate Injuries

The lunate is located in the proximal row of carpal bones and sits between the capitate distally and the distal radius proximally. Lunate fractures account for 3.9% of all carpal bone fractures.[39] Isolated lunate fractures are uncommon except in the case of Kienböck's disease, also known as idiopathic avascular necrosis of the lunate. Associated injuries of the radius, carpals, or metacarpals occur 50% of the time.[38]

The typical mechanism of injury for a lunate fracture involves a fall on an outstretched hand. Patients with lunate fractures will present with pain over the dorsum of the wrist that is exacerbated by palpation of the dorsal aspect of the lunate. Axial loading of the third metacarpal can also accentuate the pain.

Standard wrist radiographs of the lunate often fail to demonstrate the fracture because visualization of the lunate is often obscured by superimposed bones.[31] CT has been found to be more sensitive than plain radiography at identifying fractures of the lunate.[18]

Early identification and management of these fractures is essential to prevent AVN, carpal instability, and nonunion. Patients with suspected or diagnosed lunate fractures should be immobilized in a thumb spica splint with the hand and thumb in neutral position. Lunate fractures require a hand-specialist follow-up in 1 to 2 weeks.[39]

Trapezium Injuries

The trapezium is located on the radial side of the distal row of carpal bones and forms a double-saddle articulation with the base of the first metacarpal. Fractures of the trapezium account for 4.3% of all carpal bone fractures and can be divided into fractures of the trapezial body and fractures of the trapezial ridge.[39]

Fractures of the trapezial body are most common and are often the result of an axial load through the thumb or forced hyperextension and abduction of the thumb. Fractures of the trapezial ridge are most often the result of a fall on an outstretched hand resulting in a direct blow to the trapezium or by avulsion of the trapezium by the transverse carpal ligament. Physical examination demonstrates point tenderness at the volar base of the thumb just distal to the scaphoid and pain with axial loading of the thumb. Pain may be exacerbated by resisted wrist flexion and pinch grasp.

Trapezial fractures are most easily identified on the oblique view because complete visualization of the trapezium is obscured by superimposed bones in the PA and lateral views. Specialized radiographs, including a pronated anteroposterior view, may better help visualize the trapeziometacarpal articulation.[38] The carpal tunnel view is the best view for identifying fractures of the trapezial ridge. CT can be used to diagnose suspected fractures that are not identified on plain radiographs.[18]

Treatment of trapezial fractures is dependent on the type of fracture and presence of displacement. Nondisplaced triquetral body fractures can be immobilized in a short-arm thumb spica for 4 to 6 weeks. All other types of fractures should be immobilized and referred for hand-specialist follow-up.[39]

Trapezoid Injuries

The trapezoid is located in the distal row of carpal bones and positioned between the second metacarpal, capitate, scaphoid, and trapezium. Because it is well protected, it is the least commonly fractured carpal bone, accounting for only 0.4% of all carpal bone fractures.[30] The most common mechanism of injury is a high-energy axial load to a flexed second metacarpal, which most often produces a dorsally displaced fracture/dislocation of the trapezoid.

Physical examination of these patients demonstrates point tenderness over the dorsum of the wrist at the base of the second metacarpal. Pain can be exacerbated with movement of the second metacarpal. Using standard radiographs of the wrist, a fracture/dislocation of the trapezoid is most easily identified on the PA view as loss of the normal joint space between the distal scaphoid and the trapezium and trapezoid.[42] CT has superior sensitivity when compared with plain radiographs and may be necessary to diagnose trapezoid injury.[18]

Identification of a trapezoid injury is essential because complications of an untreated injury may lead to AVN of the trapezoid. Nondisplaced fractures may be treated with a short-arm thumb spica for 4 to 6 weeks. Displaced fractures and fracture/dislocations require prompt hand-specialist consultation.[39]

Carpal Instability

Carpal instability resulting from forced wrist hyperextension has been described as a progressive spectrum of injury ranging from scapholunate dissociation (Stage I) to perilunate dislocation (Stage II) to lunotriquetral disruption (Stage III) and finally to lunate dislocation (Stage IV).[43] The typical mechanism of injury is a fall on an outstretched hand or a high-impact force, such as might occur in a motor vehicle collision.

Physical examination typically shows a swollen tender wrist with limited range of motion secondary to pain. There is also the possibility of reduced grip strength. Median nerve palsy secondary to compression of the median nerve in the carpal tunnel by the lunate can be seen in Stage III and Stage IV injuries. Standard PA and lateral radiographs may be diagnostic of carpal instability, but the findings can be subtle. Nearly 25% of injuries were missed in a study of 166 cases of perilunate dislocations and fracture dislocations.[44]

Scapholunate dissociations (Stage I) involve disruption of the scapholunate interosseous ligament, which is sometimes associated with a fracture of the scaphoid waist. In patients with scapholunate dissociation, the PA radiograph will demonstrate a widening of scapholunate space of more than 3 mm. This widening is sometimes referred to as the Terry Thomas sign (**Fig. 9**). Another finding on the PA view is the cortical ring sign, which reflects the distal pole of the scaphoid seen on end. On lateral views, scapholunate dissociation is evidenced by an increased scapholunate angle of more than 60°.[31] Stress views can be used for diagnosis confirmation by accentuate widening of the scapholunate joint. These radiographs include anteroposterior (AP) views taken with a clenched fist and with ulnar deviation.

Perilunate dislocations (Stage II) involve disruption of the radius-lunate-capitate axis. The capitate, the entire distal row of carpal bones, and the radial portion of the proximal row of carpal bones displace dorsally with respect to the lunate. Sometimes this can be associated with a fracture of the scaphoid waist and is then referred to as a transscaphoid perilunate dislocation. Standard radiograph findings in patients with a perilunate dislocation include loss of congruity of the 3 carpal

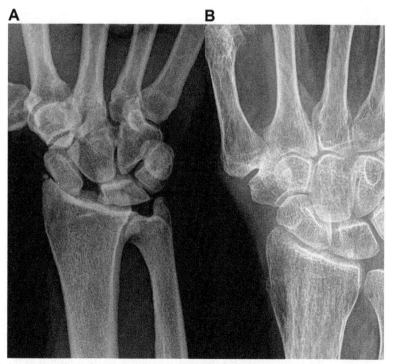

Fig. 9. (*A*) PA radiograph showing a scapholunate dissociation. (*B*) When compared with normal PA it clearly shows an increase of greater than 3 mm in the scapholunate space.

arcs and an abnormal triangular configuration of the lunate on AP view. Perilunate dislocation can be identified more easily on lateral radiographs, which show normal alignment of the lunate and distal radius, with all the other carpal bones located posterior to the lunate (**Fig. 10**).[39]

Lunotriquetral disruptions (Stage III) are caused when the triquetrum exerts torque on the lunotriquetral ligament leading to a tear in the ligament or an avulsion fracture of the triquetrum. Standard radiographs appear similar to a perilunate dislocation but include a dislocation of the triquetrum that is most easily identified on the PA view as overlap of the triquetrum on the lunate or hamate.

Lunate dislocations (Stage IV) are the result of dorsal radiocarpal ligament disruption, which allows the displaced capitate to push the lunate in a volar direction into the carpal tunnel. Lateral radiographs of lunate dislocations result in a spilled-teacup appearance, which is a reflection of the lunate tilting so that its distal articular surface faces the palm (see **Fig. 10**). PA views of the hand have a similar appearance to radiographs demonstrating perilunate dislocations.[45]

Management of perilunate and lunate dislocations in the ED requires emergent hand-specialist consultation for immediate reduction and immobilization. Although closed reduction could be attempted in the ED to reduce compression on the median nerve, the best results for long-term recovery are achieved with open reduction and internal fixation.[46]

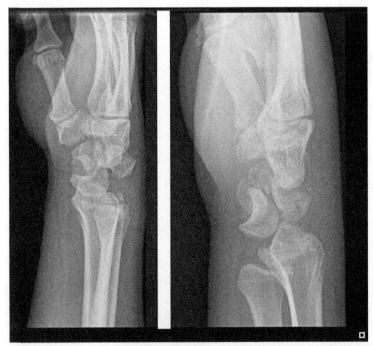

Fig. 10. The image on the left shows a perilunate dislocation. The entire distal row of carpal bones is dislocated dorsally. The lunate, however, remains articulated to the radial head. Note the ulnar styloid fracture, which often occurs in conjunction with a perilunate dislocation. In comparison, the image on the right shows a lunate dislocation and a scaphoid fracture, which shows the classic spilled-tea-cup sign, where the lunate is pushed in the volar direction into the carpal tunnel.

FRACTURES OF THE DISTAL RADIUS AND ULNA

Fractures of the distal radius and ulna are the most common type of fractures in patients younger than 75 years of age.[47] Historically eponyms have been used to describe these fractures, and although eponyms are still in use today, several more recent classification systems have been developed to better characterize these fracture patterns relative to their management and prognosis.[48]

A fall on an outstretched hand is a common mechanism of injury for a transverse fracture of the distal radial metaphysis, with dorsal displacement and angulation. This fracture is commonly referred to as a Colles fracture and can be associated with a fracture of the ulnar styloid.

Patients with this type of injury often complain of pain and swelling over the dorsum of the wrist and on physical examination demonstrate a dinner-fork deformity caused by the dorsal displacement and angulation of the fracture. Median nerve injury can occur with this fracture and a careful neurovascular examination both on initial presentation and following treatment is essential. Standard radiographs of the wrist will demonstrate the fracture through the radial metaphysis. The lateral radiograph is the best view to appreciate the degree of dorsal displacement and angulation and typically demonstrates loss of the normal volar tilt of the distal radial articular surface.

Management of Colles fractures should include closed reduction, which can be facilitated by the use of a hematoma block and finger traps. After successful reduction patients should be immobilized in a long-arm splint in neutral position or pronation with orthopedic follow-up in 7 to 10 days. Emergent orthopedic consultation is necessary if initial attempts at closed reduction are unsuccessful, if there is neurovascular compromise, or if there is an open fracture.[39]

A fall onto the dorsum of the hand with the wrist in flexion is the typical mechanism of injury for a transverse fracture of the metaphysis of the distal radius, with associated volar displacement and volar angulation. This fracture is commonly referred to as a reverse Colles fracture or a Smith fracture.

Patients with this type of fracture often present with pain and swelling of the wrist. On physical examination they have fullness noted on the volar aspect of the wrist. Like the Colles fracture, median nerve injury can occur with this type of fracture and a careful neurovascular examination both on initial presentation and following treatment is essential. Standard PA radiographs will demonstrate the fracture line through the distal radius, but the degree of volar angulation will be best appreciated on the lateral view.

Like the Colles fracture, the Smith fracture is treated with closed reduction. Following reduction, patients should be placed in a long-arm splint in supination.[49] Emergent orthopedic/hand-specialist consultation is recommended for these fractures because they are more likely to be unstable and urgent surgical management is more often necessary.[39]

A distal radius fracture with dislocation of the radiocarpal joint is commonly referred to as a Barton fracture. This fracture generally occurs from a high-energy impact to the radiocarpal joint. If the impact occurs while the wrist is volarly flexed, the fracture affects the volar rim of the radius and is referred to as a volar Barton fracture. If the impact occurs while the wrist is in dorsiflexion, the fracture affects the dorsal rim of the radius and is referred to as a dorsal Barton fracture.

Patients with this type of fracture will present with wrist pain and swelling, and on physical examination will have deformity of the wrist. Standard radiographs will demonstrate the fracture, which is distinguished from a Smith or Colles fracture by the radiocarpal dislocation. The lateral radiograph is the best view for demonstrating the degree of articular surface involvement and the amount of associated displacement. These fractures require emergency orthopedic/hand-specialist consultation for early operative management.[49]

An intraarticular fracture through the radial styloid process caused by a direct blow or a fall on the radial side of the wrist is commonly termed a Hutchinson fracture. Patients with this type of fracture will typically present with pain and swelling of the wrist. Standard radiographs of the wrist demonstrate the fracture best on PA view as a transverse fracture of the radial metaphysis with extension through the radial styloid. Nondisplaced fractures can be managed with a short-arm splint and routine orthopedic/hand-specialist follow-up. Displaced fractures require reduction and immobilization. Accurate anatomic alignment following reduction is essential because multiple ligaments of the wrist attach to the radial styloid process and inappropriate alignment can cause future complications.

DISTAL RADIOULNAR JOINT DISRUPTION

Disruption of the distal radioulnar joint (DRUJ) may be seen as an isolated injury, or more commonly, in association with distal radius fractures. In the former, the injuries are typically the result of a traumatic dislocation of the distal ulna and can be characterized as either volar or dorsal dislocations.

Table 1
Recommended splints for selected fractures

Fracture	Splint	Referral
Phalanx Distal Dorsal Volar Middle Proximal	Splinted in FULL extension Slight flexion Radial/ulnar gutter Radial/ulnar gutter	Nonemergent referral
Metacarpal First Second Third Fourth Fifth	Thumb spica Volar/radial gutter Volar/radial gutter Ulnar gutter Ulnar gutter	Nonemergent referral necessary for all fractures with good anatomic alignment after reduction Emergent referral for nonreducible fractures or neurovascular involvement
Scaphoid	Thumb spica: long or short	Definite fracture: emergent referral Suspected fracture: nonemergent referral
Hamate Hook Body	Thumb spica with wrist flexed and MCP at 90° Short-arm cast	Specialist referral within 1 week
Lunate	Short-arm splint	Referral in 1 to 2 weeks
Triquetral	Short-arm splint	Nonemergent
Pisiform	Short-arm splint	Emergent if signs of ulnar neuropathy
Capitate	Short-arm thumb spica	Emergent referral if associated with a dislocation
Trapezium	Short-arm thumb spica	Nonemergent
Trapezoid	Short-arm thumb spica	Emergent if displaced, otherwise nonemergent

Dorsal dislocations are the most common and are typically the result of a fall on to an outstretched arm with a rotational pronation force to the impact. Physical examination reveals excessive prominence of the ulnar head and lack of forearm rotation secondary to pain when the wrist is supinated. Standard radiographs demonstrate overlap of the distal ulna with the distal radius on the PA view with the ulnar head displaced in the dorsal direction on the lateral projection.

Volar dislocations are typically the result of a fall on an outstretched arm with a rotational supination force to the impact. Physical examination demonstrates loss of the typical dorsal prominence of the ulnar head and lack of forearm rotation secondary to pain when the wrist is pronated. Standard radiographs demonstrate overlap of the distal ulna with the distal radius on the PA view with the ulnar head displaced in the volar direction on lateral projection.

Displaced distal radius fractures can also be associated with injury to the ulnar side of the wrist, causing disruption in the supporting structures of the DRUJ. Radiographic signs of DRUJ instability are[50]

- Ulnar styloid fracture involving the base with more than 2 mm displacement
- Irreducible dislocation of the DRUJ
- Fractures involving the sigmoid notch of the radius
- Wide displacement of the DRUJ
- Radial shortening.

If DRUJ instability is suspected based on clinical examination or radiographic studies an emergent orthopedic/hand-specialist consultation should be obtained for reduction and immobilization **(Table 1)**.[49]

SUMMARY

The intricate anatomy of the hand and wrist, which allows for significant functionality, also allows for several complex fractures and dislocations. Despite the complexity of these injuries, a complete history, thorough physical examination, and pertinent imaging studies can prevent delays in diagnosis. Particular attention should be given to the neurovascular examination and mechanical function of the structures in question. If an injury is suspected based on the history and physical examination, but is not supported by standard radiographs, further imaging studies, such as CT or MRI, may be needed or empiric treatment provided until orthopedic/hand-specialist follow-up can be obtained. Careful and complete evaluation of patients presenting to the ED with injuries of the hand and wrist is essential because missed diagnoses can cause significant pain and long-term disability.

REFERENCES

1. Alderman AK, Storey AF, Chung KC. Financial impact of emergency hand trauma on the health care system. J Am Coll Surg 2008;206:233.
2. Chung KC, Spilson SV. The frequency and epidemiology of hand and forearm fractures in the United States. J Hand Surg Am 2001;26:908.
3. Hart RG, Kleinert HE, Lyons K. A modified thumb spica splint for thumb injuries in the ED. Am J Emerg Med 2005;23:777.
4. Juiter JB, Belsky MR. Fractures and dislocations of the hand. In: Bruce D, Browner JB, Levine AM, et al, editors, Skeletal trauma: basic science, management, and reconstruction, vol. II. Philadelphia: W. B Saunders; 2008. p. 1262.

5. Lee SG, Jupiter JB. Phalangeal and metacarpal fractures of the hand. Hand Clin 2000;16:323.

6. Jahss S. Fractures of the metacarpals – a new method of reduction and immobilization. J Bone Joint Surg Am 1938;20:178.

7. Hardy MA. Principles of metacarpal and phalangeal fracture management: a review of rehabilitation concepts. J Orthop Sports Phys Ther 2004;34:781.

8. Waterbrook AL, Germann CA, Southall JC. Is epinephrine harmful when used with anesthetics for digital nerve blocks? Ann Emerg Med 2007;50:472.

9. Coons MS, Green SM. Boutonniere deformity. Hand Clin 1995;11:387.

10. Bendre AA, Hartigan BJ, Kalainov DM. Mallet finger. J Am Acad Orthop Surg 2005;13:336.

11. Brzezienski MA, Schneider LH. Extensor tendon injuries at the distal interphalangeal joint. Hand Clin 1995;11:373.

12. Allen GM, Drakonaki EE, Tan ML, et al. High-resolution ultrasound in the diagnosis of upper limb disorders: a tertiary referral centre experience. Ann Plast Surg 2008;61:259.

13. Drape JL, Tardif-Chastenet de Gery S, Silbermann-Hoffman O, et al. Closed ruptures of the flexor digitorum tendons: MRI evaluation. Skeletal Radiol 1998;27:617.

14. Redler MR, McCue FC 3rd. Injuries of the hand in athletes. Vasc Med 1988; 115:331.

15. Aronowitz ER, Leddy JP. Closed tendon injuries of the hand and wrist in athletes. Clin Sports Med 1998;17:449.

16. Newland CC. Gamekeeper's thumb. Orthop Clin North Am 1992;23:41.

17. Hong E. Hand injuries in sports medicine. Prim Care 2005;32:91.

18. Welling RD, Jacobson JA, Jamadar DA, et al. MDCT and radiography of wrist fractures: radiographic sensitivity and fracture patterns. AJR Am J Roentgenol 2008;190:10.

19. Perron AD, Brady WJ. Evaluation and management of the high-risk orthopedic emergency. Emerg Med Clin North Am 2003;21:159.

20. Ring D, Jupiter JB, Herndon JH. Acute fractures of the scaphoid. J Am Acad Orthop Surg 2000;8:225.

21. Krasin E, Goldwirth M, Gold A, et al. Review of the current methods in the diagnosis and treatment of scaphoid fractures. Postgrad Med J 2001;77:235.

22. Gooding A, Coates M, Rothwell A. Cost analysis of traditional follow-up protocol versus MRI for radiographically occult scaphoid fractures: a pilot study for the Accident Compensation Corporation. N Z Med J 2004;117:U1049.

23. Parvizi J, Wayman J, Kelly P, et al. Combining the clinical signs improves diagnosis of scaphoid fractures. A prospective study with follow-up. J Hand Surg Br 1998;23:324.

24. Adey L, Souer JS, Lozano-Calderon S, et al. Computed tomography of suspected scaphoid fractures. J Hand Surg Am 2007;32:61.

25. Ty JM, Lozano-Calderon S, Ring D. Computed tomography for triage of suspected scaphoid fractures. Hand (N Y) 2008;3:155.

26. Sakuma M, Nakamura R, Imaeda T. Analysis of proximal fragment sclerosis and surgical outcome of scaphoid non-union by magnetic resonance imaging. J Hand Surg Br 1995;20:201.

27. Beeres FJ, Hogervorst M, Kingma LM, et al. Observer variation in MRI for suspected scaphoid fractures. Br J Radiol 2008;81:950.

28. Memarsadeghi M, Breitenseher MJ, Schaefer-Prokop C, et al. Occult scaphoid fractures: comparison of multidetector CT and MR imaging–initial experience. Radiology 2006;240:169.

29. Gellman H, Caputo RJ, Carter V, et al. Comparison of short and long thumb-spica casts for non-displaced fractures of the carpal scaphoid. J Bone Joint Surg Am 1989;71:354.
30. Garcia-Elias M. Carpal bone fractures. In: Watson HK, editor. The wrist. Philadelphia: Lipincott, Williams, and Wilkins; 2001. p. 174.
31. Singh AK. Extremity trauma. In: Soto JA, editor. Emergency radiology: the requisites. 1st edition. Philadelphia: Mosby; 2009. p. 112.
32. Bishop AT, Beckenbaugh RD. Fracture of the hamate hook. J Hand Surg Am 1988;13:135.
33. Marchessault J, Conti M, Baratz ME. Carpal fractures in athletes excluding the scaphoid. Hand Clin 2009;25:371.
34. Andresen R, Radmer S, Sparmann M, et al. Imaging of hamate bone fractures in conventional X-rays and high-resolution computed tomography. An in vitro study. Invest Radiol 1999;34:46.
35. You JS, Chung SP, Chung HS, et al. The usefulness of CT for patients with carpal bone fractures in the emergency department. Emerg Med J 2007;24:248.
36. Yamazaki H, Kato H, Nakatsuchi Y, et al. Closed rupture of the flexor tendons of the little finger secondary to non-union of fractures of the hook of the hamate. J Hand Surg Br 2006;31:337.
37. Rettig ME, Dassa GL, Raskin KB, et al. Wrist fractures in the athlete. Distal radius and carpal fractures. Clin Sports Med 1998;17:469.
38. Vigler M, Aviles A, Lee SK. Carpal fractures excluding the scaphoid. Hand Clin 2006;22:501.
39. Woolfrey KG, Eisenhauer MA. Wrist and forearm. In: Marx JA, Hockberger RS, Walls RM, et al, editors. Rosen's emergency medicine. 7th edition. Philadelphia: Mosby; 2009. p. 491–560.
40. Rand JA, Linscheid RL, Dobyns JH. Capitate fractures: a long-term follow-up. Clin Orthop Relat Res 1982;165:209–16.
41. Minami M, Yamazaki J, Chisaka N, et al. Nonunion of the capitate. J Hand Surg Am 1987;12:1089.
42. Stein AH Jr. Dorsal dislocation of the lesser multangular bone. J Bone Joint Surg Am 1971;53:377.
43. Mayfield JK, Johnson RP, Kilcoyne RK. Carpal dislocations: pathomechanics and progressive perilunar instability. J Hand Surg Am 1980;5:226.
44. Herzberg G, Comtet JJ, Linscheid RL, et al. Perilunate dislocations and fracture-dislocations: a multicenter study. J Hand Surg Am 1993;18:768.
45. Rogers LF, Taljanovic MS, Boles CA. In: Adam AD, editor. Grainger and Allison's diagnostic radiology. 5th edition. Philadelphia: Churchill Livingstone; 2008. p. 999.
46. Grabow RJ, Catalano L 3rd. Carpal dislocations. Hand Clin 2006;22:485.
47. Kreder HJ, Hanel DP, Agel J, et al. Indirect reduction and percutaneous fixation versus open reduction and internal fixation for displaced intra-articular fractures of the distal radius: a randomised, controlled trial. J Bone Joint Surg Br 2005; 87:829.
48. Wulf CA, Ackerman DB, Rizzo M. Contemporary evaluation and treatment of distal radius fractures. Hand Clin 2007;23:209.
49. Benjamin HJ, Hang BT. Common acute upper extremity injuries in sports. Clin Pediatr Emerg Med 2007;8:15.
50. Mulford JS, Axelrod TS. Traumatic injuries of the distal radioulnar joint. Orthop Clin North Am 2007;38:289.

The Emergency Department Evaluation, Management, and Treatment of Back Pain

Brian N. Corwell, MD

KEYWORDS

• Back pain • Epidural abscess • Spinal stenosis • Diskitis

Back pain is one of the most common symptom-related complaints for visits to primary care physicians (PCPs) and is the most common musculoskeletal complaint that results in visits to the emergency department (ED).[1–3] Most adults (almost 90%) experience back pain at some time in their lives.[1,3,4] It contributes to high levels of lost work days, disability, and health care use.[5–7] It is the primary cause of work-related disability in persons less than 45 years of age. In 2005, back complaints prompted 139 million visits at a cost of $17.6 billion.[8] Although in the past higher use of the ED was primarily by a sicker, more disabled, and chronically ill population, recent trends suggest that EDs may be welcoming more patients who have traditionally sought care from their PCP. The 2006 Massachusetts Health Care Reform legislation sought to move state residents toward universal health care coverage and improve access to primary care medicine. Following this, ED visits soared. However, almost half (44%) of ED users noted that their visit could have been managed by their PCP had one been available.[9] This suggests that, with recent national health care initiatives moving in a similar direction, an increasing number of patients with common complaints such as back pain will visit the ED.

Although back pain has a benign course in more than 90% of patients, physicians must be vigilant and comfortable looking for warning signs of a neurologically impairing or life-threatening cause. As with many common complaints that have an overwhelmingly benign etiology, there may be a tendency toward complacency. The first goal of ED assessment of patients with back pain is to evaluate for potentially

---

Financial disclosures: None.
Department of Emergency Medicine, University of Maryland School of Medicine, 110 South Paca Street, 6th Floor, Suite 200, Baltimore, MD 21201, USA
E-mail address: bcorwell@som.umaryland.edu

Emerg Med Clin N Am 28 (2010) 811–839
doi:10.1016/j.emc.2010.06.001
0733-8627/10/$ – see front matter © 2010 Elsevier Inc. All rights reserved.

dangerous causes that, if not promptly recognized, could result in significant morbidity and mortality. The standard recommended approach is to obtain from all patients with lower back pain a careful and comprehensive history and to perform a thorough physical examination, and to rely on the presence of so-called "red flags" or alarm symptoms to guide further diagnostic tests, specialty evaluation, and treatment. This methodical approach helps to identify the small percentage of patients who have serious pathology as the underlying cause of their pain. This article focuses on the essential elements of an efficient and effective evaluation of patients with back pain in the ED, with special emphasis on epidural abscess, epidural compression syndrome, malignancy, spinal stenosis, and back pain in children.

CLINICAL HISTORY

The importance of a thorough and accurate clinical history cannot be overemphasized. As with any patient who complains of pain, symptoms should be characterized by the basic historical elements of the episode, such as the intensity, onset, character, severity, location, exacerbating and alleviating factors, and the presence of radiation. Further questions related to red flags must also be asked to identify patients at high risk. A summary of the red flag signs and symptoms can be found in **Table 1**.

Different causes of acute low back pain have different distinguishing characteristics. Typical nonspecific back pain is unilateral. It may radiate to the buttocks or posterior thigh but not past the knee. This pain is increased with movement, better with rest, and there are no complaints of numbness, weakness, or bowel or bladder dysfunction. Peripheral nerve pain may be described as a pins and needles sensation or burning, as opposed to nerve root pain, which is transient and sharp, relieved with recumbent positioning, and exacerbated by Valsalva maneuvers. Discogenic pain is typically worse with flexion, whereas pain from spondylolysis is aggravated by facet loading, which occurs in extension. Inflammatory back pain (spondyloarthritis) is insidious in onset, affects younger patients (<40 years of age), improves with exercise but not with rest, and causes increased pain at night with improvement on arising. Sciatica is sharp or burning and radiates laterally or posteriorly down the leg distal to the knee, usually to the foot or ankle. There may also be associated numbness or weakness. Epidural compression syndromes (spinal cord compression, cauda equine syndrome, and conus medullaris syndrome) are associated with numbness, weakness, bilateral leg pain, incontinence, and saddle anesthesia.

The age of the patient is an important initial consideration. Physicians must be especially cautious if the patient is less than 18 or more than 50 years of age because there

Table 1	
History and physical examination red flags	
Historical Red Flags	**Physical Red Flags**
Age <18 or >50 y	Fever
Pain lasting more than 6 wk	Writhing in pain
History of cancer	Bowel or bladder incontinence
Fever and chills	Saddle anesthesia
Night sweats, unexplained weight loss	Decreased or absent anal sphincter tone
Recent bacterial infection	Perianal or perineal sensory loss
Unremitting pain despite rest and analgesics	Severe or progressive neurologic defect
Night pain	Major motor weakness
Intravenous drug users, immunocompromised	
Major trauma	
Minor trauma in the elderly	

is a higher likelihood of serious pathology as the cause for the back pain. Tumors and infection occur with higher frequency in these age groups.[10–12] Younger patients are also at increased risk of spondylolysis and spondylolisthesis.[13,14] In the older patient, an abdominal aortic aneurysm (AAA) must always be considered as a potential cause. The presence of hematuria can make this entity resemble the classic kidney stone. Isolated low back pain is a common presentation of a contained rupture of an AAA.

The elderly may sustain fractures, including pathologic fractures, with minor trauma. This condition is likely secondary to osteoporosis. Chronic steroid users are also at increased risk for fracture, even with minor mechanisms. The immunocompromised, intravenous drug abusers (IVDAs), and those with a recent bacterial infection (eg, pneumonia or urinary tract infection) are at increased risk of spinal bacterial infections. Any patient with back pain and a history of IVDA should be assumed to have an abscess or vertebral osteomyelitis until proven otherwise.[15,16] Recent gastrointestinal or genitourinary procedures may also cause a transient bacteremia leading to an infectious cause of the patient's back pain. Patients with cancer are another high-risk group. The spine is the third most common site for cancer to metastasize.[17,18] Most patients with systemic cancer have spinal metastasis. Cancers that are known to most commonly metastasize to the spine are breast, lung, and prostate, but also include kidney, thyroid, and multiple myeloma.[19] These patients are at greater risk of epidural compression syndrome and pathologic vertebral fractures.

Most episodes of lower back pain resolve or significantly improve within 4 to 6 weeks, therefore lack of significant improvement in 6 to 8 weeks is a red flag.[20,21] It should then be established whether the patient is primarily describing back or leg symptoms. Radicular pain in a dermatomal distribution, often into the lower hamstring, knee, and foot, indicates nerve root compression or irritation (sciatica). The more common nonspecific back pain without true radiculopathy may still radiate into the buttocks or upper thighs but not past the knee, implying muscle or ligamentous strain or disc disease without associated nerve involvement.

The clinician should attempt to elicit historical features that are suggestive of infection or malignancy, such as unintentional weight loss (more than 4.5 kg in 3 months), fevers, chills, and night sweats. Back pain associated with chest, abdominal, or urinary complaints is suggestive of an extraspinal cause. Because most benign back pain is tolerable, worsened with activity, and improved with rest or lying still, symptoms such as severe night pain (especially deep bony pain) and severe unrelenting pain that is not relieved by rest, recumbency, or appropriate analgesic treatment should raise a red flag for malignancy or infection.[22–24]

Symptoms that are suggestive of epidural compression syndrome are mainly neurologic in origin, and include any loss of bowel or bladder function, urinary retention, erectile dysfunction, saddle anesthesia, or progressive distal leg numbness or weakness.[21,25] In older patients, typically those greater than 60 years of age, spinal stenosis is suggested by lower back pain with radiculopathy that is worsened with walking, prolonged standing, and back extension (standing) but is relieved with rest and forward flexion (sitting).[26–28] Pain from disc herniation is relieved by lying supine and is worsened by Valsalva maneuvers, coughing, sneezing, and positions that produce increased pressure on annular fibers, such as prolonged sitting, standing, and bending postures.[29,30]

PHYSICAL EXAMINATION

The purpose of the physical examination is to evaluate neurologic complaints discovered in the history, identify potential neurologic defects, and to uncover any red flags.

Carefully evaluate the patient's vital signs, general appearance, and back, then perform a complete neurologic examination of the legs. Lumbar spine pathology is frequently manifested in the lower extremities as an alteration in the patient's reflexes, sensation, and/or muscle strength. The neurologic examination systematically tests the clinical relationship between the reflexes and the motor and sensory components of the most commonly affected nerve roots.

First and foremost, the clinician must account for any abnormal or unstable vital signs, which may indicate an extraspinal cause of the back pain such as an AAA. Fever, present in approximately 50% of patients with osteomyelitis or spinal epidural abscess, is a red flag for infection.[12,22] The absence of fever, equally common, does not rule out a spinal infection.

Next, consider the general appearance of the patient. In most cases, patients with back pain prefer to lie still because movement worsens their pain. Those individuals in extreme pain or writhing in pain may have an underlying emergent cause. This would include both spinal causes, such as epidural abscess and osteomyelitis, and extraspinal causes such as intra-abdominal (ie, mass), retroperitoneal (ie, nephrolithiasis or hemorrhage), or vascular (ie, AAA) causes. Next, the patient's back should be fully exposed and inspected for signs of infection. The midline spinous processes should be palpated for tenderness suggesting fracture or infection (sensitivity 86%, specificity 60%).[26] Pain during lumbar flexion suggests discogenic pain, whereas pain on lumbar extension suggests facet disease. Secondary findings of paraspinal muscle spasm or edema should be noted.

A detailed distal neurologic examination must be performed that targets the 3 most common locations for disc herniation: L4, L5, and S1. More than 95% of herniated discs affect the L4 to L5 or L5 to S1 interspaces, causing impingement on the L5 and S1 nerve roots, respectively.[31,32] Patients with these radiculopathies complain of acute back pain and pain radiating down the lateral (L5) or posterior (S1) leg to the ankle or foot. Pathology at the higher lumbar spine (L1, L2, L3) causes acute back pain with anterior thigh radiation, weakness with hip flexion (iliopsoas muscle action), and anterior thigh sensory changes in the corresponding dermatome. This may be seen in older patients with symptoms of spinal stenosis. There are no individual reflexes for the L1 to L3 lumbar levels. Those with pathology at the lower sacral levels (S2–S5) have sacral or buttock pain that radiates down the posterior leg or into the perineum and can have difficulties with penile erection (S2–S4), abnormal perianal sensation (S3–S5), anal wink (S2–S4), rectal tone (S2–S5), and bladder function (S2–S4).

An understanding of the key physical components of the targeted L4 to S1 neurologic examination is essential. At each level, the corresponding muscle strength, sensation, and reflex needs to be tested and documented. True sensory loss is best tested with pinprick rather than light touch. Sensory fields can have considerable overlap so areas that are exclusively served by an individual nerve must be examined. Similarly, because many muscles have innervation from multiple roots, preserved strength may be found despite significant involvement of a single nerve root. The L4 neurologic level strength is tested with knee extension, ankle inversion, and dorsiflexion (sensitivity 49%–63%, specificity 52%–89%).[31,33,34] Sensation is tested from the medial leg down to the medial surface of the great toe (not including the first web space). The corresponding reflex is the patellar reflex (sensitivity 15%–50%, specificity 67%–93%).[34,35] The L5 neurologic level strength is tested with great toe dorsiflexion (extensor hallucis longus) (sensitivity 37%–61%, specificity 55%–71%) and heel walking.[35,36] Sensation is tested from the lateral leg, dorsum of the foot, and the first web space. There is no reliable reflex to test L5, which is the most commonly compressed nerve root. The S1 neurologic level strength is tested with foot eversion (peroneals) and toe walking (ankle plantar flexion) (sensitivity 13%–47%, specificity 76%–100%).[33,35] Sensation is tested from the lateral foot and ankle. The corresponding reflex is the Achilles reflex (sensitivity 47%–56%, specificity 57%–90%).[31,34–36] Ankle reflexes become increasingly absent with age, lost in nearly 50% of those more than 80 years of age.[37] This loss is usually symmetric, thus unilateral absence may signify pathology.[38] The overall sensitivity and specificity of the sensory examination in the diagnosis of lumbar disc herniation is 16% to 50% and 62% to 86% respectively.[33–35]

Although impractical and unnecessary for office practice, urinary catheterization can be helpful in evaluating select patients in the ED. Measurement of a postvoid bladder residual volume tests for the presence of urinary retention with overflow incontinence. This finding is sensitive and specific for cauda equina syndrome.[6] Large postvoid residual volumes (>100 mL) indicate a denervated bladder with resultant overflow incontinence and suggest significant neurologic compromise.[26,39,40] This finding warrants immediate evaluation for epidural compression syndrome. A negative postvoid residual volume is reassuring and effectively rules out significant bilateral neurologic compromise.

Digital rectal examination is not a routine part of the physical examination in most patients with back pain but should be performed in select individuals. Appropriate patients include anyone with red flags, severe pain, and those in whom epidural compression syndrome is being considered, such as those individuals with severe pain and progressive neurologic findings. The rectal examination can aid in the assessment of sphincter tone and perianal sensation (S3–S5), anal wink (S2–S4), and in checking for masses or a possible perirectal abscess. A Babinski test should also be performed in patients with findings concerning for neurologic compromise. A positive test involves extension of the great toe with flexion and splaying of the other toes, and suggests a lesion affecting the upper motor neurons or corticospinal tract.

The straight leg raise (SLR), which tests for the presence of a herniated disc causing nerve root compression, is one of the most important tests for evaluating back pain. This examination technique is approximately 80% sensitive for a herniated disc cause of pain (sensitivity 72%–97%, specificity 11%–66%).[41] The SLR has a positive predictive value (PPV) of 67% to 89% and a negative predictive value (NPV) of 33% to 57% in patients with a high probability of having a disc herniation versus a PPV of 4% in those patients with a low probability (based on the absence of neurologic symptoms or sciatica).[41,42] A positive test causes or reproduces radicular pain below the knee of the affected leg when the leg is elevated between 30° and 70°. A positive finding also occurs if radicular symptoms are elicited when the leg is then lowered until pain is eased and the ipsilateral ankle is dorsiflexed (Braggard sign).[43] Pain below 30°, above 70°, or with reproduction of pain only in the back, hamstring, or buttock region does not constitute a positive test. Care should be taken that the patient is not actively helping in lifting the leg and that the knee remains straight throughout the examination. Pain referred to the affected leg when the opposite asymptomatic leg is tested, called a positive crossed SLR, strongly indicates nerve root irritation from a herniated disc. This finding has a high specificity (85%–100%), but low sensitivity (29%), with a PPV of 79% to 92% and NPV of 22% to 44%.[41,42]

If the patient is reluctant or unwilling to lie supine for SLR testing, the seated SLR or slump test should be attempted. The traditional supine SLR is more sensitive than the seated SLR (sensitivity of 0.67 vs 0.41).[44] To perform the slump test, the patient sits at the edge of the examination table and slumps forward while flexing the neck and trunk. This movement is followed by knee extension and ankle dorsiflexion. A positive test reproduces radicular pain. The slump test was positive in 94% of patients with frank disc herniation, 78% of patients with bulging discs, and 75% of patients without radiographic findings.[45] The SLR and slump test demonstrate good correlation ($\kappa = 0.69$).[46] The slump test has greater sensitivity than the SLR (0.84 vs 0.52) with slightly lower specificity (0.83 vs 0.89).[47]

The clinician must also be able to distinguish between true pathologic back pain and nonorganic back pain. Waddell signs are physical examination findings that can aid in making this distinction, and can be remembered by the acronym DORST (distraction, over-reaction, regional disturbances, simulation tests, and tenderness).[48] Superficial, nonanatomic, or variable tenderness during the physical examination suggests a nonorganic cause. The clinician may also simulate back pain through provocative maneuvers such as axial loading of the head or passive rotation of the shoulders and pelvis in the same plane. Neither maneuver should elicit low back pain. There may be a discrepancy between the symptoms reported during the supine and sitting SLR. The seated version of the test, sometimes termed the distracted SLR, can be performed while distracting the patient or appearing to focus on the knee. Further, radicular pain elicited at a leg elevation of less than 30° is suspicious because the nerve root and surrounding dura do not move in the neural foramen until an elevation of more than 30° is reached. Sensory and motor findings suggestive of a nonorganic cause include stocking, glove, or nondermatomal sensory loss or weakness that can be characterized as give-away, jerky, or cogwheel. Gross overreaction is suggested by exaggerated, inconsistent, painful responses to a non-offensive stimulus.

Traditionally Waddell signs, especially if 3 or more are present, were believed to correlate with not only functional complaints (physical findings without anatomic cause) and decreased likelihood of return to work but also with malingering. The association between Waddell signs and malingering has been misinterpreted, falsely propagated, misused both clinically and medicolegally, and ignores the caveats about the interpretation and application of the signs from the original study article.[49] As originally conceived, Waddell signs were not intended for use in detecting malingering or sincerity of effort. Subsequent studies have found that Waddell signs are associated only with poorer treatment outcome, decreased functional performance, decreased likelihood of return to work, higher levels of pain intensity and duration, psychological distress, and perceived disability.[50–53] However, there has been little evidence to support the association between Waddell signs and secondary gain or malingering.[51,52] When combined with shoulder motion and neck motion producing lower back pain, Waddell signs predict a decreased probability of the individual returning to work.[54] There is poor interobserver agreement in the assessment of Waddell signs.[55] Another test worth noting is the Hoover test, which assesses the patient's voluntary effort. Patients are instructed to lift their leg while their heels are cupped by the examiner. True volitional effort results in increased downward pressure on the untested heel. ED staff may also note inconsistency in observed spontaneous activity during time of care, such as with dressing, undressing, and getting off the examination table. Although these signs can be used in the evaluation of select patients, they are merely a component of a comprehensive examination. Waddell signs should never be used independently because they lack the sensitivity to be able to distinguish nonorganic problems from true organic pathology.[51]

DIAGNOSTIC TESTING

In general, if the history and physical examination do not reveal any concerning findings or red flags for emergent pathology, no further testing is required. Diagnostic testing is indicated only if it will help guide specific patient management strategies. Blind diagnostic testing (so-called "shotgunning") may lead to a cascade of further testing and false-positive results, which themselves will beget further testing and possibly unnecessary interventions. Such an approach may foster the patient's inaccurate belief that there is true pathology present, which can increase their anxiety and medical expenses. However, if red flags are uncovered in the history and physical examination, further evaluation with appropriate diagnostic testing is warranted.

Routine laboratory studies are rarely needed for the initial evaluation of nonspecific acute low back pain. Laboratory testing, consisting of a white blood cell (WBC) count, erythrocyte sedimentation rate (ESR), and C-reactive protein (CRP) is indicated in cases of suspected infection or malignancy. In cases of spinal infection, the sensitivity of an increased WBC count (35%–61%), ESR (76%–95%), and CRP (82%–98%) may help guide further evaluation or consideration of other entities.[56–58] An increased ESR also has a role in the diagnostic evaluation of occult malignancy (sensitivity 78%, specificity 67%).[59] Urinalysis is useful for atypical presentations of pyelonephritis. Other tests such as blood cultures, prostate-specific antigen, calcium, and alkaline phosphatase may be considered in appropriate cases.

Imaging, like laboratory testing, is not indicated in the absence of red flags or concerns for malignancy, fracture, infection, or epidural compression syndrome. Unnecessary imaging only serves to increase the cost of the visit and the length of stay, and subjects the patient to unnecessary radiation. Although the added diagnostic value of modern neuroimaging is significant, there is concern that these studies may be overused in patients with lower back pain presenting to the ED.[60,61] Patients who receive radiography are more likely to be satisfied with their care, and up to 80% of patients with low back pain would accept plain radiographs if given the choice, despite the lack of benefit associated with routine imaging.[62] This suggests a need for the ED physician to address patient preferences and expectations. Educational interventions may be effective for reducing the proportion of patients who expect routine imaging for their low back pain.[63]

Most patients in the ED with lower back pain do not require plain radiographs. Studies show that plain radiographs rarely reveal any helpful information.[20,64,65] Radiographic studies have not been shown to help diagnose uncomplicated lower back pain and rarely alter clinical decision making.[61,62] Plain radiographs (anteroposterior and lateral views) should be the first step only in cases of suspected infection, fracture, malignancy, or neurologic compromise.[66] Additional views are only indicated if spondylolysis or spondylolisthesis is suspected. They otherwise add unnecessary cost and radiation.[60] The amount of gonadal radiation from a single 2-view plain radiograph series of the lumbar spine is equivalent to being exposed to daily chest radiographs for 1 year.[67] Negative plain radiographs do not rule out disease such that, if sufficient pretest probability of a potential neurologic emergency exists, the ED physician should proceed with further imaging (computed tomography [CT] or magnetic resonance imaging [MRI]) regardless of plain radiograph results.[20] In these cases, if these studies can easily and quickly be obtained, there is no need for plain radiographs because they do not offer unique information. A bone scan can be useful when looking for spinal stress fractures, infectious processes, and spinal metastatic disease, especially in the patient without neurologic symptoms.[20] However, it is not typically ordered from the ED and has largely been replaced by MRI.[68]

In the absence of a serious or progressive neurologic deficit, or concern for epidural compression syndrome, neoplasm, or spinal infection; CT or MRI should not be part of the diagnostic evaluation in the ED. Isolated sensory loss or the absence of a reflex is not considered to be a progressive neurologic deficit. CT is superior to plain radiographs for the detection of vertebral fractures and other bony pathology, especially fractures involving posterior spine structures, bone fragments within the spinal canal, or spinal malalignment.[69,70] CT is increasingly used as a primary screening modality for moderate to severe spine trauma. CT with myelography (or with intravenous [IV] gadolinium) may be used in those patients with concern for epidural abscess, epidural compression, or vertebral osteomyelitis who are otherwise unable to have MRI. Evaluation of vertebral body bony destruction seen on plain radiograph is best visualized by CT. However, if a neurologic deficit is present, MRI is more appropriate.

With the exception of the evaluation of acute trauma, MRI is the most informative investigative modality and identifies almost all pathologic states that benefit from surgical management. MRI is the modality of choice for evaluation of spinal infectious lesions (sensitivity 96%, specificity 92%), malignancy (sensitivity 83%–93%, specificity 90%–97%), disc herniation, and epidural compression syndrome (sensitivity 93%, specificity 97%).[71] In acute disc herniation without progressive neurologic symptoms, MRI can be delayed for 4 to 6 weeks and coordinated by the patient's PCP.[60,61,72,73] Disc disease is a component of normal aging and a nonspecific finding[74–76]; 1 in 4 of all asymptomatic persons younger than 60 years have MRI findings of a herniated disc.[77] That number increases to 1 in 3 in people older than the age of 60 years.[77] In one study, more than 50% of asymptomatic patients were identified as having a bulging disc on MRI.[78]

PHARMACOTHERAPY

One of the most important goals of treatment is to provide an acceptable level of analgesia while the underlying condition resolves or to ameliorate the suffering of those patients who await definitive therapy. When considering a particular pharmacologic therapeutic agent, recall that physicians notoriously underestimate, and subsequently undertreat, pain.[79]

First-line pharmacologic therapy should include nonopioid analgesic agents such as acetaminophen or nonsteroidal anti-inflammatory drugs (NSAIDs), both of which are excellent analgesics with comparable efficacy.[65,80,81] Some clinicians consider acetaminophen superior because of its low cost, efficacy, and lower side effect profile.[80] Given the increasing recognition of acetaminophen's role in hepatotoxicity, patients should be cautioned not to take acetaminophen in any form (eg, over-the-counter preparations) in addition to opiate-acetaminophen combination narcotics.[82] NSAIDs have well-known renal and gastrointestinal side effects that should also be considered. NSAIDs may be a better option for younger patients who are less likely to have these potential complications, whereas acetaminophen may be more appropriate for older patients.[80,81] NSAIDs are slightly superior to acetaminophen for pain relief from osteoarthritis not limited to the back.[81] Ketorolac (either intramuscular or IV) may provide early improved analgesia in those unable to tolerate oral medication in the acute setting. There does not seem to be a specific NSAID that is clearly more effective than others.[80]

Opioid analgesics should be considered a third-line alternative, and best used for those experiencing severe acute back pain with inadequate control with non-narcotic analgesics.[81] Though counterintuitive from clinical experience, the data for opioid superiority compared with other analgesics, such as NSAIDs or acetaminophen, is sparse and inconclusive. Opioids have not been shown to be more effective than either NSAIDs or acetaminophen for initial treatment of acute lower back pain, nor do they increase the likelihood of return to work.[65,81,83–85] When prescribed, opioids should be combined with an NSAID, taken on a fixed dosing schedule, and only for a limited time.[86,87] The physician should always consider the known side effects of opioids (constipation, confusion, and sedation) especially in the elderly population. There is good evidence that muscle relaxants reduce pain and that different types are equally effective.[81,88–90] However, the high incidence of significant side effects such as dizziness and sedation limits prolonged use. Muscle relaxants seem to confer the most benefit to patients with back pain and associated muscle spasm who can tolerate the side effect profile. Benzodiazepines are second-line muscle relaxants because of concerns for their abuse potential. Both types of muscle relaxants may be beneficial in an every-bedtime capacity, thereby limiting side effects. Opioid and muscle relaxant use is not compatible with most workplace responsibilities. There is no role for starting any long-acting chronic pain medication (ie, oxycontin, methadone, fentanyl patches) in the ED. A regimen of NSAIDs, acetaminophen, and skeletal muscle relaxants may suffice for most patients.

Epidural glucocorticoid injections seem to have the best effect in patients with radiculopathy caused by a herniated disc, but do not provide benefit beyond 4 to 6 weeks.[91] Further, they do not delay surgery in those who are already surgical candidates.[92] Steroid injections do not seem to be effective for other entities such as nonspecific low back pain or spinal stenosis.[91,93] Lumbar epidural steroid injections are never indicated for acute or emergent treatment and thus have no role in the ED management of back pain. In general, this procedure is part of an outpatient pain management regimen for the patient with radiculopathy who fails to respond to several weeks of conservative therapy.

There is no clear benefit to oral glucocorticoids for patients with lower back pain, with or without sciatica.[65,81,94,95] However, some practitioners continue to use glucocorticoids for back pain with lumbosacral radiculopathy, acknowledging that the benefit is likely modest and transient.[96,97] The practitioner should always consider the negative side effect profile of steroids, including hyperglycemia, gastrointestinal bleeding, and an increased risk of infection. Nonpharmacologic analgesia can include the use of heat or cold externally applied to the lower back. There is better evidence for the use of heat than ice for treatment of lower back pain.[98,99] Anecdotal evidence suggests that cold packs may be beneficial early in symptom treatment and moist heat may help with pain and muscle spasm in the first 1 to 2 weeks. However, actual care rendered rarely reflects these evidence-based practice guidelines and recommendations.[100] Notable deviations from established treatment guidelines include infrequent inclusion of advice, education, and reassurance (20.5%) in addition to infrequent prescription of simple analgesics (17.7%). In a study of more than 3500 patients with a new episode of lower back pain, providers demonstrated an overreliance on opioids (19.6%) and early imaging (25.3%).[100] More patients were referred to imaging than received advice and education. Such usual practice is unlikely to lead to the best patient outcomes and clearly contributes to the high cost of managing lower back pain.

SUMMARY

An individual red flag does not necessarily correspond to a specific pathology; it indicates a higher probability of a serious underlying condition that may require further investigation. However, multiple red flags always require further investigation that is often initiated in the ED. Following the history and physical examination, patients with acute low back pain can be divided into 3 main categories: (1) patients with nonspecific lower back pain, (2) patients with nerve root or radicular pain, and (3) patients with serious or emergent spinal pathology, including red flag conditions such as tumor, infection, or epidural compression syndrome. The first priority is to make sure that the back pain is of musculoskeletal origin and to rule out nonspinal pathology such as from an AAA. The next step is to exclude the presence of serious spinal pathology such as epidural compression syndrome or epidural abscess. The physician must determine whether the patient has nerve root pain. In the absence of radicular pain, the pain is classified as nonspecific low back pain.

NONSPECIFIC LOWER BACK PAIN

Most people (80%–90%), and most patients in the ED, have nonspecific lower back pain, which is pain without a clear origin and not caused by a specific disease or spinal abnormality.[65] These patients have low back pain and an otherwise negative history and physical examination.[26] This diagnosis of exclusion is made only after ruling out the more worrisome causes of back pain.[20] Typically, patients have mild to moderate pain, localized asymmetrically in the lumbar or sacral paraspinous muscles. Pain, typically characterized as an ache or spasm, may radiate into the buttocks or thigh, and is worsened with activity and relieved with rest. At times, this reported radiation can elicit an improper diagnosis of radiculopathy or disc herniation as opposed to true radicular symptoms, which radiate below the knee in a dermatomal distribution, and may be associated with sensory loss, weakness, or reflex changes. Physical examination may reveal mild to moderate paraspinal muscle tenderness and/or paravertebral muscle spasm but will not reveal any red flags or neurologic abnormalities. Because most patients with nonspecific lower back pain experience symptomatic resolution within 4 to 6 weeks, only conservative management is needed.[65] No further diagnostic testing is required beyond the history and physical examination.[29] Conservative management includes continuation of daily activities as tolerated, ice, heat, analgesia, and/or muscle relaxants, patient education, and referral for close follow-up with their PCP to ensure that the problem resolves.[81]

Persistent pain for more than 4 to 6 weeks, including a prolonged exacerbation of chronic back pain, should be evaluated with the previously mentioned laboratory tests (CBC, ESR, and/or CRP) and a 2-view plain radiograph of the lower back. Prior imaging, such as CT or MRI, should also be reviewed if possible. The ED physician should perform a thorough (re)review of red flags in the history and physical examination that may have been missed on the initial evaluation or have developed in the interim. If there are any new concerning findings, the patient should be approached like any new patient with the same findings. In the absence of new findings, chronic back pain is often regarded as one of the most challenging clinical scenarios. The underlying cause of chronic back pain is complex and multifactorial, making proper assessment and treatment nearly impossible in the ED setting. These patients usually require a multidisciplinary treatment approach for the greatest chance for success. The prescription of narcotics to these patients must be an individualized decision in accordance with the ED physician's assessment of the clinical scenario. The risk of providing narcotics to a drug-seeking patient must be carefully weighed against the risk of denying pain medicine to a patient with true pain in true need.

COCCYDYNIA

Coccydynia is another common back condition presenting to the ED. It is more common in adults, women, and the obese. It commonly occurs from acute trauma, usually caused by a fall backward into a sitting position that results in a bruised, broken, or sometimes dislocated coccyx. Other causes include repetitive minor trauma; for example, prolonged sitting on hard, ill-fitting, or narrow surfaces such as a bicycle seat. Those with poor posture are also at increased risk because leaning backward excessively puts an increased load on the coccyx. Patients complain of pain in the tailbone that is worse with sitting, especially when leaning backward, and on standing. They may report pain with sexual intercourse or with defecation. Rectal examination is essential and the only way to fully palpate the coccyx. The ED physician will find tenderness localized to the coccyx both with external palpation in the gluteal crease and when the coccyx is grasped between the forefinger and the thumb. Differential diagnosis should included prostatitis, pelvic inflammatory disease, and rectal abscess. Imaging is only useful if considering infection, cancer, or other pathology, as confirmation of a coccygeal fracture is not always necessary because of the risks of radiation exposure and the unlikely event that imaging will change management. ED attempts at reduction are not recommended. Treatment involves protecting the tailbone from further trauma, such as by advising the patient to sit leaning forward and prescribing a donut or wedge cushion that distributes weight away from the coccyx. Heat or ice is advised, allowing the patient to choose whichever is most effective. Hot sitz-type baths may also be helpful. Analgesic medications should be selected based on symptoms, and, if opioids are chosen, a stool softener should also be provided to avoid pain with constipation and straining.

Lumbosacral Disc Disease and Radiculopathy

Lumbar radiculopathy is a clinical diagnosis of nerve root irritation and compression leading to symptoms in the distribution of the affected lumbar or sacral nerve root, such as numbness, weakness, or paresthesias. The most common causes are from disc herniation and spondylotic degeneration causing foraminal stenosis. Disc herniation is unusual before 18 years of age and is rare in the fibrotic discs of the elderly. Disc herniation occurs when the tough outer disc layer (the annulus fibrosis) tears, and the inner gelatinous material (the nucleus pulposus) prolapses, inflames, and compresses a nerve root. This herniation may be anywhere on the continuum from asymptomatic to severely painful. Disc herniation is most common at the L4 to L5 and L5 to S1 levels, causing L5 and S1 radiculopathies, respectively. Clinical symptoms are typically self-limited with a high rate of spontaneous improvement and low likelihood of progression to a neurologic emergency.

Although patients complain of pain in their lower back, unilateral lower extremity pain and radicular symptoms predominate because of the anatomic distribution of the nerve roots involved. Pain radiating below the knee is more likely to represent true radiculopathy than pain radiating only to the gluteal region or posterior thigh. Motor findings, such as focal weakness, occur less frequently than focal sensory or reflex changes. Patients typically report a combination of pain and a constellation of sometimes vague sensory symptoms such as anesthesia, dysesthesia, hyperesthesia, or paresthesia. A dermatomal pattern of sensory loss or a reduced or absent deep tendon reflex is more suggestive of a specific root lesion than the pattern of radicular pain.[38,101] Symptoms tend to become worse with Valsalva maneuvers and better with recumbent positioning. Diagnosis consists of localizing the pain and neurologic dysfunction to an isolated nerve root, as discussed earlier. In addition to disc herniation, other causes for radiculopathy should always be considered, including cord compression, spinal stenosis, tumor, and infection. Multinerve root pathology and/ or the presence of bilateral symptoms are potential indicators of a spinal mass lesion or large central disc herniation that compresses multiple descending nerve roots within the spinal canal.

The natural history of disc herniation is that pain from pressure and nerve irritation improves as the local inflammation subsides. The size of the disc protrusion may naturally decrease with time. A bulging disc is a common entity, likely a component of normal aging that may be an incidental finding on a MRI.[74,75,77,78] Although disc herniation and radiculopathy are commonly considered together, herniation is usually asymptomatic and likely only occasionally causes symptoms of sciatica.

It may be helpful for the ED practitioner to classify the typical patient with lumbar radiculopathy into one of the 3 main groups of common presentations. The first is the patient with painful radicular symptoms and a pure sensory dysfunction without other neurologic deficits. The next patient category has the same symptoms but includes a mild nonprogressive identifiable motor deficit with or without an associated reflex change. The third patient group includes severe or worsening motor deficits. Patients who have a herniated disc with symptoms in a single nerve root distribution and an otherwise normal examination do not require an urgent or emergent MRI or even specialty referral.[3,65,102] Many patients who have a herniated disc can be managed conservatively as outpatients by their PCP with follow-up and re-evaluation in 1 week. Because clinical symptoms are typically self-limited and unlikely to progress to a neurologic emergency, the ED evaluation of patients with stable symptoms is focused on pain control and activity modification and does not require emergent diagnostic testing. These patients must not have any red flags such as urinary retention or saddle anesthesia that would suggest another emergent condition (eg, epidural compression), and they must be neurologically intact (no progressive or bilateral neurologic deficits). Urgent neuroimaging and consultation initiated from the ED is necessary for patients with acute lumbar radiculopathy and red flags that suggest rapidly progressive or bilateral neurologic deficits, urinary retention or saddle anesthesia, or suspected epidural abscess or neoplasm. Patients with intractable pain should be admitted for pain control.

Patients with the common symptoms of back pain with radiculopathy should receive appropriate analgesics, be advised to avoid bed rest, and be treated like those with nonspecific lower back pain.[65,103] Patients should be reassured that most people experience symptomatic resolution within 4 to 6 weeks with conservative, nonsurgical management.[65,104] If the pain from disc herniation does persist for longer than 6 weeks, outpatient MRI is indicated.[60,65] Corticosteroid injections into the epidural space may relieve some of the inflammation associated with disc herniation and represent another outpatient option for patients in severe pain. Although some reduction of symptoms may be obtained initially, no long-term benefit or reduction in the need for later surgery has been documented.[91,92] There is also no clear benefit to the use of systemic steroids in cases of disc herniation with radiculopathy.[81] With a documented herniation, some patients with prolonged intractable pain may benefit from surgical discectomy compared with conservative management, although this remains controversial.[105–107] Other indications for surgery include worsening motor or sensory deficits.

EPIDURAL ABSCESS

Spinal epidural abscess, now diagnosed in 1 in 10,000 hospital admissions, remains a rare disease despite a doubling of the overall incidence in the past 2 decades.[12] Although traditional risk factors such as diabetes, alcoholism, and human immunodeficiency virus (HIV) remain unchanged, the aging population, increased IVDA, and the increasing use of spinal instrumentation and indwelling devices (epidural catheters, spinal stimulators, and vascular access) may help to explain this increased incidence. Another possible explanation involves the improved diagnostic sensitivity of modalities such as MRI that allow for early detection.

Epidural abscesses may originate from either remote spread (25%–50%) via the bloodstream or local contiguous spread (15%–30%) from infected adjacent skin and soft tissue such as from a psoas abscess or infected vertebral body.[12] An emerging cause is via direct inoculation into the spinal canal (eg, during spinal surgery or with implantable spinal devices). The source of infection is not identified in up to one-third of cases.[12] There are several proposed mechanisms of bacterial damage to the spinal cord, including direct mechanical compression of neural elements or blood supply, or thrombosis and thrombophlebitis of nearby veins.[12,108]

The most common isolated pathogen is *Staphylococcus aureus*, accounting for up to two-thirds of epidural abscess cases.[31] Empiric antibiotics should target the most commonly identified organisms: *S aureus* (with an increasing prevalence of methicillin-resistant *S aureus*), gram-negative bacteria (*Escherichia coli*), streptococci, coagulase-negative staphylococci (*Staphylococcus epidermidis*), and, rarely, anaerobes.[108–110]

Prompt recognition and proper management are imperative to avoid disastrous complications including sepsis, paralysis, or death. Spinal epidural abscess remains a challenging diagnosis to make, and almost half of cases are initially misdiagnosed.[12] In one study, the mean duration between symptom onset and the first ED visit was 5 days, and between symptom onset and hospital admission was 9 days. Patients averaged 2 ED visits before admission.[111] The difficulty in initially making this diagnosis likely stems from the relative infrequency of traditionally accepted signs and symptoms. The classic symptom triad of epidural abscess consists of fever, back pain, and neurologic deficits. As with most triads, few patients (<15%) have all 3 components at the time of presentation. Almost 75% have back pain and 50% are febrile initially.[12] The rate of neurologic progression is highly variable, and up to 67% of patients have a normal initial neurologic examination. Only 60% have a WBC count greater than 12,000 cells/mm^3.[15,110,112,113] These data underscore the need for a high index of clinical suspicion. Early diagnosis and treatment are imperative because the extent of preoperative neurologic deficit is an important predictor of the final neurologic outcome. Therefore, in cases in which the ED physician has a moderate to high pretest probability of disease, further workup should be pursued despite a normal WBC count, a normal initial neurologic examination, and the absence of fever.

Spinal epidural abscess commonly presents with fever and severe back pain that is usually aggravated by movement or palpation. Signs of nerve root injury or spinal cord compression may be present but are typically late findings. Left untreated, an epidural abscess will cause symptoms that progress in a typical sequence.[114] Providers see patients somewhere on this continuum. The disease starts with general malaise and a possible fever, followed by a backache that progresses to back pain and becomes severe. Patients may subsequently complain of nerve root pain and shooting pain in the distribution of the affected nerve. Many patients at this stage, characterized by nonspecific symptoms, may be misdiagnosed without a high index of clinical suspicion. These symptoms are then followed by motor weakness, sensory changes, bowel and bladder dysfunction, and, eventually, paralysis (4%–22%) or death (5%).[12,114] Patients may progress rapidly through these symptomatic stages, and some stages may be missed. Despite being initially present only half of the time, fever does help distinguish epidural abscess from other causes of back pain. If findings on the history or physical examination are worrisome for a spinal epidural abscess, patients urgently require MRI. With a low index of suspicion, including normal results of serum WBC count, ESR, CRP, and lumbosacral plain radiographs, patients can be discharged with close follow-up.

Epidural abscesses occur more commonly in the thoracolumbar area because of a larger epidural space and more infection-prone fat tissue. Because the epidural space is a vertically oriented sheath, longitudinal extension occurs so that infection at one level frequently tracks to adjacent spinal levels. Laboratory studies including blood cultures should be obtained. Lumbar puncture (LP) and direct needle aspiration have no role in the ED management of epidural abscesses. LP has a low diagnostic yield, with a Gram stain that is usually negative and cultures that are rarely positive.[12,114] MRI is the diagnostic test of choice because it aids in surgical planning and is the best test for early detection allowing for the diagnosis of small abscesses before the development of cord impingement.[12,115,116] For patients unable to have MRI, CT with gadolinium contrast is the next alternative. Plain films are rarely diagnostic early in disease.

The patient's final neurologic outcome is best predicted by their presurgical neurologic condition, highlighting the importance of timely diagnosis.[12,111,117,118] Standard treatment involves a combination of surgical and medical management.[12,15] Surgical treatment involves decompression and drainage of purulent material. Medical treatment focuses on systemic intravenous antibiotic therapy. The choice and timing of antibiotics and the decision to give steroids should be discussed with consultants from infectious disease and spine surgery if time allows. Initial antibiotics are broad spectrum, and should include vancomycin because of the increased prevalence of methicillin-resistant S aureus. Additional agents include metronidazole plus a third- or fourth-generation cephalosporin (eg, cefotaxime).[12] Subsequent antibiotic therapy will be based on culture and sensitivity results of blood cultures or needle aspirate. Because of the difficulty in predicting the progression of neurologic deficits, surgical consultation should be initiated from the ED with direct physician-to-physician communication.

Recent literature suggests that a subset of patients who are hemodynamically stable, neurologically intact, and at low overall risk of bad outcomes may be treated nonsurgically, although this is not the current standard of care.[119-123] These patients may include those who have serious underlying medical conditions making them an unacceptably high operative risk, those who refuse surgery, those with panspinal infection, or those with advanced neurologic deficits who are considered unlikely to improve with surgery. This last group consists of those with complete paralysis present for more than 36 to 48 hours before diagnosis and treatment. These patients may still benefit from nonemergent surgery to prevent a source of subsequent sepsis.[12,124] Some patients with small abscesses and no neurologic deficits may benefit from needle aspiration (to identify the organism) plus antibiotic therapy without surgical decompression.[119] Medical-only treatment is based on case reports and retrospective analysis that may be subject to reporting bias and does not represent the standard of care. Treatment decisions are best made by a team of consultants involving spine surgeons, internists, infectious disease specialists, and interventional radiologists.

EPIDURAL SPINAL CORD COMPRESSION

Epidural compression syndrome is a collective term encompassing spinal cord compression, cauda equina syndrome, and conus medullaris syndrome. These pathologic entities are grouped together because they share similar ED presentation, evaluation, and management. The only difference is the level of neurologic deficit at the time of presentation. The most common cause of epidural compression syndrome is a massive midline disc herniation, usually at the L4 to L5 disc level.[125] Other causes include tumor, epidural abscess, spinal canal hematoma, or lumbar spine spondylosis.

As in epidural abscess, the primary determinant of ultimate neurologic outcome is the neurologic status at the time of diagnosis, so making an early diagnosis is critical. However, delayed diagnosis is common. Back pain with a progressive increase in intensity is often the first symptom. Unlike other causes of back pain, pain from epidural spinal cord compression is worse with recumbent positioning secondary to epidural venous plexus distention. In time, associated unilateral or bilateral radiculopathy may develop. There may be more complaints of leg pain or neurologic symptoms than of back pain in many patients. Weakness is also commonly present at the time of diagnosis. It is usually symmetric and may have progressed to the point of significant gait disturbance or paralysis. Cauda equina lesions are also associated with decreased lower extremity reflexes.

Although less common than motor findings, abnormal sensory findings may include lower extremity paresthesia and anesthesia. One of the most frequent sensory deficits is saddle region anesthesia, which denotes loss of sensation around the anus, genitals, perineum, buttocks, and posterior-superior thighs. Patients may complain about bowel, bladder, or sexual dysfunction, and may also have decreased anal sphincter tone (60%–80%) on physical examination.[26] Urinary retention with overflow incontinence (sensitivity of 90%, specificity of 95%) is a common, though late, finding.[26] The probability of cauda equina syndrome in patients without urinary retention is approximately 1 in 10,000. An attempt may be made to localize the lesion by noting the level of the neurologic deficits, such as with the loss of bowel or bladder function (S2–S5) or the loss of the ankle jerk reflex (S1–S2). Such an exercise may not be necessary because MRI scans through the entirety of the lumbosacral spine. With presumed cauda equina syndrome, a sensory level deficit or a positive Babinski reflex suggests involvement of the conus medullaris. This terminal region of the spinal cord lies in close proximity to the nerve roots. Pathology to this region can therefore yield both upper and lower motor neuron signs; a mixture of both spinal cord and nerve root dysfunction.

Similar to the pathologic appearance of spinal epidural abscess on MRI, multiple locations of pathology often coexist. Imaging should include the entire spine if there is concern of metastatic compression or infection. In other cases, regional MRI may be appropriate. Information obtained from the MRI helps the admitting team with prognosis and treatment planning. CT with myelography should be used in patients who are not candidates for MRI.

General treatment guidelines involve providing analgesia and steroids. Pain control is the most pressing need from the patient's perspective and often requires opioid analgesics. One must only imagine a patient with vertebral metastases lying on his/her back for a long MRI study to appreciate the importance of effective analgesia. Early and effective pain control also helps the physician complete the history, physical examination, and diagnostic testing in a more effective and timely manner. The administration of glucocorticoids can minimize ongoing neurologic damage from compression and edema until definitive therapy can be initiated. The optimal initial dose and duration of therapy is controversial, with a recommended dose range of dexamethasone anywhere from 10 to 100 mg intravenously.[126,127] The ED physician should administer the first dose as soon as the diagnosis is suspected, rather than waiting for confirmatory diagnostic testing that often takes hours to complete. High-dose steroids are associated with serious side effects but have proven efficacy, whereas low-dose steroids have a lower side effect profile but no randomized controlled data to support their use.[126] Traditional dosing (dexamethasone 10 mg) can be used in patients with minimal neurologic dysfunction, reserving the higher dose (dexamethasone 100 mg) for patients with profound or rapidly progressive symptoms, such as paraparesis or paraplegia.[126,127] Some specialists may omit or delay gluco-corticoids in patients with small epidural lesions without any associated neurologic abnormalities.

As previously stated, final neurologic outcomes may be predicted by the functional status of the patient on arrival. Most patients who require a catheter on arrival will continue to do so. Patients who are ambulatory on arrival will likely remain ambulatory. Patients who are too weak to walk but not paraplegic have an approximately 50% chance of walking again. Those patients who are paraplegic on arrival are unlikely to walk again.[128] These statistics highlight the need for early detection and give insight to probable prognosis. All patients with evidence of neoplastic epidural cord compression should be administered glucocorticoids, provided adequate analgesia, and be admitted to the hospital with urgent consultation and evaluation for possible operative decompression and/or radiation therapy. On average, outcome is improved if decompression takes place within 24 to 48 hours of symptom onset.[129–131] Consultation with surgery and radiation oncology initiated in the ED facilitates more timely intervention.

CANCER

Both benign and malignant tumors can cause myelopathy as a result of external compression or intramedullary growth. The most common syndrome involves metastatic spread to the epidural space, causing spinal cord compression. The thoracic spine is the most common site of bony metastasis.[132] Back pain is the initial symptom of spinal metastasis in most presentations. Patients present with pain at the site of the lesion that is often described as dull, constant, and aching. Unlike the pain associated with mechanical low back pain and disc herniation, which improves with rest, cancer-related back pain tends to be unrelieved by rest and may even worsen with recumbency. Severe nighttime pain is also characteristic. Pathologic compression fractures may present with abrupt worsening of back pain. Patients with neoplastic epidural spinal cord compression may report radicular symptoms and progressive weakness with accompanying sensory loss and bladder dysfunction. Rapid progression to paraplegia can occur secondary to vascular compression. Similarly to epidural abscess, timely diagnosis and treatment is essential because the ultimate neurologic prognosis depends on the neurologic function at the time of intervention.

Plain radiographs may or may not show destructive lesions in 1 or multiple vertebral bodies. MRI is the imaging modality of choice to assess for spinal metastasis and neoplastic epidural spinal cord compression. CT is a better imaging modality than MRI for cortical bone destruction. Although any tumor may involve the bone, the most common cancers that metastasize to the spine are breast, lung, and prostate.[133]

A systematic approach to the patient with cancer and back pain is accomplished by categorizing patients into 3 groups based on signs and symptoms. The first patient group has had a sudden or rapid change in their back pain and developed new or progressive signs or symptoms suspicious for epidural compression, such as bowel or bladder incontinence, weakness, loss of reflexes, or the development of bilateral or multiroot findings. These patients are at high risk for rapid deterioration and should be evaluated and treated as previously discussed for possible emergent epidural compression syndrome in the ED. In addition to high-dose corticosteroids, patients with a vertebral neoplasm may also benefit from radiation therapy. The second patient group has back pain with stable neurologic signs or symptoms present for days to weeks. These findings include an isolated Babinski sign or mild and stable unilateral neurologic symptoms such as weakness, sensory changes, or radiculopathy in a single nerve root without evidence of cord compression. The presence of bilateral or multi-root involvement excludes patients from this group. Patients in group 2 should have plain radiographs performed in the ED and should also have MRI within 24 hours that can be done as an inpatient or outpatient. Considering the risk of myelopathic progression, it is safest to initiate the first dose of dexamethasone in the ED and admit these patients for pain control. With consensus and comfort between patient, ED physician, and PCP, patients can be discharged to their homes. The third patient group involves patients who have stable back pain without neurologic complaints or abnormalities suggestive of cord compression. These patients do not require treatment with dexamethasone. The ED evaluation should include plain radiographs. If there is any bony pathology, advanced imaging with MRI or CT is indicated as an outpatient within the next several days. If the plain radiographs are normal, further evaluation is not emergent. Patients must be closely followed by their PCP for improvement and lack of progressive symptoms. Follow-up appointments should occur within 1 week.

Some patients without known cancer have red flag signs and symptoms that are merely suggestive of malignancy, such as unexplained weight loss or back pain that is worse at night. As previously discussed, these patients require further risk stratification with plain radiographs and laboratory testing, including a WBC count, ESR, and CRP. With normal test results, these patients can be referred to their PCP for further workup and evaluation. With abnormal diagnostic results, such as a bone lesion on plain radiographs or an extremely increased ESR, urgent CT or MRI should be performed on an outpatient basis within the next week.

Unlike cauda equina syndrome, which usually requires only focal MRI of the lumbosacral spine, evaluation for malignancy requires screening MRI of the entire spine to evaluate for falsely localizing lesions, because clinically silent multilevel involvement is common and there is a 10% risk of distant asymptomatic metastases, which may affect subsequent treatment.[134] Additional imaging can be ordered from the ED and performed urgently from the hospital floor. Neoplastic epidural spinal cord compression is a true emergency and requires prompt diagnosis and treatment for the best possible patient outcome. Treatment in the ED would include high-dose corticosteroids with specialty consultation for radiation therapy and/or surgical decompression.

LUMBAR SPINAL STENOSIS

Lumbar spinal stenosis is usually secondary to degenerative arthritis (spondylosis). Stenosis of the vertebral canal occurs from a combination of loss of intervertebral disc height with bulging, facet joint hypertrophy and thickening of the ligamentum flavum.[27] Considering the aging population of the United States, ED physicians should expect to see this condition more frequently and increase our comfort with its diagnosis and treatment. Lumbar stenosis, in isolation, is frequently asymptomatic. Similarly to degenerative disc disease, there is poor correlation between the severity of symptoms and the degree of spinal canal stenosis seen on MRI. Neurologic symptoms are believed to be caused by both direct mechanical compression and nerve root ischemia. The classic and most common symptoms of lumbar spinal stenosis are that of neurogenic claudication: burning pain in the back that radiates to the buttocks and posterior-lateral legs.[26,27] Some patients may only note symptoms when active and not at rest. There are associated bilateral sensory changes, such as numbness or tingling and/or mild weakness affecting the legs, that are often asymmetric. Focal weakness, sensory loss, or reflex changes may occur when spinal stenosis is associated with radiculopathy. The physical examination may reveal single or multiple lumbosacral radiculopathies with sensory loss, areflexia, and/or focal weakness in the distribution of the involved nerve roots.[28] Symptoms are usually bilateral and aggravated by walking, prolonged standing, or spinal extension, and relieved with sitting, lying, or waist flexion.[27,28] This is because erect posture narrows the cross-sectional area of both the central canal and neural foramina. Neurogenic claudication (also called pseuodoclaudication) is differentiated from vascular claudication by etiology and symptomatology. Neurogenic claudication is caused by neurologic compression, not by arterial insufficiency.[26] Unlike vascular claudication, symptoms are often provoked by standing erect without walking, and may persist while at rest.[28]

Diagnosis is made with clinical findings that suggest spinal stenosis and with a neuroimaging study that shows structural narrowing. A history and physical examination can allow a presumptive diagnosis of spinal stenosis; however, a positive neuroimaging study without clinical correlation (ie, an incidental finding of canal narrowing) is insufficient for diagnosis. Just as in degenerative disc disease, radiographic spinal stenosis is an age-related population norm. More than 20% of asymptomatic persons greater than 60 years of age may have findings of spinal stenosis on imaging studies.[27] MRI is the study of choice and CT myelography is a second option in those in whom MRI is contraindicated. ED management of patients with spinal stenosis should be conservative and focus on pain control with acetaminophen, NSAIDs, and opiates. In the absence of alarming red flag findings (progressive neurologic deficit or evidence of cauda equina syndrome), these patients do not require laboratory or radiographic studies in the ED. Data supporting the role of epidural injection are sparse and inconclusive.[27] There is no role for epidural injection in the ED. Evaluation should also include outpatient referral to the patient's PCP to maximize medical management. The ED physician can consider an outpatient surgical referral for those patients with symptoms that are either severe or functionally disabling or for those in whom maximal medical therapy does not relieve symptoms sufficiently to allow for activities of daily living.

BACK PAIN IN CHILDREN

Although back pain represented only 0.4% of all visits to an inner-city pediatric department,[135] a brief mention of pediatric pathology causing back pain is warranted in this discussion. Most cases of back pain in children and adolescents receive no definitive diagnosis. However, children with back pain are more likely than their adult counterparts to have an underlying pathologic cause for their pain. Common identifiable causes include trauma (up to 25%) and nonspecific/benign musculoskeletal pain (24%–50%).[136–139] Other causes included idiopathic pain (13%), infections such as urinary tract infection (5%), viral illness (4%), and other miscellaneous causes (6%).[135]

The standard approach of the history and physical examination is to evaluate for red flags, just as in adults. Although age less than 18 years is considered a red flag, close attention should be paid to children less than 10 years old, particularly those less than 5 years old. Tumor, discitis, and malignancy occur with greater frequency in this age group.[140] Osteoid osteoma is the most common tumor in children who present with back pain. This tumor classically presents as intense nocturnal pain relieved with NSAIDs.[141] Protracted (>3–4 weeks) or worsening pain is also more concerning in children.[140] Inquire as to whether the pain interferes with activity and play. Pain preventing child play should raise concern. Inflammatory disease is suggested by morning stiffness and limited mobility that improves with a hot shower and activity and returns with rest. Inquire about recent febrile or bacterial illness. Young athletes with back pain represent a special subpopulation with a high incidence of structural injuries to the posterior spinal elements such as spondylolysis.[14] If the child participates in sports, ask about training intensity, duration, frequency, and especially recent increases that may suggest overuse injury. Children with sickle cell disease may have avascular necrosis of vertebral bodies. Caution should be exercised when attributing back pain to scoliosis in children because it is rarely a painful condition.

Physical examination should include physician-observed ambulation and a focused lower extremity neurologic evaluation, just as in adults. Pain with flexion suggests muscle injury/spasm or injury to the anterior spinal elements. Pain with extension indicates injury to the posterior elements or sacroiliac joint. Refusal to walk may suggest occult trauma, discitis, or osteomyelitis. As in adults, the clinical evaluation should direct the laboratory and radiologic evaluation. Children with a short symptom duration who appear well, with a normal neurologic examination in the absence of any red flags, can be conservatively managed without further diagnostic testing. They can be discharged with good-quality discharge instructions and follow-up with their pediatrician. Children with concerning signs or symptoms should proceed with a WBC count and ESR. Other tests, such as urinalysis and blood cultures, should be ordered if clinically appropriate. Plain radiographs of the lower back should also be obtained, with consideration of oblique views if spondylolysis is a consideration. Routine oblique views should not be performed. Children with suspected malignancy, spine infection, or progressive neurologic findings benefit from MRI. Timing and location of the study should be coordinated with the pediatrician or hospitalist.

Spondylolysis is a unilateral or bilateral defect in the pars interarticularis portion of the vertebrae. It is a stress fracture mostly seen in the lumbar vertebrae, and most commonly L5. Spondylolisthesis can occur when bilateral spondylolytic defects allow the forward translation of 1 vertebral body on another, occurring at L5 on S1 most frequently. It is graded based on the percentage of the lower vertebral body that is now uncovered (eg, 25%), termed slippage. Repetitive microtrauma to the bone from lumbar hyperextension or repeated lumbar flexion and extension leads to pars defects and eventual spondylolysis. Progression to spondylolisthesis occurs during the growth spurt and is correlated with persistent pain and lack of healing.[142] Spondylolysis is common in adolescent athletes and presents with acute lower back pain.[14] Sports that involve lumbar hyperextension, repetitive flexion/extension, or torsion have the highest incidence (eg, gymnastics, dance, figure skating).[140,143] ED diagnosis of back strain in this population should only occur following careful consideration of more serious pathology, including spondylolysis or spondylolisthesis. The typical patient is an active adolescent who complains of insidious onset of aching lower back pain that may radiate into the gluteal region, usually with activity. Pain is relieved with rest and worsened by extension or lateral bending.[139] On physical examination, patients may be focally tender to palpation and have pain worse with lateral bending or extension than with lumbar flexion. The neurologic examination is frequently normal. Clinical suspicion may be increased with a positive single-legged hyperextension test (stork test) in which the child stands on 1 leg and bends backward, thereby exacerbating ipsilateral lower back pain.[140,144] If neurologic symptoms and/or radiculopathy are present, an alternative diagnosis should be considered, because they are rarely associated with spondylolysis. There is no role for diagnostic laboratory tests.

Diagnostic imaging should start with plain radiographs with added oblique views. Classically, oblique views show the "Scotty dog" sign with a crack on the dog's neck/collar, the pars.[145] The Scotty dog's head (superior articular facet), nose (transverse process), eye (pedicle), neck (pars interarticularis), and body (lamina) should be easily identified on the oblique radiograph. A defect in the pars may indicate an acute fracture or an old nonunion. Bony sclerosis may be seen if healing has begun. ED management includes pain control, cessation of offending activities, particularly extension activities, and rest. Outpatient follow-up with an orthopedic specialist should be made. Inconclusive ED workup should involve discharge with close follow-up with the patient's pediatrician for consideration of single-photon emission computed tomography (SPECT) scan or MRI.[144,146] Spondylolisthesis is managed by observation. Progression usually stops when the child achieves skeletal maturity. Current recommendations are for limited contact sports in children with less than 30% to 50% slippage and surgical stabilization for children with slippage greater than 30% to 50%. Treatment becomes more aggressive if the child is symptomatic.

In addition to the infectious pathology discussed earlier, children are prone to inflammation and infection of the intervertebral discs, particularly in the lumbar region. Untreated, this may spontaneously resolve or progress to vertebral osteomyelitis or abscess formation. In comparison with children with osteomyelitis, children with discitis tend to be younger (2.8 vs 7.5 years of age), are less likely to be febrile (28% vs 78%), have a shorter duration of symptoms (22 vs 33 days) and are clinically less toxic in appearance.[10] Parents bring their young child to the ED noting irritability and reported back pain (27%), often associated with a limp or refusal to crawl or walk (63%).[147] Physical examination findings are nonspecific and may include an inability to flex the lower back (50%), loss of lumbar lordosis (40%), a tendency to lie still, and percussion tenderness over the involved spine.[140,147] Asking the child to pick up an object from the ground may be a helpful part of the physical examination. Fever is absent or low grade. Early in the disease course, systemic toxicity is rare and, if present, suggests osteomyelitis. WBC count can be normal early in the disease course, but the ESR is increased in more than 90% of patients.[10] The imaging study of choice is MRI. Children with MRI findings of discitis should be admitted, provided with pain control, and started on empiric antibiotics to cover the most common isolate, S aureus, in addition to other less common isolates including coagulase-negative Staphylococcus and Kingella kingae.[148] Appropriate initial antibiotics to be started in the ED include vancomycin and a third-generation cephalosporin such as ceftriaxone.

ADDITIONAL INFORMATION

In general, the recommended role of the ED physician in the management of acute lower back pain is to rule out significant pathology and obtain a correct diagnosis while avoiding excessive investigation. Subsequent goals include initiating appropriate treatment, providing analgesia, and patient education. Although patients should avoid vigorous exercise and provocative or high-impact activities after treatment, complete rest is not recommended. Bed rest has been proved to be deleterious to successful recuperation from back pain, leading to less functional recovery and slightly increased pain than in those advised to remain ambulatory.[149] Remaining active also helps with muscle spasm and atrophy. The ED physician should recommend that patients continue their daily activities and gradually increase specific exercises as tolerated. Patients should understand that back pain does not need to be totally alleviated before returning to work. Issues of return to work should be based on consideration of the work duties of the patient. Unlike a white-collar desk job, the patient with a job involving heavy manual labor may benefit from time away from work if no light-duty options are available. The ED work note should make this distinction clear.

Patients should understand that emergent evaluation by a back surgeon (neurosurgeon or orthopedic surgeon) is indicated for patients who are having back emergencies such as severe or progressive motor weakness, epidural abscess, or signs and symptoms of epidural compression syndrome. Outpatient referral for entities such as persistent disabling symptoms, including severe pain and radiculopathy, are elective and should be done only after attempts at maximal medical treatment have failed, and made by a patient's PCP. Carefully selected and presented advice and information about back pain can have a positive effect on patients' beliefs and clinical outcomes. The ED physician should reassure the patient by acknowledging their pain and being supportive. Care should be taken to avoid negative or confusing messages. An example of this would be avoiding language (eg, ruptured disc) that may frighten the medically naive patient and that may imply a serious abnormality when none exists.[150]

It is important to provide a full explanation of the diagnosis, evaluation, treatment plan, and anticipated time course for expected recovery in terms that the patient understands. For example, patients should be educated about why they are not undergoing laboratory tests or radiographic studies of their lower back and should be reassured of the likely benign course of the pain. Most patients can be convinced by education and an explanation of radiation dosing and associated deleterious effects. This approach helps avoid misperceptions of substandard care or subsequent unnecessary return visits within 48 hours when symptoms are still present. Patients should be reassured that back pain is common, that the pain does not indicate ongoing harm or serious pathology, and that the outlook is good. As mentioned earlier, the ED physician should avoid making unnecessary presumptive diagnoses and avoid the medicalization of benign conditions by ordering unnecessary tests. This behavior, coupled with the overprescription of analgesics (particularly opiates), fosters a belief on the part of the patient of the existence of serious pathology for an otherwise benign condition. If the facility evaluating the patient is unable to obtain an appropriate imaging study (eg, MRI) when needed, consider transfer to another facility with ready radiology access and specialty consultation for the patient with suspected spinal infection or epidural compression syndrome.

Patients may ask the ED physician about complementary and alternative treatments. Some supplemental treatment modalities have been shown to be of debatable efficacy in the management of acute and chronic low back pain. These treatments include acupuncture, physiotherapy, chiropractic manipulation, massage, ultrasound, traction, and transcutaneous nerve stimulation.[65,151] These treatments may be useful adjuncts to the ED physician's armamentarium for the outpatient treatment of many back conditions and may be of particular help for patients with acute flares of chronic or subacute back pain. The greatest benefit of these modalities has been found in patients who have belief in, and higher expectations of, the efficacy of a specific treatment modality, or who have had a favorable response to a particular modality in the past. These patients are more likely to derive benefit in the future and to demonstrate greater functional improvement at 12-week follow-up.[152] These treatments are generally safe and do not involve harm, so patients can be encouraged to pursue them as an outpatient. These modalities tend to cost more than conventional medical supportive care but, like most alternative treatments, are associated with enhanced patient satisfaction. Physical therapy may be beneficial for those patients with symptoms present for 4 to 6 weeks, although not in the acute setting.[153] Spinal manipulation involves moving a joint, in this case the spinal column, beyond its usual end range of motion but not past its anatomic range of motion. There is controversial benefit, with studies showing mixed results, although it may be as effective as conventional treatment.[154,155] Acupuncture and massage do not show clear data for acute treatment, but may be helpful for chronic back pain.[156,157]

Perhaps the most important aspect of ED management of acute back pain involves the discharge instructions. All patients with back pain evaluated in the ED who are not admitted should be given clear instructions with unambiguous indications to return or go to the nearest ED with symptoms such as new or progressive leg weakness, bowel or bladder dysfunction, or saddle anesthesia. Although not practical considering the available time for patient encounters in the ED setting, time spent discussing prevention is time well spent. This discussion may take the form of pre-printed written discharge instructions. The future of ED medicine likely involves a greater number of uninsured and primary care patients, so there are invaluable benefits to providing information detailing the benefits of exercise, weight loss, staying active, and avoidance of activities that involve repetitive twisting or bending or high-impact activities that increase spinal stress. Proper bending and lifting techniques should be included.

Almost all patients with nonspecific lower back pain can be discharged from the ED with follow-up with their PCP. In rare circumstances, severe ongoing pain despite treatment and/or inadequate support at home for recovery may preclude discharge. Patients with cancer and intractable bony pain may also require admission for pain control. For patients who have a red flag diagnosis of cauda equina syndrome or epidural abscess, immediate neurosurgical consultation is required for emergent surgical decompression. Patients with epidural abscess also require administration of intravenous antibiotics.

The clinical pitfall to avoid is diagnosing an emergent back pain episode as just a back strain. The ED physician should always check for the presence of red flags in all patients who have back pain. To summarize, the patients who have low back pain emergencies are: (1) those who have a past medical history of malignancy and new back pain with neurologic findings, (2) those who have back pain and symptoms of epidural compression syndrome, (3) those who have back pain with symptoms suggesting an infectious cause, (4) those who have back pain with gross muscle weakness or paralysis, and (5) those who have back pain and bilateral or multiple nerve root involvement.

REFERENCES

1. Andersson GB. Epidemiological features of chronic low-back pain. Lancet 1999; 354:581–5.
2. Hart L, Deyo R, Cherkin D. Physician office visits for low back pain. Frequency, clinical evaluation, and treatment patterns from a U.S. national survey. Spine 1995;20:11–9.
3. Wipf J, Deyo R. Low back pain. Med Clin North Am 1995;79:231–46.
4. Frymoyer J, Cats-Baril W. An overview of the incidences and costs of low back pain. Orthop Clin North Am 1991;22:263–71.
5. Agency for Healthcare Research and Quality, U.S. Department of Health & Human Services. 2009. Available at: http://ahrq.gov/about/cj2000/cjhelp00. htm#back. Accessed December 20, 2009.
6. Guo H, Tanaka S, Halperin W, et al. Back pain prevalence in US industry and estimates of lost workdays. Am J Public Health 1999;89:1029–35.
7. Dagenais S, Caro J, Haldeman S. A systemic review of low back pain cost of illness studies in the United States and internationally. Spine J 2008;8:8–20.
8. AHRQ News and Numbers. U.S. Department of Health & Human Services. 2008. Available at: http://www.ahrq.gov/news/nn/nn030608.htm. Accessed November 17, 2009.

9. Long S, Stockley K. Emergency department visits in Massachusetts. Urban Institute policy brief. 2009. Available at: http://www.rwjf.org/publichealth/product.jsp?id=48929. Accessed November 22, 2009.
10. Fernandez M, Carrol CL, Baker CJ. Discitis and vertebral osteomyelitis in children: an 18-year review. Pediatrics 2000;105:1299–304.
11. Turner P, Green J, Galaskl C. Back pain in childhood. Spine 1989;14:812–4.
12. Darouiche R. Spinal epidural abscess. N Engl J Med 2006;355:2012–20.
13. King HA. Back pain in children. Orthop Clin North Am 1999;30:467–74.
14. Micheli LJ, Wood R. Back pain in young athletes. Significant differences from adults in causes and patterns. Arch Pediatr Adolesc Med 1995;149:15–8.
15. Rigamonti D, Liem L, Sampath P, et al. Spinal epidural abscess: contemporary trends in etiology, evaluation, and management. Surg Neurol 1999;52: 189–97.
16. Sampath P, Rigamonti D. Spinal epidural abscess: a review of epidemiology, diagnosis and treatment. J Spinal Disord 1999;12:89–93.
17. Schiff D, O'Neill B, Suman V. Spinal epidural metastasis as the initial manifestation of malignancy: clinical features and diagnostic approach. Neurology 1997; 49:452–6.
18. Witham T, Khavkin Y, Gallia G, et al. Surgery insight: current management of epidural spinal cord compression from metastatic spine disease. Nat Clin Pract Neurol 2006;2:87–94.
19. Sioutos PJ, Arbit E, Meshulam CF, et al. Spinal metastases from solid tumors. Analysis of factors affecting survival. Cancer 1995;76:1453–9.
20. Bigos S, Bowyer O, Braen G, et al. Acute lower back problems in adults. Clinical practice guideline. AHCPR Pub. No. 95-0643. Rockville (MD): US Department of Health and Human Services, Public Health Service, Agency for Health Care Policy and Research; 1994.
21. Deyo RA, Weinstein J. Primary care: low back pain. N Engl J Med 2001;344: 363–70.
22. Reihsaus E, Waldbaur H, Seeling W. Spinal epidural abscess: a meta-analysis of 915 patients. Neurosurg Rev 2000;23:175–204.
23. Schmidt R, Markovchick V. Nontraumatic spinal cord compression. J Emerg Med 1992;10:189–99.
24. Abdu W, Provencher M. Primary bone and metastatic tumors of the cervical spine. Spine 1998;23:2767–77.
25. Helweg-Larsen S, Sørensen P. Symptoms and signs in metastatic spinal cord compression: a study of progression from first symptom until diagnosis in 153 patients. Eur J Cancer 1994;30A:396–8.
26. Deyo RA, Rainville J, Kent DL. What can the history and physical examination tell us about low back pain? JAMA 1992;268:760–5.
27. Katz JN, Harris MB. Clinical practice. Lumbar spinal stenosis. N Engl J Med 2008;358:818–25.
28. Hall S, Bartleson JD, Onofrio BM, et al. Lumbar spinal stenosis. Clinical features, diagnostic procedures, and results of surgical treatment in 68 patients. Ann Intern Med 1985;103:271–5.
29. Gregory D, Seto C, Wortley G, et al. Acute lumbar disk pain: navigating evaluation and treatment choices. Am Fam Physician 2008;78:835–42.
30. Morris E, Di Paola M, Vallance R, et al. Diagnosis and decision making in lumbar disc prolapse and nerve entrapment. Spine 1986;11:436–9.
31. Sprangfort EV. The lumbar disc herniation. A computer-aided analysis of 2504 operations. Acta Orthop Scand Suppl 1972;142:1–95.

32. Jonsson B, Stromqvist B. Symptoms and signs in degeneration of the lumbar spine. A prospective, consecutive study of 300 operated patients. J Bone Joint Surg Br 1993;75:381–5.

33. Kerr RS, Cadoux-Hudson TA, Adams CB. The value of accurate clinical assessment in the surgical management of the lumbar disc protrusion. J Neurol Neurosurg Psychiatry 1988;51:169–73.

34. Knutsson B. Comparative value of electromyographic, myelographic and clinical-neurological examinations in diagnosis of lumbar root compression syndrome. Acta Orthop Scand 1961;49(Suppl):1–134.

35. Lauder TD. Physical examination signs, clinical symptoms, and their relationship to electrodiagnostic findings and the presence of radiculopathy. Phys Med Rehabil Clin N Am 2002;13:451–67.

36. Hakelius A, Hindmarsh J. The comparative reliability of preoperative diagnostic methods in lumbar disc surgery. Acta Orthop Scand 1972;43:234–8.

37. Bowditch MG, Sanderson P, Livesey JP. The significance of an absent ankle reflex. J Bone Joint Surg Br 1996;78:276–9.

38. McGee S. Evidence-based physical diagnosis. Philadelphia: WB Saunders; 2001.

39. Podnar S, Trsinar B, Vodusek D. Bladder dysfunction is patients with cauda equina lesions. Neurourol Urodyn 2006;25:23–31.

40. Della-Giustina D. Emergency department evaluation and treatment of back pain. Emerg Med Clin North Am 1999;17:877–93.

41. Andersson GB, Deyo RA. History and physical examination in patients with herniated lumbar discs. Spine 1996;21(Suppl 24):10–185.

42. Deville WL, van der Windt DA, Dzaferagic A, et al. The test of Lasègue: systematic review of the accuracy in diagnosing herniated discs. Spine 2000;25: 1140–7.

43. Cyriax J. Perineuritis. Br Med J 1942;1:578–80.

44. Rabin A, Gerszten P, Karausky P, et al. The sensitivity of the seated straight-leg raise test compared with the supine straight-leg raise test in patients presenting with magnetic resonance imaging evidence of lumbar nerve root compression. Arch Phys Med Rehabil 2007;88:840–3.

45. Stankovic R, Johnell O, Maly P, et al. Use of lumbar extension, slump test, physical and neurological examination in the evaluation of patients with suspected herniated nucleus pulposus. A prospective clinical study. Man Ther 1999;4: 25–32.

46. Walsh J, Hall T. Agreement and correlation between the straight leg raise and slump tests in subjects with leg pain. J Manipulative Physiol Ther 2009;32: 184–92.

47. Majlesi J, Togay H, Unalan H, et al. The sensitivity and specificity of the slump and straight leg raising tests in patients with lumbar herniation. J Clin Rheumatol 2008;14:87–91.

48. Waddell G, McCulloch JA, Kummel E, et al. Nonorganic physical signs in low-back pain. Spine 1980;5:117–25.

49. Main C, Waddell G. Behavioral responses to examination. A reappraisal of the interpretation of "nonorganic signs". Spine 1998;23:2367–71.

50. Scalzitti D. Screening for psychological factors in patients with low back problems: Waddell's nonorganic signs. Phys Ther 1997;77:306–12.

51. Fishbain D, Cole B, Cutler R, et al. A structured evidence-based review on the meaning of nonorganic physical signs: Waddell signs. Pain Med 2003; 4:141–81.

52. Fishbain D, Cutler R, Rosomoff H, et al. Is there a relationship between nonorganic physical findings (Waddell signs) and secondary gain/malingering? Clin J Pain 2004;20:399–408.

53. Carleton R, Kachur S, Abrams M, et al. Waddell's symptoms as indicators of psychological distress, perceived disability, and treatment outcome. J Occup Rehabil 2009;19:41–8.

54. Kummel BM. Nonorganic signs of significance in low back pain. Spine 1996;21: 1077–81.

55. Fritz J, Wainner R, Hicks G. The use of nonorganic signs and symptoms as a screening tool for return-to-work in patients with acute low back pain. Spine 2000;25:1925–31.

56. Chelsom J, Solberg CO. Vertebral osteomyelitis at a Norwegian university hospital 1987–97: clinical features, laboratory findings and outcome. Scand J Infect Dis 1998;30:147–51.

57. Kapeller P, Fazekas F, Krametter K, et al. Pyogenic infectious spondylitis: clinical, laboratory, and MRI features. Eur Neurol 1997;38:94–8.

58. Beronius M, Bergaman B, Anderson R. Vertebral osteomyelitis in Goteborg, Sweden: a retrospective study of patients during 1990–95. Scand J Infect Dis 2001;33:527–32.

59. Deyo RA, Diehl AK. Cancer as a cause of back pain: frequency, clinical presentation, and diagnostic strategies. J Gen Intern Med 1988;3:230–8.

60. Jarvik J, Deyo R. Diagnostic evaluation of low back pain with emphasis on imaging. Ann Intern Med 2002;137:586–97.

61. Chou R, Fu R, Carrino J, et al. Imaging strategies for low-back pain: systematic review and meta-analysis. Lancet 2009;373:463–72.

62. Kendrick D, Fielding K, Bentley E, et al. Radiography of the lumbar spine in primary care patients with low back pain: randomized controlled trial. BMJ 2001;322:400–5.

63. Deyo R, Diehl A, Rosenthal M. Reducing roentgenography use. Can patient expectations be altered? Arch Intern Med 1987;147:141–5.

64. Liang M, Komaraff A. Roentgenograms in primary care patients with acute low back pain. Arch Intern Med 1982;142:1108–12.

65. Chou R, Qaseem A, Snow V, et al. Diagnosis and treatment of low back pain: a joint clinical practice guideline from the American College of Physicians and the American Pain Society. Ann Intern Med 2007;147(7):478–91.

66. Suarez-Almazor M, Belseck E, Russell A, et al. Use of lumbar radiographs for the early diagnosis of low back pain. JAMA 1997;277:1782–6.

67. Jarvik JG. Imaging of adults with low back pain in the primary care setting. Neuroimaging Clin N Am 2003;13:293–305.

68. Algra P, Bloem J, Tissing H, et al. Detection of vertebral metastases: comparison between MR imaging and bone scintigraphy. Radiographics 1991;11: 219–32.

69. McAfee P, Yuan H, Fredrickson B, et al. The value of computed tomography in thoracolumbar fractures. An analysis of one hundred consecutive cases and a new classification. J Bone Joint Surg Am 1983;65:461–73.

70. Campbell S, Phillips C, Dubovsky E, et al. The value of CT in determining potential instability of simple wedge-compression fractures of the lumbar spine. Am J Neuroradiol 1995;16:1385–92.

71. Oland G, Hoff TG. Intraspinal cross-section areas measured on myelography—computed tomography. The relation to outcome in nonoperated lumbar disc herniation. Spine 1996;21:1985–9.

72. Cox J. Low back pain: mechanisms, diagnosis, and treatment. 6th edition. Philadelphia: Lippincott Williams & Wilkins; 1999. p. 406.

73. Jarvik J, Hollingworth W, Martin B, et al. Rapid magnetic resonance imaging vs radiographs for patients with low back pain: a randomized controlled trial. JAMA 2003;289:2810–8.

74. Jensen MC, Brant-Zawadzki MN, Obuchowski N, et al. Magnetic resonance imaging of the lumbar spine in people without back pain. N Engl J Med 1994; 331:69–73.

75. Biering-Sørensen F, Hansen F, Schroll M, et al. The relation of spinal x-ray to low-back pain and physical activity among 60-year-old men and women. Spine 1985;10:445–51.

76. Kalichman L, Li L, Kim D, et al. Facet joint osteoarthritis and low back pain in the community-based population. Spine 2008;33:2560–5.

77. Boden S, McCowin P, Davis D, et al. Abnormal magnetic-resonance scans of the cervical spine in asymptomatic subjects. A prospective investigation. J Bone Joint Surg Am 1990;72:1178–84.

78. Weinreb J, Wolbarsht L, Cohen J, et al. Prevalence of lumbosacral intervertebral disk abnormalities on MR images in pregnant and asymptomatic nonpregnant women. Radiology 1989;170:125–8.

79. Donovan M, Dillon P, McGuire L. Incidence and characteristics of pain in a sample of medical-surgical inpatients. Pain 1987;30:69–78.

80. Roelofs P, Deyo R, Koes B, et al. Non-steroidal anti-inflammatory drugs for low back pain. Cochrane Database Syst Rev 2008;1:CD000396.

81. Chou R, Huffman LH. Medications for acute and chronic low back pain: a review of the evidence for an American Pain Society/American College of Physicians clinical practice guideline. Ann Intern Med 2007;147:505–14.

82. Larson A, Polson J, Fontana R, et al. Acetaminophen-induced acute liver failure: results of a United States multicenter, prospective study. Hepatology 2005;42: 1364–72.

83. Martell B, O'Connor P, Kerns R, et al. Systematic review: opioid treatment for chronic back pain: prevalence, efficacy, and association with addiction. Ann Intern Med 2007;146:116–27.

84. Deshpande A, Furlan A, Mailis-Gagnon A, et al. Opioids for chronic low-back pain. Cochrane Database Syst Rev 2007;3:CD004959.

85. Volinn E, Fargo J, Fine P. Opioid therapy for nonspecific low back pain and the outcome of chronic work loss. Pain 2009;142:194–201.

86. Fordyce W, Brockway J, Bergman J, et al. Acute back pain: a control-group comparison of behavioral vs traditional management methods. J Behav Med 1986;2:127–40.

87. Caldwell J, Hale M, Hague, et al. Treatment of osteoarthritis pain with controlled release oxycodone or fixed combination oxycodone plus acetaminophen added to nonsteroidal anti-inflammatory drugs: a double blind, randomized, multicenter, placebo controlled trial. J Rheumatol 1999;26:862–9.

88. Browning R, Jackson J, O'Malley P, et al. Cyclobenzaprine and back pain. Arch Intern Med 2001;161:1613–20.

89. Van Tulder M, Touray T, Furlan A, et al. Muscle relaxants for nonspecific low back pain: a systemic review within the framework of the Cochrane collaboration. Spine 2003;28:1978–92.

90. Chou R, Peterson K, Helfand M. Comparative efficacy and safety of skeletal muscle relaxants for spasticity and musculoskeletal conditions: a systematic review. J Pain Symptom Manage 2004;28:140–75.

91. Armon C, Argoff CE, Samuels J, et al. Assessment: use of epidural steroid injections to treat radicular lumbosacral pain: report of the Therapeutics and Technology Assessment Subcommittee of the American Academy of Neurology. Neurology 2007;68:723–9.

92. Carette S, Leclaire R, Marcoux S, et al. Epidural corticosteroid injections for sciatica due to herniated nucleus pulposus. N Engl J Med 1997;336: 1634–40.

93. Koes BW, Scholten RJ, Mens JM, et al. Efficacy of epidural steroid injections for low-back pain and sciatica: a systematic review of randomized clinical trials. Pain 1995;63:279–88.

94. Friedman B, Holden L, Esses D, et al. Parenteral corticosteroids for emergency department patients with non-radicular low back pain. J Emerg Med 2006;31: 365–70.

95. Haimovic I, Beresford H. Dexamethasone is not superior to placebo for treating lumbosacral radicular pain. Neurology 1986;36:1593–4.

96. Finckh A, Zufferey P, Schurch MA, et al. Short-term efficacy of intravenous pulse glucocorticoids in acute discogenic sciatica. A randomized controlled trial. Spine 2006;31:377–81.

97. Holve R, Barkan H. Oral steroids in initial treatment of acute sciatica. J Am Board Fam Med 2008;21:469–74.

98. French SD, Cameron M, Walker BF, et al. Superficial heat or cold for low back pain. Cochrane Database Syst Rev 2006;1:CD004750.

99. Nadler SF, Steiner DJ, Erasala GN, et al. Continuous low-level heatwrap therapy for treating acute nonspecific low back pain. Arch Phys Med Rehabil 2003;84: 329–34.

100. Williams C, Maher C, Hancock M, et al. Low back pain and best practice care: a survey of general practice physicians. Arch Intern Med 2010;170:271–7.

101. Engstrom J. Back and neck pain. In: Fauci A, Braunwald E, Kasper D, et al, editors. Harrison's principles of internal medicine. 17th edition. New York: McGraw-Hill; 2008. p. 94–100.

102. Della-Giustina D, Nolan R. Evaluation and management of acute low back pain. Emerg Med 2004;36:20–8.

103. Hilde G, Hagen K, Jamtvedt G, et al. Withdrawn: advice to stay active as a single treatment for low-back pain and sciatica. Cochrane Database Syst Rev 2007;2: CD003632.

104. Weber H. The natural history of disc herniation and the influence of intervention. Spine 1994;19:2234–8.

105. Weinstein J, Tosteson T, Lurie J, et al. Surgical vs nonoperative treatment for lumbar disk herniation: the Spine Patient Outcomes Research Trial (SPORT): a randomized trial. JAMA 2006;296:2441–50.

106. Chou R, Baisden J, Carragee E, et al. Surgery for low back pain: a review of the evidence for an American pain society guideline. Spine 2009;34:1094–109.

107. Peul W, van Houwelingen H, van den Hout W, et al. Surgery verses prolonged treatment for sciatica. N Engl J Med 2007;356:2245–56.

108. Gellin BG, Weingarten K, Gamache FW Jr, et al. Epidural abscess. In: Scheld WM, Whitley RJ, Durack DT, editors. Infections of the central nervous system. 2nd edition. Philadelphia: Lippincott-Raven; 1997. p. 507.

109. Danner RL, Hartman BJ. Update on spinal epidural abscess: 35 cases and review of the literature. Rev Infect Dis 1987;9:265–74.

110. Nussbaum ES, Rigamonti D, Standiford H, et al. Spinal epidural abscess: a report of 40 cases and review. Surg Neurol 1992;38:225–31.

111. Davis DP, Wold RM, Patel RJ, et al. The clinical presentation and impact of diagnostic delays on emergency department patients with spinal epidural abscess. J Emerg Med 2004;26:285–91.
112. Akalan N, Ozgen T. Infection as a cause of spinal cord compression: a review of 36 spinal epidural abscess cases. Acta Neurochir (Wien) 2000;142:17–23.
113. Soehle M, Wallenfang T. Spinal epidural abscesses: clinical manifestations, prognostic factors, and outcomes. Neurosurgery 2002;51:79–85.
114. Darouiche RO, Hamill RJ, Greenberg SB, et al. Bacterial spinal epidural abscess. Review of 43 cases and literature survey. Medicine (Baltimore) 1992;71:369–85.
115. Parkinson J, Sekhon L. Spinal epidural abscess: appearance on magnetic resonance imaging as a guide to surgical management. Report of five cases. Neurosurg Focus 2004;17:E12.
116. Wong D, Raymond N. Spinal epidural abscess. N Z Med J 1998;111:345–7.
117. Hlavin M, Kaminski H, Ross J, et al. Spinal epidural abscess: a ten-year perspective. Neurosurgery 1990;27:177–84.
118. Lu C, Chang W, Lui C, et al. Adult spinal epidural abscess: clinical features and prognostic factors. Clin Neurol Neurosurg 2002;104:306–10.
119. Wheeler D, Keiser P, Rigamonti D, et al. Medical management of spinal epidural abscess: case report and review. Clin Infect Dis 1992;15:22–7.
120. Siddiq F, Chowfin A, Tight R, et al. Medical vs surgical management of spinal epidural abscess. Arch Intern Med 2004;164:2409–12.
121. Curry W, Hoh B, Amin-Hankani S, et al. Spinal epidural abscess: clinical presentation, management, and outcome. Surg Neurol 2005;63:364–71.
122. Savage K, Holtom P, Zalavras CG. Spinal epidural abscess: early clinical outcome in patients treated medically. Clin Orthop Relat Res 2005;439:56–60.
123. Sørensen P. Spinal epidural abscesses: conservative treatment for selected subgroups of patients. Br J Neurosurg 2003;17:513–8.
124. Sendi P, Bregenzer T, Zimmerli W. Spinal epidural abscess in clinical practice. QJM 2008;101:1–12.
125. Podnar S. Epidemiology of cauda equina and conus medullaris lesions. Muscle Nerve 2007;35:529–31.
126. Loblaw DA, Laperriere NJ. Emergency treatment of malignant extradural spinal cord compression: an evidence-based guideline. J Clin Oncol 1998;16:1613–24.
127. Byrne TN. Spinal cord compression from epidural metastases. N Engl J Med 1992;327:614–9.
128. Helwig-Larsen S. Clinical outcome in metastatic spinal cord compression: a prospective study of 153 patients. Acta Neurol Scand 1996;94:269–75.
129. Ahn U, Ahn N, Buchowski J, et al. Cauda equina syndrome secondary to lumbar disc herniation: a meta-analysis of surgical outcomes. Spine 2000;25:1515–22.
130. Kohles S, Kohles D, Karp A, et al. Time-dependent surgical outcomes following cauda equina syndrome diagnosis: comments on a meta-analysis. Spine 2004; 29:1281–7.
131. Shapiro S. Medical realities of cauda equina syndrome secondary to lumbar disc herniation. Spine 2000;25:348–52.
132. Posner J. Back pain and epidural spinal cord compression. Med Clin North Am 1987;71:185–205.
133. Portenoy R. Cancer pain. Epidemiology and syndromes. Cancer 1989;63: 2298–307.
134. Portenoy R, Lipton R, Foley K. Back pain in the cancer patient: an algorithm for evaluation and management. Neurology 1987;37:134–8.

135. Selbst SM, Lavelle JM, Soyupak SK, et al. Back pain in children who present to the emergency department. Clin Pediatr (Phila) 1999;38:401–6.
136. Combs JA, Caskey PM. Back pain in children and adolescents: a retrospective review of 648 patients. South Med J 1997;90:789–92.
137. Feldman DS, Hedden DM, Wright JG. The use of bone scan to investigate back pain in children and adolescents. J Pediatr Orthop 2000;20:790–5.
138. Bhatia NN, Chow G, Timon SJ, et al. Diagnostic modalities for the evaluation of pediatric back pain: a prospective study. J Pediatr Orthop 2008;28:230–3.
139. Kim HJ, Green DW. Adolescent back pain. Curr Opin Pediatr 2008;20:37–45.
140. Hollingworth P. Back pain in children. Br J Rheumatol 1996;35:1022–8.
141. Cohen MD, Harrington TM, Ginsburg WW. Osteoid osteoma: 95 cases and a review of the literature. Semin Arthritis Rheum 1983;12:265–81.
142. Morita T, Ikata T, Katoh S, et al. Lumbar spondylolysis in children and adolescents. J Bone Joint Surg Br 1995;77:620–5.
143. Baker RJ, Patel D. Lower back pain in the athlete: common conditions and treatment. Prim Care 2005;32:201–29.
144. Masci L, Pike J, Malara F, et al. Use of the one-legged hyperextension test and magnetic resonance imaging in the diagnosis of active spondylolysis. Br J Sports Med 2006;40:940–6.
145. Ginsburg GM, Bassett GS. Back pain in children and adolescents: evaluation and differential diagnosis. J Am Acad Orthop Surg 1997;5:67–78.
146. Takemitsu M, El Rassi G, Woratanarat P, et al. Low back pain in pediatric athletes with unilateral tracer uptake at the pars interarticularis on single photon emission computed tomography. Spine 2006;31:909–14.
147. Brown RA, Hussain K, McHugh K, et al. Discitis in young children. J Bone Joint Surg 2001;83:106–11.
148. Cushing AH. Diskitis in children. Clin Infect Dis 1993;17:1–6.
149. Vroomen PC, de Krom MC, Wilmink JT, et al. Lack of effectiveness of bed rest for sciatica. N Engl J Med 1999;340:418–23.
150. Deyo RA. Clinical strategies for controlling costs and improving quality in the primary care of low back pain. J Back Musculoskeletal Rehabil 1993;3:1–13.
151. Pengel HM, Maher CG, Refshauge KM. Systematic review of conservative interventions for subacute low back pain. Clin Rehabil 2002;16:811–20.
152. Myers SS, Phillips RS, Davis RB, et al. Patient expectations as predictors of outcome in patients with acute low back pain. J Gen Intern Med 2008;23:148–53.
153. Sinclair SJ, Hogg-Johnson SH, Mondloch MV, et al. The effectiveness of an early active intervention program for workers with soft-tissue injuries. The Early Claimant Cohort Study. Spine 1997;22:2919–31.
154. Assendelft WJ, Morton SC, Yu EI, et al. Spinal manipulative therapy for low back pain. A meta-analysis of effectiveness relative to other therapies. Ann Intern Med 2003;138:871–81.
155. Eisenberg DM, Post DE, Davis RB, et al. Addition of choice of complementary therapies to usual care for acute low back pain: a randomized controlled trial. Spine 2007;32:151–8.
156. Furlan AD, Brosseau L, Imamura M, et al. Massage for low-back pain: a systematic review within the framework of the Cochrane Collaboration Back Review Group. Spine 2002;27:1896–910.
157. Furlan AD, van Tulder MW, Cherkin DC, et al. Acupuncture and dry-needling for low back pain: an updated systematic review within the framework of the Cochrane Collaboration. Spine 2005;30:944–63.

Management and Treatment of Pelvic and Hip Injuries

Jean Williams-Johnson, MBBS, MSc, DM[a],*,
Eric Williams, MBBS, MSc, DM[a], Harold Watson, MBBS, MSc, DM[b]

KEYWORDS

• Angiography • Pelvic stabilization • Avascular necrosis
• Pelvic packing • Hip reduction • Falls

PELVIC FRACTURES

Pelvic fractures are a disruption of the bony structures of the pelvis and can be life threatening. The incidence of pelvic injuries in the United States is estimated to be more than 100,000 per annum.[1] Intrapelvic and abdominal hemorrhages remain the main cause of death in patients, with an overall mortality rate between 6% and 35% in large series of high-energy pelvic fractures.[2] Although the mortality rate has been decreasing, management of these complex injuries requires prompt diagnosis and appropriate intervention. Improvement in outcomes are attributed to advances in prehospital and hospital emergency care, interventional radiology, and surgical and critical care The main mechanism of this injury is blunt trauma to the pelvis, for which injury from motorcycle crashes, pedestrian injuries, side impact motor vehicle collisions, and falls are the most common causes. Because of the tremendous force necessary to cause a pelvic fracture, these fractures frequently involve injuries to the pelvic organs as well as extrapelvic structures such as the head, thorax, and abdomen. Therefore, a complete assessment is mandatory.[3] Mortality rates approach 50% when associated with hemodynamic instability.[4] To date, the best predictor for determining the likelihood of mortality is the Injury Severity Score and not the type of pelvic injury.[5]

RELEVANT ANATOMY AND INJURY PATTERN

The pelvis consists of the medial sacrum, the coccyx, and the bilateral innominate bones. The bilateral innominate bones are formed by the fusion of 3 separate bones:

[a] Emergency Medicine Division, Department of Surgery, Radiology, Anaesthesia and Intensive Care, University of the West Indies and the University Hospital of the West Indies (Mona), Kingston, Jamaica, West Indies
[b] Faculty of Medical Sciences, The University of the West Indies, Cave Hill Campus and Queen Elizabeth Hospital, Bridgetown, Barbados, West Indies
* Corresponding author.
E-mail address: jeanjohnson@cwjamaica.com

Emerg Med Clin N Am 28 (2010) 841–859
doi:10.1016/j.emc.2010.07.002
0733-8627/10/$ – see front matter © 2010 Elsevier Inc. All rights reserved.

emed.theclinics.com

the ilium, ischium, and pubis. The acetabulum is located at the center of the fusion site and forms the fossa or socket of the hip joint.

The pelvis is arranged in a ring, with the pubis at the base of this circular structure that is joined to the wing-shaped ilium by the ischium. The right and left pubic bones articulate in the midline forming the pubic symphysis. The symphysis is a true amphiarthrosis, which is separated by a fibrocartilage disk. In women, the flexibility of the symphysis is influenced by progesterone allowing the birth canal to widen. The upper borders of either halves of the pubis can be used as an estimation of joint disruption.[6]

The posterior portion of the pelvis is formed by the sacrum, which is located between the right and left iliac portions of the innominate bones, resulting in the sacroiliac (SI) joint on either side. The stability of the posterior pelvis is maintained by the SI joints. The sacrospinous ligament runs from the sacrum to the ischial spine, whereas the sacrotuberous ligament attaches the sacrum to the ischial tuberosity.[7] These ligaments along with the others oppose the rotational effect of gravity at the SI joint and provide the strength of the pelvic ring as a unit. A significant force is required to fracture or disrupt the pelvic ring, and therefore intra-abdominal injuries are associated with ring disruption as a result of the huge transfer of energy and absorbed forces.[8] In the trauma patient, the correlation of injury pattern with pelvic fractures cannot be overemphasized. The urethra and bladder are closely associated posteriorly to the pubic symphysis, whereas the rectum lies immediately anterior to the sacrum. The female patient needs special consideration with regard to the gynecologic organs, including the gravid uterus when present.

The pelvis is enriched with extensive vasculature, which poses problems that can lead to significant hemorrhage. Fractures, dislocation of the SI joint, and tearing of the pelvic ligaments can involve the internal iliac vessels, resulting in life-threatening bleeding. The common iliac artery branches into the external iliac artery, which exits the pelvis anteriorly over the pelvic brim. The internal iliac artery lies over the pelvic brim. These arteries along with their associated veins can be injured during pelvic disruption. Hemorrhage directly attributed to pelvic injuries is mostly of a venous origin[9] (90%), which may cease through the body's normal hemostatic mechanisms but sometimes requires direct or indirect vascular compression, supplemental blood products, and/or interventional coagulation.[10] In selected patients this pathophysiology of hemorrhage in the traumatic pelvis can justify stabilization without surgical intervention.

The injury pattern usually determines mechanical stability, which plays a key role in deciding definitive orthopedic treatment (operative vs nonoperative). There are several fracture classification systems that are used to describe pelvic injuries, and most classification systems are based on the direction of forces and the nature and stability of the pelvic disruption.

The Tile classification system is based on the integrity of the posterior SI complex and attempts to predict the need for surgical intervention. Type A pelvic injuries are stable because the SI complex is intact and do not require surgery, whereas type B fractures involve partial disruption of the complex and are unstable. Type C fractures involve a complete disruption of the posterior SI complex and are also unstable.[9]

The classification system developed by Young and Burgess is based on the observation that the direction of the force or energy determines the pattern of the fracture.[7] The classification takes into account the mechanism of injury and divides pelvic disruptions into anteroposterior compression (APC), lateral compression (LC), vertical shear (VS), and a separate category called combined mechanisms (**Fig. 1**).

This classification is based on the use of a routine series of pelvic views including anteroposterior (AP) and inlet and outlet views, and thin-cut (3 mm) computed tomographic (CT) scans.[10,11]

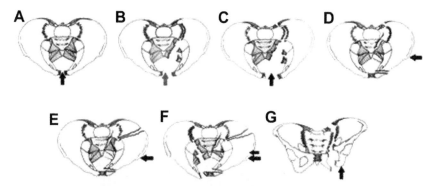

Fig. 1. The Young and Burgess classification of pelvic fracture. (*A*) APC type I. (*B*) APC type II. (*C*) APC type III. (*D*) LC type I. (*E*) LC type II. (*F*) LC type III. (*G*) VS. The arrow in each panel indicates the direction of force producing the fracture pattern. (Copyright © Jesse B. Jupiter, MD and Bruce D. Browner, MD.)

The posterior pelvic ring defines ultimate stability. VS injuries are unstable fractures (**Fig. 2**). LC fractures are the most commonly encountered injuries.[7] APC fractures are commonly termed "open-book" pelvic fractures. There is widening of the anterior pelvis, usually with separation of the pubis (**Fig. 3**). The APC and LC categories are further divided into types I, II, and III, based on the increasing severity and the mechanism of injury.[12]

The main objective of the Young and Burgess classification is to predict associated injuries and resuscitation needs along with the mortality associated with these groups of fractures.[12]

EPIDEMIOLOGY

Pelvic fractures account for approximately 3% of skeletal trauma.[13] These injuries consist of pelvic ring and acetabular fractures as well as avulsion injuries. Single pubic ramus and avulsion fractures are most common. Pelvic fractures are classified as stable if the pelvis has one break point in the ring and these tend to have minimal bleeding, with the bones staying in place.[14] Unstable pelvic fractures have 2 or

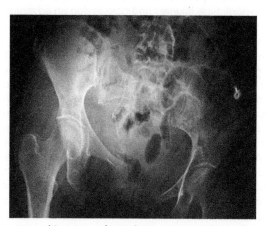

Fig. 2. VS fracture pattern. (*Courtesy of* eMedicine, Omaha, NE; with permission.)

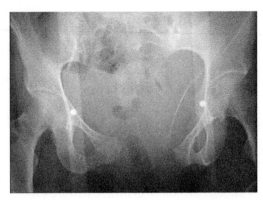

Fig. 3. AP fracture pattern.

more disruptions in the pelvic ring and are often associated with moderate to severe bleeding. Either categories can be closed (skin intact) or open. The latter is associated with a higher mortality.[15,16] The mechanism of injury is often related to age, with motor vehicle crashes being more prevalent in adults, and car-pedestrian injuries more notorious in children. Elderly patients tend to have pubic rami fractures without associated internal injuries as the result of minimal trauma. The mortality rate for severe trauma in the elderly patient is also high.[17,18] In 2007, a study examining the trauma registry in the United Kingdom reported that 58% of the patients with pelvic ring fracture were males.[19]

PREHOSPITAL CARE

In general, as in all severe trauma cases, safe and efficient transfer of the patient to the emergency department (ED) is paramount. Prehospital transport protocols are essential. Close attention must be paid to spinal immobilization, airway protection, and circulatory support. Compression of sites of external hemorrhages and splinting of long bone fractures should be done where appropriate. These activities not only control bleeding in the vicinity of a fracture but also improve pain control. The role of the pneumatic antishock garment (MAST) in the prehospital emergency medical care of adult and pediatric patients is limited.[20] Although a stabilizer of the pelvis (especially for open-book type injuries) and possessing an advantageous mechanical effect for venous return in the hypotensive pelvic trauma patient, MAST does have significant disadvantages that outweigh the benefits.[10,12,21]

Compartment syndrome, skin necrosis, and the need for removal to attain access in the event of abdominal exploration are significant drawbacks. Many prehospital protocols no longer use MAST. Although MAST is still useful for stabilization of patients with these injuries, commercially available pelvic binders and hospital sheets have largely replaced it. These devices provide circumferential compression around the pelvis and are simple, quick, and easy to apply, cost-effective, and noninvasive.[22] Pelvic binders are equipped with an adjustable buckle to achieve the recommended tension of about 180 N.[23] The use of these devices has resulted in a decrease in the need for transfusions, length of admission, and mortality, particularly with APC injuries.[24] **Fig. 4** is an example of a pelvic force-controlled circumferential pelvic sling belt, which can be easily applied and controlled by means of a buckle with a fabric hook-and-loop fastener release. Expedient transportation is the key to survival and should be the main focus in the prehospital setting as soon as the devices are applied.

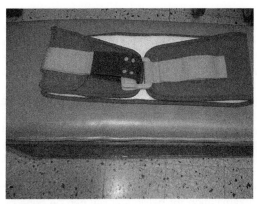

Fig. 4. A standard emergency room pelvic binder. (*Courtesy of* SAM Medical Products, Portland, OR, USA. Available at: http://www.sammedical.com/sam_sling. Accessed May 5, 2010; with permission.)

ED MANAGEMENT

Contemporary recommendations for pelvic fractures and hemorrhage include stabilization fixation, angiography, and exploratory laparotomy with packing.[24,25] The patient's condition must dictate what is done and when. No clear recommendations can be made because the published studies have different inclusion and exclusion criteria, and clinical presentations vary over a wide spectrum.[26,27] As a result, contemporary management strategies are usually based on algorithmic guidelines.

Patients with pelvic trauma should be quickly assessed using the Advanced Trauma Life Support guidelines.[9,10,12]

The primary survey focuses on identification and treatment of any life-threatening injury. A focused history at the appropriate time should be sought to identify any comorbid illness, allergy, and the mechanism of injury.

All patients should be given oxygen and intravenous fluids. Spine immobilization is important. For adequate pain control, narcotics (morphine sulfate) should be titrated intravenously to the desired effects. Antibiotics should be administered if there is any evidence of bowel rupture, vaginal or urinary tract injuries, and open fractures. Tetanus prophylaxis should also be considered when appropriate. Stabilization of the pelvis can be done with a sheet. The key to using a sheet wrap is to apply this device around the center of the trochanter and not the iliac crest. Stabilization of the patient takes priority over obtaining plain radiographs.

Hypotensive patients who are unresponsive to initial fluid resuscitation (2 L crystalloids) may require massive amounts of fluid, exposing the patient to additional complications (ie, coagulopathy and pulmonary edema). In general, most of these patients require transfusions of platelets and fresh frozen plasma (FFP). As a general guideline, 2 or 3 U of FFP and 7 to 8 U of platelets are needed for every 5 L of volume replacement.[12] Massive blood transfusion and the administration of recombinant factor VIIa may be required in life-threatening hemorrhage, if other measures to control the pelvic bleeding fail.[28,29] In general, a high index of suspicion is needed for pelvic fractures in unconscious patients or those who complain of pelvic pain. Multitrauma patients inclusive of those with head and spinal injuries can pose a challenge, and the physical examination plays a pivotal role. Attention to details and a routine approach to examination cannot be oversimplified. Inspection for active bleeding, deformities, and even contusions and abrasions in the lower abdomen, pelvis, and lower limbs should be done. The pattern of injury is often useful to predict an otherwise unnoticed pelvic injury. For example, patients with a head or neck injury with a lower limb injury must have the pelvis carefully scrutinized because the pelvis is sandwiched between these proximal and distal anatomic sites. These sandwiched injuries are particularly useful in heightening the suspicion of pelvic trauma in a comatose patient with no obvious immediate clinical findings.

The presence of blood at the urethral meatus is a sign of urethral injury. Similarly, scrotal or labial ecchymosis or hematoma should suggest a pelvic injury. Rectal or vaginal bleeding warrants further evaluation. The goals of a rectal examination are to identify bleeding and to determine the position of the prostate (a high-riding prostate suggests urethral disruption). However, the digital rectal examination in isolation has a low sensitivity for diagnosing this injury.[30] Suspected urethral injuries should be evaluated with a retrograde urethrogram to confirm an intact urethra before inserting a urinary catheter. Examination for pelvic stability can be done by applying manual compression to the anterosuperior iliac spines or iliac crests. A positive finding results in significant pains or rotational instability. Caution should be exercised because the application of this maneuver may aggravate the injury and cause further bleeding.[31] Although physical examination is specific for pelvic stability, it has a low sensitivity.[17] In the patient in advanced stage of pregnancy, physiologic stretching of the pelvic ligaments may mimic bony instability.[28]

Hemodynamic instability is a distinct red flag in the ED. Physicians should search for the source of shock, which in most cases is caused by active hemorrhage. There are five potential sites of hemorrhage: external regions, long bones, chest, abdomen, and retroperitoneum.

Provided that the patient is hemodynamically stable and not comatose, some investigators suggest that the routine use of AP pelvic radiography is not necessary.[32] The sensitivity of plain radiographs for fracture detection is less than 80%.[33] Plain radiographs are most appropriate for hemodynamically unstable patients to allow for rapid diagnosis of pelvic fractures and the consideration for early interventional radiology. Therefore, in the hemodynamically unstable patient, plain radiographs do have a role in planning for definitive management, where CT is time consuming and may also require risky transportation to the radiology suite.

CT provides a superior image with better resolution than plain radiographs, and may augment the identification of small fractures, soft tissue injuries in proximity to the pelvis, and active arterial bleeding.[34,35] CT is extremely valuable for defining posterior ring instability as well as the detection of retroperitoneal and intraperitoneal bleeding. CT can also confirm hip dislocations associated with acetabular fracture. Contrast-enhanced CT is an option in the hemodynamically stable trauma patient and has been reported to be fairly accurate in determining the presence or absence of ongoing bleeding. Cerva and colleagues[35] compared CT with angiography and showed that CT was 90% accurate in detecting bleeding. CT is also useful in assessing the volume of pelvic hemorrhage as well as in planning the strategy for definitive fixation of the fractures.

The focused abdominal sonography for trauma (FAST) is a useful investigative modality. This technique was first introduced in Europe in the 1980s (Fig. 5).[36] The purpose of this technique is to identify free fluid. FAST is unable to detect retroperitoneal hemorrhage or bowel injury.[9]

If FAST is equivocal and there is clinical suspicion of continuous or ongoing intraperitoneal hemorrhage, diagnostic peritoneal lavage (DPL) can be considered. DPL is also useful in the evaluation of the hemodynamically unstable patient in the ED. A supraumbilical approach should be used to minimize the possibility of inadvertent entry into

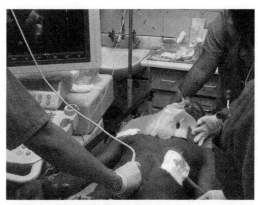

Fig. 5. The use of FAST in a multiple trauma patient. In FAST, ultrasound technology is used to detect the presence of hemoperitoneum in a pelvic fracture. (*Courtesy of* University Hospital of the West Indies, West Indies, Jamaica; with permission.)

a pelvic hematoma, which may result in a false-positive interpretation. Grossly positive results are indications for exploration (>8 mL of aspirated blood from the peritoneal cavity or obvious enteric contents).[10]

External fixation can prevent dislodgment of clots and reopposes bleeding osseous surfaces, thereby promoting clot formation and decreasing ooze. The timing of application, the location of pin placement on the patient's pelvis, and the contra-indications for using this procedure remain controversial.[37] However, this procedure can be done quickly even in the angiography suite. The choice of external fixation or pelvic compression as opposed to angiography is often based on an initial assessment of the fracture pattern and resources available at each institution. The use of an external pelvic fixation device can help reduce hemorrhage by compression and immobilization of the pelvis prior to exploratory laparotomy.

There are 2 main types of external fixation: anterior frames and the C-clamp. A posteriorly applied C-clamp provides adequate posterior ring stabilization. The C-clamp should be applied under fluoroscopic guidance to avoid iatrogenic injury.[38] Potential drawbacks to the use of external fixators are the need for orthopedic surgeons to be readily available and the need for specific training. Because there are other readily available devices, including sheets, the role of external fixators for the persistently hemodynamically unstable patient with an unstable fracture is not universally accepted.[10]

After initial stabilization with pelvic compression and the exclusion of any life-threatening injuries, the options available for the hemodynamically unstable patient are laparotomy with packing and interventional radiology. Clinical features that indicate the possibility of ongoing pelvic fracture hemorrhage include prehospital hypotension, recurrent hypotension during resuscitation, or transfusion of more than 6 U of packed red blood cells during the first 24 hours. Failure to stabilize the patient hemodynamically may require pelvic packing.

Most (85%–90%) pelvic hemorrhages associated with fractures are venous in origin, and the tamponading effect of packing is a treatment option.[39] This approach is particularly useful in patients in extremis. Extraperitoneal packing allows stabilization of the unstable patient in the operating room and can stabilize the patient enough to allow transport to the angiography suite where embolization can be performed. Totterman and colleagues[40] concluded that extraperitoneal packing can provide a significant increase in systolic blood pressure. This procedure is fast and easy to perform and has been shown to decrease the need for emergent angiography.[41]

Immediate access to angiography along with a skilled radiologist makes angiography an institution-dependent decision. Although angiography is an important tool in the management of severe pelvic injuries, the precise early timing of this procedure is crucial. Furthermore, angiography and embolization are not effective in controlling bleeding from venous injuries and bony sites.[12] There has been a trend toward the use of angioembolization as opposed to surgical intervention to control hemorrhage.[42,43]

One of the other challenges in pelvic injuries is to address open pelvic fractures. Suspicions of rectal or vaginal injury should be considered. Because there is increased morbidity and mortality with these injuries, early diagnosis and specific treatment is mandatory.[10]

Specific pelvic injuries (urethral, gynecologic, and rectal injuries) need appropriate specialist referral, highlighting that these injuries require a multidisciplinary approach.

Fig. 6 is an algorithm recommended by Durkin and colleagues[10] on the contemporary management of pelvic injuries.[28]

SUMMARY

Pelvic fractures are serious injuries, and successful management is best accomplished by a team approach. In the ED, a quick primary survey and rapid stabilization of the pelvis with a sheet, a commercial binder, or an external fixation device are essential.

HIP INJURIES

The occurrence of hip injuries is recognized as being a major public health problem for both the developing and developed world. Injuries that occur to the hip are commonly either dislocations or fractures. Projections from a group of reviewers have shown that there will be an increase in the number of hip fractures occurring worldwide from 1.66 million in 1990 to 6.26 million by 2050.[44,45] Hip fractures alone account for more than 250,000 hospital visits per year in the United States.[44] The main causes for these visits include the preponderance of high-velocity trauma, falls, and increasing life expectancy.[46] The proportion of men to women for all types of hip fractures is approximately 1:3.[47] The incidence doubles each decade after 50 years, and nearly half the fractures occur after the affected person's 80th birthday.[48] Late identification is a recognized cause of increased morbidity and mortality. Among the hip fracture patients, 1 in 5 die within a year of injury, and as much as 50% of these patients never regain their premorbid levels of independence and functioning.[48–50] In the United States, the annual cost for hip fractures can be as high as $8.68 billion (these costs are related to inpatient care, nursing home care, and outpatient services).[51]

The ability to recognize and act appropriately to patients who present with a hip injury to the ED is essential for an emergency provider. This section examines the different types of hip injuries and their management.

Anatomy of the Hip

An understanding of the anatomy of the hip joint as it relates to the bony and vascular architecture is essential for the efficient management of these injuries.

The femoral head has a flattened ellipsoid shape and articulates with the acetabulum to form a ball and socket joint. The head is connected to the shaft of the femur by the femoral neck and creates the appearance of an oblique strut between a vertical beam, the femoral shaft, and a horizontal beam, the pelvis.[52] The head is situated

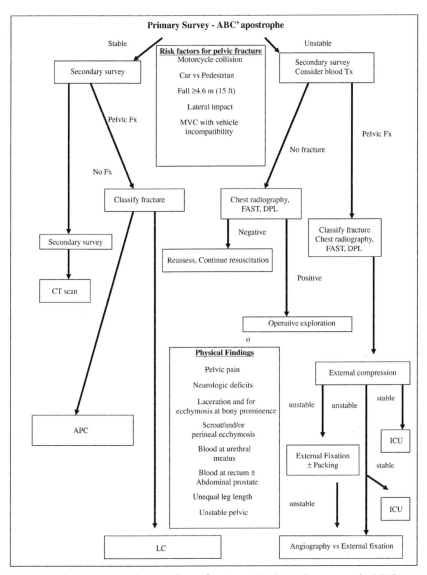

Fig. 6. Pelvic fracture algorithm. Fx, bone fracture; ICU, intensive care unit; MVC, motor vehicle collision; Tx, treatment. (*Reprinted from* Durkin A, Sagi HC, Durham R, et al. Contemporary management of pelvic fractures. Am J Surg 2006;192:222; with permission from Elsevier.)

deep within the acetabular socket, which is further enhanced by a cartilaginous labrum. In the inferior aspect of the acetabulum is the acetabular notch, which is bridged by the transverse acetabular ligament. This articulation with the acetabulum is supported by a joint capsule, which is further strengthened by muscular and ligamentous attachments. Therefore, it requires significant force to disrupt the joint. The iliofemoral ligament (the Y ligament of Bigelow) is the largest of these ligaments and reinforces the hip anteriorly.[52,53] The pubofemoral ligament reinforces the hip inferiorly and the ischiofemoral ligament, the thinnest ligament, reinforces the hip joint posteriorly. The ligamentum teres plays a minor role in the stability of the hip joint but carries the foveal artery to the head of the femur.[52]

The femoral neck facilitates a wide range of movement at the hip and is susceptible to fracture because of its narrow circumference, length, and angle (**Fig. 7**).[52] There are 5 trabecular networks of cancellous bone, which provide the mechanical strength across the proximal femur. Ward's triangle is an area of diminished density in this trabecular pattern and is the weakest point of the femoral neck, which results in this area being the site for many femoral neck or subcapital fractures.[54]

The tenuous blood supply to the proximal femur is the cause of high incidence of avascular necrosis of the femoral head after fractures of the femoral neck.[52] The blood supply is from the retinacular or epiphyseal arteries, which arise from the lateral and posterior medial circumflex arteries (**Fig. 8**). These arteries form a ring around the femoral neck called the trochanteric anastomosis (these circumflex arteries arise from the profunda femoris or deep femoral arteries). The arteries then travel under the synovium of the femoral neck and provide most of the blood supply to the femoral head, forming the cruciate anastomosis.[52,53] The femoral head also receives blood from the foveal artery (a branch of the obturator artery). The foveal artery runs through the ligamentum teres into the fovea; however, the foveal artery alone is not thought to provide enough to meet the metabolic needs of the femoral head.[53] Finally, the area receives additional nutrients from the metaphyseal arteries.

An understanding of the neuroanatomy of the hip joint is important for assessing injuries and providing early local analgesia. The 2 major nerves supplying the hip joint are the femoral and the sciatic nerves.[52] The femoral nerve is important for knee extension, knee deep tendon reflexes, and sensation above and medial to the patella.

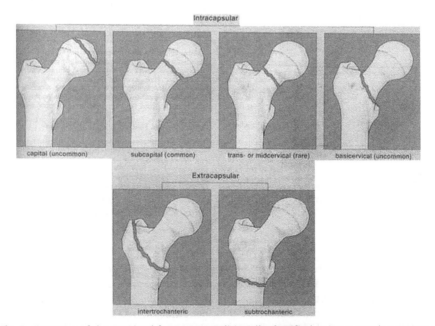

Fig. 7. Fractures of the proximal femur are traditionally classified as intracapsular or extracapsular. (*From* Greenspan A. Orthopedic radiology. Philadelphia: JB Lippincott; 1988. p. 5.17; with permission.)

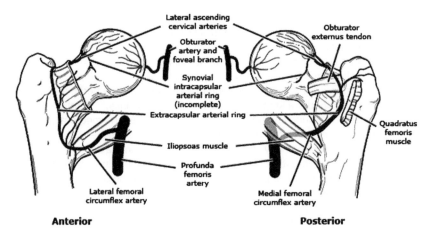

Anterior   **Posterior**

Fig. 8. The lateral ascending cervical arteries provide the blood supply to most of the femoral head. Foveal vessels may supply a varying area directly adjacent to the insertion of the ligamentum. (*From* Baumgaertner MR, Higgins TF. Femoral neck fractures. In: Bucholz RW, Heckman JD, editors. Rockwood and Green's fractures in adults, vol. 2. 5th edition. Philadelphia: Lippincott Williams & Wilkins; 2002. Copyright © 2002 Lippincott Williams & Wilkins; with permission.)

Of importance, sensation to the midshaft of the femur and distal femur is exclusively from the femoral nerve. Injury to the sciatic nerve is seen in up to 10% of patients with hip dislocations, and results in weakness in the hamstrings and all muscles inferior to the knee. Injury to the sciatic nerve is also associated with the absence of ankle deep tendon reflexes and sensation loss below the knee and to the back of the thigh.[53,55]

Hip Fractures

The anatomy of the hip joint and its blood supply in particular can lead to disastrous consequences if the patient's injuries are not attended to urgently. Femoral neck fractures are more common in the elderly.[52,56] Intertrochanteric fractures are also common in the elderly, with an average age ranging between 75 and 81 years.[52] In the elderly, the mortality rate is 4% to 11.5% and can go up to 36% during the first year after the fracture.[44] There is also significant morbidity, which is often secondary to various factors such as immobilization, which can lead to deep vein thrombosis, pulmonary embolism, pneumonia, and muscular atrophy.[45] Other factors that can lead to morbidity include surgical problems such as anesthetic morbidity, postoperative infection, loss of fixation, malunion, or nonunion. The inability to return to prefracture level of functioning results in loss of independence, reduction in quality of life, and depression and other psychiatric problems in the elderly.[44]

In patients younger than 44 years, significant kinetic energy is required to cause a hip fracture, and 75% of these injures are femoral head fractures.[52] The most common cause is motor vehicle collision. In the elderly, cigarette smoking, institutional living, maternal history of hip fractures, previous hip fracture, previous Colles fracture, low weight, tall stature, and alcohol abuse contribute to the incidence of hip fracture.[45] Osteoporosis also features strongly among the causes.[50] Fractures seldom occur in the elderly who do not fall. Researchers suggest that the act of falling and not the presence of osteoporosis is important for the occurrence of hip fractures.[49,56] A United States survey done on persons older than 65 years reported that falls were equally common between men and women but were more likely to result in injury in women.[57] Internationally, falls tend to occur more commonly in nursing homes, with a frequency of 1.6 to 2 falls per patient per year The causes of falls are myriad and preventable for the most part and can be looked at in terms of intrinsic and extrinsic factors.[58] Extrinsic factors include slippery surfaces such as wet bathroom floors, loose rugs, objects left lying on the floor, poor lighting, low-lying objects such as low beds, and low toilet seats. Poorly maintained walking aids also predispose to falls.[49,56] Intrinsic factors include age, visual or hearing impairment, arthritis, dementia, and medication use.[49,56]

Patients who present with hip injuries must first be assessed in the standard fashion, with attention paid to their airway, breathing, and circulation status. In particular, the patient's blood pressure must be monitored continuously because up to 3 L of blood loss can be hidden in the pelvis and 1.5 L in the thigh.[28] In the emergency room, the patient's clothing should be removed, and stability of the hip and pelvis should be assessed and maintained. Distal pulses must be assessed and the compartments of the leg palpated to check for compartment syndrome. If the pulses are neither equal nor palpable, a bedside Doppler may be necessary. Analgesics should be administered early.

Laboratory studies should include a complete blood cell count, typing, and cross-matching, and plain radiographs of the hip. Standard films include AP and lateral views of the hip. An AP view of the pelvis with the hip internally rotated 15° to 20° optimally images the femoral acetabulum. The integrity of Shenton line, which is a line traced along the inner aspects of the femoral head and inner pubic ramus, as well as the trabecular pattern of the femoral neck should be assessed, and there should be no transverse area of sclerosis.[6,7] If the fracture is not identified and still suspected, modalities such as a bone scan, CT, magnetic resonance imaging (MRI), and Judet views (oblique views of the hip) can be done to aid in the evaluation.[7] Clinical features that may increase the possibility for nondisplaced fractures include inability to bear weight (pain on axial loading) and pain on range-of-motion maneuvers (internal and external rotation and straight leg raise).[59,60] The absence of these signs alone or in combination, however, does not exclude a fracture. CT has the same challenge as with plain radiography, in that the resolution of osteoporotic trabecular bone is limited and fractures that run parallel to the trabecular plane may be hidden. MRI is the preferred modality, especially useful for the nondisplaced or occult hip fracture.[47,61] One study demonstrated that the use of coronal-weighted T1 MRI resulted in 100% accuracy with regard to the confirmation of hip fractures.[62] MRI also has the advantage of being noninvasive and able to detect fractures within 24 hours (some sources quote as early as 4 hours) of them occurring.[63,64]

Pain control is essential. Parental analgesia and muscle relaxants may be necessary. For the multitrauma patient for whom systemic analgesia would prevent further examination, the emergency provider may perform a femoral nerve blockade to prevent unwanted depression of the sensorium that can occur with the use of parenteral analgesics.[65] Orthopedic consultation is necessary for all hip fractures, especially in cases in which there is neurovascular compromise. The patient should also receive tetanus prophylaxis and intravenous antibiotics as appropriate.

Hip fractures involve any aspect of the proximal femur from the head to the first 4 to 5 cm of the subtrochanteric area. Hip fractures can be broadly categorized as being intracapsular or extracapsular, depending on whether or not the fracture is located within the capsule of the hip joint (see **Fig. 7**). Intracapsular hip fractures can be further subdivided into 2 groups: femoral head and femoral neck fractures (subcapital, trans- or midcervical, or basicervical). Femoral head fractures may be simple (type I) or comminuted (type II). These fractures are not common and may be associated with hip dislocations. Posterior dislocations are associated with inferior femoral head fractures, whereas anterior dislocations are associated with superior femoral head fractures. These fractures are usually simple type I fractures. Comminuted femoral head fractures are usually caused by direct trauma and may be associated with severe injuries such as pelvic or upper extremity fractures on the same side.[52] Whenever posterior fractures or dislocations are noted, there may be sciatic nerve injuries, associated pelvic fractures, and lower limb fractures on the same side.[54]

The intracapsular femoral neck fractures require emergency reduction and internal fixation within 6 hours to decrease the risk of avascular necrosis.[66] These procedures are important because the potential for avascular necrosis of the femoral head after a femoral neck fracture ranges from 5% to 50%, depending on the degree of displacement and the time to fracture reduction.[66] Femoral neck fractures are classified by the Garden classification, which describes 4 types of femoral neck fractures.[7,67] Type I is an incomplete or impacted fracture. Type II is a nondisplaced complete fracture, and types III and IV are partially displaced or completely displaced fractures, respectively. The diagnosis of femoral neck fractures types I and II are challenging, and more than just a plain radiograph may be needed to make the diagnosis.

Extracapsular fractures are further classified by virtue of their relationship to the greater and lesser trochanters as intertrochanteric, greater trochanteric, lesser trochanteric, and subtrochanteric fractures.

Intertrochanteric fractures tend to occur in the elderly as a result of a fall, and most cases have to be repaired surgically (**Fig. 9**). These fractures involve the cancellous bone between the region of the greater and lesser trochanters. There can be extensive bleeding into this fracture because of the good vascular environment of the cancellous bone. Intertrochanteric fractures are classified as stable or unstable. For stable fractures, there is a single fracture line between the 2 trochanters and no displacement. For unstable fractures, there are multiple fracture lines or comminution with associated displacement.[52] The patient's limb is usually externally rotated and shortened. There is a risk of complications from these fractures, including a mortality rate of up to 15%, a rate of osteomyelitis up to 8%, and an increased risk of thromboembolism if the patient is not mobilized early.[52] There is also a risk of nonunion and avascular necrosis from these injuries. If clinically the patients have suspected fractures but plain radiographs are normal, CT or MRI may be needed to make the diagnosis.

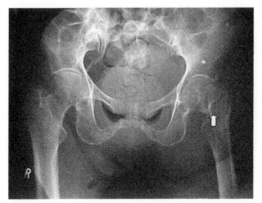

Fig. 9. Radiograph showing intertrochanteric fracture of the left femur. (*Courtesy of* the University Hospital of the West Indies, West Indies, Jamaica; with permission.)

Subtrochanteric fractures involve injuries occurring within 5 cm of the lesser trochanter. These fractures are seen in the elderly with bone pathology (eg, Paget disease) and metastatic cancer, which predispose this region to fractures from minor trauma.[7,52] Subtrochanteric fractures also occur in younger individuals who sustain great force to the area. The patient presents in significant pain, and the thigh may be swollen. There is a risk of extensive blood loss into the area, and early traction resulting in a change in shape from a cylinder to a sphere may result in significantly less blood loss. These fractures most often require orthopedic fixation, and the emergency physician refers the patient as an emergency to the on-call orthopedic service.

Greater trochanteric fractures are rare and, when seen in adults, require a significant force and are caused by avulsion at the insertion of the gluteus maximus muscle. The patient may present with a limp, and plain radiographs will reveal the fracture. Fractures of the lesser trochanter are seen in young adults, and the mechanism of injury is usually a forceful contraction of the iliopsoas muscle resulting in an avulsion of the trochanter.[7,52] Both these fractures are categorized as nondisplaced and displaced (types I and II, respectively). Treatment is usually conservative with good results. In the younger patient, however, a displacement greater than 1 cm for the greater trochanteric fractures and 2 cm for lesser trochanteric fractures requires surgical fixation.[7]

Because the hip joint is extremely stable, a significant force is usually needed to cause a dislocation, except in the elderly patient who may have osteoporosis and sustain dislocation from a seemingly trivial mechanism. Increased mortality is seen when there are associated injuries. Life-threatening injuries to the pelvis, abdomen, chest, and head should be specifically excluded. An approach similar to that for hip fractures should be used.

These injuries are orthopedic emergencies because of the high risk for avascular necrosis.[68] Hip dislocations can be anterior, posterior, central, or acetabular. However, in 90% of cases the dislocations are posterior and result from motor vehicle collisions (**Fig. 10**).[7,69] The typical mechanism is a flexed knee hitting the dashboard in a motor vehicle collision. The limb is held flexed, adducted, and internally rotated for posterior dislocation. For anterior dislocations the extremity is abducted, externally rotated, and flexed or extended. Femoral head fractures are sometimes associated with hip dislocation. The anterior hip dislocations are associated with femoral fractures in between 22% and 77% of cases.[70] Posterior hip dislocations are associated with

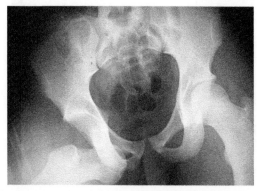

Fig. 10. Radiograph of posterior hip dislocation from teaching files. (*Courtesy of* the University Hospital of the West Indies, West Indies, Jamaica; with permission.)

femoral head fractures between 10% and 16% of the time.[52] To reduce the damage to periarticular vasculature caused by repetitive maneuvers, reduction should be performed only in a controlled setting with appropriate sedation and analgesia. It is important to perform a neurovascular assessment, because sciatic nerve injury is observed in 10% to 14% of patients with posterior hip dislocations.[54] Sciatic nerve injury is manifested by decreased muscle function below the knee, decreased ability to flex the knee, and decreased sensation on the posterolateral leg and sole of the foot.

The 3 main maneuvers used for reduction of hip dislocation are the Allis, Stimson, and Whistler maneuvers (**Fig. 11**).[69] The Allis maneuver requires at least 2 persons for success. The assistant stabilizes the pelvis. The operator stands on the stretcher and gently flexes the patient's hip to 90°. The operator then applies progressively increasing traction to the extremity along with adduction and internal rotation. The repositioning of the femur can often be detected clinically. The Stimson maneuver is performed with the patient prone, which may be impractical for the ED because the patient's airway cannot be adequately managed by this technique and a multitrauma patient cannot be positioned to lie face down. The patient's lower limbs are allowed to hang over the end of the bed. Immobilization of the pelvis is achieved by having the assistant press down on the patient's sacrum. The operator then holds the knee

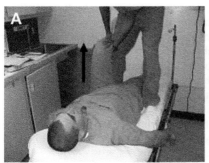
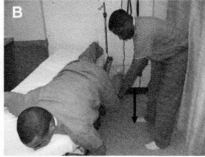
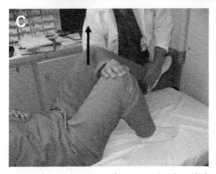

Fig. 11. (*A*) The Allis technique for reduction of a posterior hip dislocation. Anterior traction is applied to bring the femoral head into the acetabulum. An assistant is often required to stabilize the pelvis by applying downward counterpressure to the pelvis. (*B*) Stimson technique for reduction of a posterior hip dislocation. The patient can be positioned at the end of the bed with both hips over the edge of the bed. (*C*) Whistler technique for reduction of posterior hip dislocation. The operator raises his arm and shoulder, exerting upward traction on the hip while maintaining slight adduction of the leg. (*From* Newton EJ. Emergency department management of selected orthopedic injuries. Emerg Med Clin North Am 2007;25(3):781; with permission.)

and ankle flexed to 90° and applies gentle traction in a downward direction. A gentle rotation of the hip may assist in the reduction.[69]

The Whistler technique is used to reduce posterior hip dislocation in skiers and snowboarders. This technique is applicable in other scenarios as well, and is useful in that one person can perform it. After appropriate procedural sedation, the patient is placed supine on the bed with both knees flexed and the feet placed firmly on the bed. The operator places the nondominant hand under the affected knee and the other hand on the unaffected knee. By straightening his or her arm or lifting his or her shoulder, the operator adducts the patient's leg and applies gradual traction to the hip until the dislocation reduces. The advantages of this technique are that it can be performed by a single operator and the patient's airway can be monitored during the procedure. The status of the neurovascular supply to the limb must always be assessed after a reduction, and an adductor splint can be applied to limit any motion that might dislocate an unstable reduction.[69]

A superior iliac subtype is one in which the femoral head is palpable in the area of the superior iliac line; a superior pubic subtype is that in which the femoral head rests near the pubis. Finally, in the inferior or obturator subtype, the femoral head lies in the obturator canal. Anterior dislocations are usually caused by motor vehicle collisions with a severe blow to the back, or a fall. The limb is slightly abducted, externally rotated, and extended for anterior superior dislocations, and is abducted, externally rotated, and flexed for anterior inferior dislocations. An adequate neurovascular assessment is essential because of the possibility of damage to the femoral nerve, which is manifested by diminished quadriceps function, decreased knee tendon reflexes, and decreased sensation on the anterior medial thigh.

A central hip dislocation is a fracture dislocation that occurs when the femoral head lies medial to a fractured acetabulum, which occurs because of a lateral force against an adducted femur as seen in side impact motor vehicle collisions. This injury is corrected surgically.

Indications for surgery in patients with hip dislocation include an irreducible hip dislocation, a hip dislocation with a femoral neck fracture, an incarcerated fragment in the joint, and an unstable hip after reduction.[69]

SUMMARY

Patients who present to the ED with hip and pelvic injuries are at a high risk for mortality and morbidity. Early recognition of these injuries is essential to prevent disastrous outcomes.

REFERENCES

1. Lee, Feiber. Gray's anatomy. New York. 20th edition. Philadelphia; New York: BARTLEBY.COM; 1918 and 2000. p. 171–85.
2. Smith W, Williams A, Agudelo J, et al. Early predictors of mortality in hemodynamically unstable pelvis fractures. J Orthop Trauma 2007;21:31–7.
3. Papadopoulos IN, Kanakaris N, Bonovas S, et al. Auditing 655 fatalities with pelvic fractures by autopsy as a basis to evaluate trauma care. J Am Coll Surg 2006;203:30–43.
4. Gillihand M, Ward R, Borons RM, et al. Factors affecting mortality in pelvic fractures. J Trauma 1982;22:691.
5. Lunsjo K, Tadros A, Hauggaard A, et al. Associated injuries and not fracture stability predict mortality in pelvic fractures: a prospective study of 100 patients. J Trauma 2007;62(3):687–91.

6. Raby N, Berman L, de Lacey G. Accident & emergency radiology—a survival guide. London (England): WB Saunders (Harcourt Publishers Ltd -Eight Printing); 1999. p. 136.
7. Schwartz D, Reisdorff E. Emergency radiology. McGraw-Hill; 2000. Table 12.2:246.
8. Demetriades D, Karaiskakis M, Toutouzas K, et al. Pelvic fractures epidemiology and predictors of associated abdominal injuries and outcomes. J Am Coll Surg 2002;195:1–10.
9. Rice P, Melissa R. Pelvic fractures. Emerg Med Clin North Am 2007;25:795–802.
10. Durkin A, Sagi HC, Durham R, et al. Contemporary management of pelvic fractures. Am J Surg 2006;192:211–23.
11. Pennal GF, Tile M, Waddell JP, et al. Pelvic disruption: assessment and classification. Clin Orthop Relat Res 1980;151:12–21.
12. Hak D, Smith W, Takashi T. Management of hemorrhage in life-threatening pelvic fracture. J Am Acad Orthop Surg 2009;17:447–57.
13. Dalal SA, Burgess AR, Siegel JH, et al. Pelvic fracture in multiple trauma: classification by mechanism is key to pattern of organ injury, resuscitative requirements, and outcome. J Trauma 1989;29:981–1002.
14. Cedars-Sinai Orthopaedic Centre. Pelvic fractures. Available at: www.csmc.edu/6905.html. Accessed February 10, 2010.
15. Dente CJ, Felicious DV, Rozycki GS, et al. The outcome of open pelvic fractures in the modern era. Am J Surg 2005;190:830.
16. Grotz MR, Allami MK, Harwood P, et al. Open pelvic fractures: epidemiology, current concepts of management and outcome. Injury 2005;36:1.
17. O'Brien DP, Luchetle FA, Pereira SJ, et al. Pelvic fracture in the elderly is associated with increased mortality. Surgery 2002;132:710–4.
18. Kimberly BJ, Velmahos GC, Chan LS, et al. Angiographic embolization for pelvic fractures in older patients. Arch Surg 2004;139:728–32.
19. Giannoudis PV, Grotz MR, Tzioups C, et al. Prevalence of pelvic fractures, associated injuries, and mortality: the United Kingdom perspective. J Trauma 2007;63(4):857–83.
20. Cayten CG, Berendt BM, Byrne DW, et al. Efficacy of pneumatic antishock garments in severely hypotensive trauma patients. J Trauma 1993;34:728–35.
21. Brotman S, Soderstrom CA, Oster-Granite, et al. Management of severe bleeding in fractures of the pelvis. Surg Gynecol Obstet 1981;153:823–6.
22. Routt ML Jr, Falicov A, Woodhouse E, et al. Circumferential pelvic antishock sheeting: a temporary resuscitation aid. J Orthop Trauma 2002;16:45–8.
23. Bottlang M, Krieg JC, Mohr M, et al. Emergent management of pelvic ring fractures with use of circumferential compression. J Bone Joint Surg Am 2002;84(Suppl):43–7.
24. Croce MA, Menotti LJ, Savage SA, et al. Emergent pelvic fixation in patients with exsanguinating pelvic fractures. J Am Coll Surg 2007;204:935–42.
25. Pohlemann T, Bosch U, Gansslen A, et al. The Hanover experience in management of pelvic fractures. Clin Orthop Relat Res 1994;305:69–80.
26. Biffl WL, Smith WR, Moore EE, et al. Evolution of a multidisciplinary clinical pathway for the management of unstable patients with pelvic fractures. Ann Surg 2001;33:843–50.
27. Fu C, Wu S, Chen RJ, et al. Evaluation of pelvic fracture stability and the need for angioembolization: pelvic instabilities on plain film have an increased probability of requiring angioembolization. Am J Emerg Med 2009;27:792–6.
28. ATLS American College of Surgeons. Advanced trauma life support for doctors. 8th edition. Chicago: American College of Surgeons; 2008.

29. Boffard KD, Riou B, Warren B, et al. Recombinant factor V11 a as adjunctive therapy for bleeding control in severely injured trauma patients: two parallel randomized, placebo-controlled, double-blind clinical trials. J Trauma 2005;59:8–18.

30. Shlamovitz GZ, Mower WR, Bergman J, et al. Poor test characteristics for the digital rectal examination in trauma patients. Ann Emerg Med 2007;50(1):25–33.

31. Shlamovitz GZ, Mower WR, Bergman J, et al. How (un)useful is the pelvic ring stability examination in diagnosing mechanically unstable pelvic fractures in blunt trauma patients? J Trauma 2009;66(3):815–20.

32. Lunsjo K, Tadros A, Hauggard A, et al. Acute plain anteroposterior radiograph of the pelvis is not useful in detecting fractures of iliac wing and os sacrum: a prospective study of 73 patients using CT as a gold standard. Australas Radiol 2007;51(2):147–9.

33. Oboid AK, Barleben A, Porral D, et al. Utility of plain film radiographs in blunt trauma patients in the emergency department. Am Surg 2006;72(10):951–4.

34. Blackmore C, Jurkovich G, Linnau K, et al. Assessment of volume of hemorrhage and outcome from pelvic fracture. Arch Surg 2003;138:504–8.

35. Cerva DS, Mirvis SE, Shanmuganathan K, et al. Detection of bleeding in patients with major pelvic fractures: Value of contrast-enhanced CT. AJR Am J Roentgenol 1996;166:131–5.

36. Available at: http://www.trauma.org/archive/radiology/FASTintro.html. Accessed March 3, 2010.

37. Terry Conale S, American Academy of Orthopaedic Surgeon. Available at: www.aaos.org/news/aaosnow/Jul09. Accessed March 3, 2010.

38. Ganz R, Krushell RJ, Jacob RP, et al. The antishock pelvic clamp. Clin Orthop Relat Res 1991;267(20):47–51.

39. Cothren CC, Osborn PM, Moore EE, et al. Preperitoneal pelvic, packing for hemodynamic unstable pelvic fractures: a paradigm shift. J Trauma 2007;62(4):843–52.

40. Totterman A, Madsen J, Skaga N, et al. Extraperitoneal pelvic packing: a salvage procedure to control massive pelvic hemorrhage. J Trauma 2007;62(4):843–52.

41. Balogh Z, Caldwell E, Heetveld M, et al. Institutional practice guidelines on management of pelvic fracture-related hemodynamic instability: do they make a difference? J Trauma 2005;58:778–82.

42. Agolini SF, Shah K, Jaffe J, et al. Arterial embolization is a rapid and effective technique for controlling pelvic fracture hemorrhage. J Trauma 1997;43:395–9.

43. Allen C, Goslar P, Barry M, et al. Management guidelines for hypotensive pelvic fracture patients [abstract]. Am Surg 2000;66:735–8.

44. Zuckerman JD. Hip fracture. N Engl J Med 1996;334:1519–25.

45. Cooper C, Campion G, Melton LJ III. Hip fractures in the elderly a world-wide projection. Osteoporos Int 1992;2(6):285–9.

46. Kannus P, Parkkari J, Sievanen H, et al. Epidemiology of hip fractures [abstract]. Bone 1996;18:57S–63S.

47. Centers for Disease Control and Prevention (CDC). Fatalities and injuries from falls among older adults—United States 1993-2003 and 2001–2005. MMWR Morb Mortal Wkly Rep 2006;55(45):1221–4.

48. Perron AD, Miller MD, Brady WJ. Orthopedic pitfalls in the emergency department: radiographically occult hip fractures. Am J Emerg Med 2002;20(3):234–7.

49. Goddard D, Kleerekoper M. The epidemiology of osteoporosis. Practical implications for patient care. Postgrad Med 1998;104:54–76.

50. Centers for Disease Control and Prevention. Hip fractures among older adults. Available at: http://www.cdc.gov/HomeandRecreationalSafety/Falls/adulthipfx.html. Accessed December 12, 2009.

51. Brunner MD, Lance C, Eshilian-Oates L. Hip fractures in adults. Am Fam Physician 2003;67(3):537–42.
52. Rudman N, McIlmail D. Emergency department evaluation and treatment of hip and thigh injuries. Emerg Med Clin North Am 2000;18(1):29–67.
53. Abrahams P, Craven J, Lumley J. Illustrated clinical anatomy. New York: Oxford University Press; 2005.
54. Kyle RF. Fractures of the proximal part of the femur. J Bone Joint Surg Am 1994; 76:924–50.
55. Fassler PR, Swiontkowski MF, Kilroy AW, et al. Injury of the sciatic nerve associated with acetabular fracture. J Bone Joint Surg Am 1993;75:1157–66.
56. Williams-Johnson JA, Wilks RJ, McDonald AH. Falls: a modifiable risk factor for the occurrence of hip fractures in the elderly. West Indian Med J 2004;53(4): 238–41.
57. Centers for Disease Control and Prevention (CDC). Self-reported falls and fall-related injuries among persons aged $\geq$65 years-United States, 2006. MMWR Morb Mortality Wkly Rep 2008;57:225.
58. Rubenstein LZ, Josephson KR, Robbins AS. Falls in the nursing home. Ann Intern Med 1994;121(6):442–51.
59. Hossain M, Barwick C, Sinha AK, et al. Is magnetic resonance imaging (MRI) necessary to exclude occult hip fracture? Injury 2007;38(10):1204–8.
60. Cannon J, Silvestrsi S, Munro M. Imaging choices in occult hip fractures. J Emerg Med 2009;32(3):144–52.
61. Lubosky O, Liebergall M, Mattan Y, et al. Early diagnosis of occult hip fractures MRI versus CT scan. Injury 2005;36(6):788–92.
62. Oka M, Monu JU. Prevalence and patterns of occult hip fractures and mimics revealed by MRI. AJR Am J Roentgenol 2004;182:283–8.
63. Milinek EJ, Clark KC, Walker CW. Limited magnetic resonance imaging (MRI) in the diagnosis of occult hip fractures. Am J Emerg Med 1998;16:390–2.
64. Haramati N, Staron RB, Barax C, et al. Magnetic resonance imaging of occult hip fracture of the proximal femur. Skeletal Radiol 1994;23:19–22.
65. Martin B. Regional nerve block in fractured neck of the femur. Best evidence topic reports. Available at: http://www.emjonline. Accessed November 22, 2009.
66. Pallia CS, Scott RE, Chao DJ. Traumatic hip dislocation in athletes. Curr Sports Med Rep 2002;1:338–45.
67. Plancher KD, Donshik JD. Femoral neck and ipsilateral shaft fractures in the young adult. Orthop Clin North Am 1997;28:447–59.
68. Droll KP, Broekhuyse H, O'Brien P. Fracture of the femoral head [abstract]. J Am Acad Orthop Surg 2007;15(12):716–27.
69. Newton EJ, Love J. Emergency department management of selected orthopedic injuries. Emerg Med Clin North Am 2007;25:763–93.
70. DeLee JC, Evans JA, Thomas J. Anterior dislocation of the hip and associated femoral head fractures [abstract]. J Bone Joint Surg Am 1980;62:960–4.

Knee and Leg Injuries

Moira Davenport, MD[a,b]

KEYWORDS

• Knee • Leg • Neurovascular deficit • Injury

The knee plays a significant role in ambulation and the activities of daily living. During the course of these activities and its role in weight bearing, the knee is susceptible to a variety of different forces. Incidence varies greatly based on activity, but recent data report 1147.1 nonsurgical knee injuries per 100,000 people, 36.9 anterior cruciate ligament (ACL) tears per 100,000 people, and 9.1 other ligamentous injuries per 100,000 people.[1] The emergency physician should be familiar with the diagnosis and treatment of injuries resulting from these forces.

A thorough neurovascular examination should be performed upon the patient's arrival in the emergency department (ED). The detection of any neurovascular deficit is an indication for immediate reduction of a deformity in an attempt to restore normal blood flow to the injured extremity. Findings of normal neurovascular parameters should allow for a more complete evaluation before imaging studies are performed. Analgesics may be required in both cases to allow the initial examination and should be given as soon as is practical. If possible, radiographs should be performed without immobilization devices in place; however, this may not always be feasible.

KNEE ANATOMY

The knee is a hinged joint with a range of motion from 0° extension to 165° flexion and is formed by the articulation of the distal femur, proximal tibia, and the patella. Four ligaments provide most of the joint stability. The ACL and posterior cruciate ligament (PCL) prevent anterior and posterior translation of the tibia on the femur while the medial collateral ligament (MCL) and lateral collateral ligament (LCL) resist varus and valgus deformations. In recent years, a significant amount of attention has been paid to the posterolateral corner (PLC) of the knee and its role in knee stability, particularly in the varus and rotatory planes.[2,3] The anatomy of this region is complex and is

Financial Disclosures: None.
[a] Department of Emergency Medicine, Allegheny General Hospital, Drexel University College of Medicine, 320 EN Avenue, Pittsburgh, PA 15212, USA
[b] Department of Orthopedic Surgery, Allegheny General Hospital, Drexel University College of Medicine, 320 EN Avenue, Pittsburgh, PA 15212, USA
E-mail address: mdavenport72@yahoo.com

Emerg Med Clin N Am 28 (2010) 861–884
doi:10.1016/j.emc.2010.07.001
0733-8627/10/$ – see front matter © 2010 Elsevier Inc. All rights reserved.

formed by 3 tissue layers: the deep, middle and superficial layers. The deep layer contributes the most to joint stability and is composed of the popliteus muscle, the popliteofibular ligament, the LCL, the arcuate ligament, and the fabellofibular ligament (**Fig. 1**).[4–6] Isolated PLC injuries are rare; these injuries are commonly seen in conjunction with ACL and/or PCL tears.[7]

Bony injuries are described in relation to 3 distinct compartments: the medial, lateral, and patellofemoral compartments. The medial femoral condyle's articulation with the medial tibial plateau forms the medial compartment, whereas the junction of the lateral femoral condyle with the lateral tibia forms the lateral compartment. The patella is formed by the unification of several secondary centers of ossification. It sits in the midsubstance of the quadriceps and patellar tendons. The medial and lateral retinaculum and the medial patellofemoral ligament maintain patellar stability.

The tibiofemoral joint is further stabilized by the menisci; C-shaped cartilaginous rings that sit in the joint space. Each knee has a medial and lateral meniscus; in addition to their role in joint stability, these structures also contribute to shock absorption and load transfer, particularly during the gait cycle.

The popliteal artery and tibial nerve run through the popliteal fossa at the posterior aspect of the knee. These neurovascular structures are held close to the femur by the adductor magnus muscle. It is particularly important to consider this anatomic restraint during trauma because it predisposes the neurovascular bundle to injury, with disruption being the most potentially devastating consequence. The common peroneal nerve wraps around the proximal fibula and can be disrupted or damaged with injuries to the lateral aspect of the knee. This anatomic relationship further highlights the need for a complete distal neurovascular examination because chronic abnormality to this nerve can have significant morbidity (ie, foot drop).

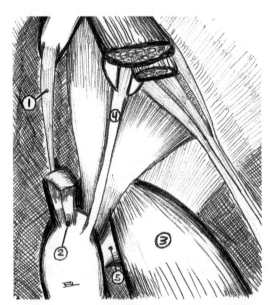

Fig. 1. Posterolateral complex. 1, LCL; 2, biceps femoris ligament; 3, popliteus muscle; 4, fabellofibular ligament; 5, popliteofibular ligament. (*Courtesy of* Benjamin Lawner, DO, University of Maryland School of Medicine, Baltimore, MD.)

Initial Evaluation

History

Individuals who have sustained knee trauma can present with a wide variety of signs and symptoms. Effusion, loss of motion, joint pain, and an inability to ambulate are all possible presentations.[8-10] Patients who have sustained significant knee injuries may present with an apparently normal appearing knee, highlighting the need for an injury-specific history. Key historical factors include the position of the extremity (particularly the knee) at the time of injury, the mechanism of injury, and the direction from which any force was applied. One should also note whether the patient has been able to ambulate since the injury and whether the knee has felt stable while attempting to ambulate. One should determine whether there is a prior history of knee injuries or surgery, and what the patient's baseline level of function is.

Physical examination

A thorough knee examination should be performed as soon as possible after injury. Again, the patient's need for analgesics should be addressed before performing the assessment. The general appearance of the knee should be noted, including the presence of any obvious deformity, effusion, erythema, ecchymosis, abrasions, and lacerations. Effusions typically are seen with intra-articular injuries including fractures and ACL tears (**Table 1**).[8-10] Palpation of all the major joint structures, including the medial and lateral joint lines, quadriceps and patellar tendons, the patella, tibial tubercule, and the MCL and LCL should be performed. Range of motion should be tested; if active motion is limited, passive motion should be assessed as well. Patellar motion within the trochlear groove should also be assessed. The patella should move in a relatively straight vertical line. Patients with patellar instability (either as a result of trauma or secondary to weak quadriceps muscles) have patellae that move laterally and then vertically in a hockey stick–like pattern. Patellar instability can also be assessed via the apprehension test by extending the knee and applying a varus force to the patella. Quadriceps tightening in an attempt to prevent dislocation is considered a positive sign, although the sensitivity and specificity of this maneuver have not been clearly elucidated.[11]

Ligamentous stability should then be assessed. Emergency physicians are typically not successful at diagnosing ACL tears via physical examination.[12] This is likely because of a lack of familiarity with examination techniques; more attention should be paid to proper examination techniques and historical details. The Lachman test examines ACL stability. The injured knee should be placed in 20° to 30° of flexion; the examiner then tries to move the tibia anterior relative to the femur.[13] The anterior drawer test can also assess ACL stability. The anterior drawer is performed similarly to the Lachman with the exception that the knee is flexed to 90°. However, with the knee at 90°, the MCL and the medial meniscus contribute to stability, making Lachman the

Table 1	
Conditions resulting in knee effusions	
Early Effusion	**Delayed Effusion**
ACL tear	Meniscal tear
Tibial plateau fracture	Cartilaginous loose bodies
PCL tear	
Femoral condyle fracture	
Patellar fracture	

more sensitive examination maneuver.[14] Lachman has a sensitivity of 85% and specificity of 94%; values for the anterior drawer are significantly lower.[15] Furthermore, the likelihood ratio of a positive Lachman indicating an ACL tear is 25 versus 3.8 for the anterior drawer.[16] The PCL is assessed via the posterior drawer test. The knee is situated as in the anterior drawer but the force applied to the tibia is directed posteriorly. MCL and LCL stability should be assessed by the application of valgus and varus forces to the knee. The tests should be performed with the knee fully extended and again with the knee 30° flexed. It is imperative to assess the 2 positions of the knee because the ACL and PCL contribute to stability when the knee is fully extended. The slightly flexed positioning effectively isolates the collateral ligaments. Laxity on any of these maneuvers may be absolute (no definitive end point detected) or relative (increased motion relative to the uninjured knee).[17,18]

The PLC of the knee is evaluated using the external recurvatum maneuver.[19] The patient should be supine on the stretcher with both legs extended. The examiner lifts the extended leg (holding the toes) and should ensure that normal knee alignment is maintained. The presence of a varus deformity (bow leg appearance) indicates a PLC disruption. A posterolateral drawer can also be performed. The patient is initially positioned as in the posterior drawer test and the foot is then externally rotated to 15°. A posterolaterally directed force is then applied to the tibia, and laxity suggests a PLC injury combined with another ligamentous injury. The maneuver should then be repeated with the knee flexed 30°; laxity in this position indicates an isolated PLC disruption. Discovery of 2 lax ligaments should raise examiner suspicion of knee dislocation and should prompt a focused neurovascular examination.

The McMurray test should be performed to assess for possible meniscal injury. The patient should be supine on the stretcher, thus allowing the examiner to lift the affected extremity and flex the knee to 90°. The examiner should have his/her thumb on either the medial or lateral joint line and the remaining fingers on the other joint line while the other hand holds the patient's lower leg. As the examiner extends and rotates the knee, a varus force is applied, effectively closing the medial joint line. As the leg is extended, the examiner is attempting to feel a clunk as the suspected meniscal fragment is extruded from the tibiofemoral joint space. The maneuver should then be applied using a valgus force to evaluate the lateral meniscus. The sensitivity and specificity of the McMurray test are 35.7% and 85.7% for detecting medial meniscus injuries and 22.2% and 100% for lateral meniscal defects.[14] However, sensitivity for both meniscal injuries decreases further with a concurrent ACL tear.[14] McMurray sensitivity also increases with the presence of joint line tenderness.[16,20] The Thessaly test has recently been developed to evaluate possible meniscal injuries. The patient stands facing the examiner, flexes the knee 20°, then internally and externally rotates the affected leg 3 times. Recreation of joint line symptoms is considered a positive test. This maneuver has a reported sensitivity of 90%, specificity of 97%, and statistical correlation with operative findings.[21] Combining the Thessaly test with McMurray also increases diagnostic sensitivity.[20]

Imaging
Although standard radiographs do not show soft tissue structures, they should be performed to evaluate for significant fractures, avulsion fractures, and effusions. Lateral, anteroposterior (AP), and sunrise views of the patella should be performed. Particular attention should be paid to the lateral view. The position of the knee should be noted; 20° to 30° of flexion is expected in a true lateral while the knee is fully extended in the cross-table lateral view. If possible, weight-bearing AP views should also be obtained to allow adequate assessment of the joint spaces. Stress radiographs (using

a commercially available device) at 30° and 80° flexion may be considered in cases of suspected PCL injury.[22,23] Oblique views should be obtained if there is suspicion for a tibial plateau fracture. However, computed tomography (CT) scan provides better bony detail, particularly for fractures with minimal to moderate depression.

The Segond fracture is a capsular avulsion of the lateral tibial plateau (**Fig. 2**). Although this injury is rare, it was considered pathognomic for ACL disruptions.[24–27] However, this fracture pattern is being seen with increasing frequency with PLC disruptions.[28]

The Pellegrini-Stieda lesion is defined as calcification of the MCL on plain radiographs (**Fig. 3**) and is classically attributed to previous MCL derangement.[29] However, recent magnetic resonance imaging (MRI) studies suggest that this lesion may also be present with PCL disruption. The forces that damage the MCL are believed to also avulse portions of the femoral periosteum, including the PCL footprint.[30–32]

Ultrasound has long been used to diagnose musculoskeletal injuries in Europe, and the practice is gaining popularity in North America. This modality has significant advantages compared with MRI, particularly in the ED setting. The dynamic nature of ultrasound imaging allows the affected joint to be examined in the position of maximal patient discomfort, thus increasing the applicability of the study. The significantly lower cost of ultrasound versus MRI also allows for real-time imaging of the contralateral joint, providing valuable information about patient-specific anatomy. Ultrasound also can correct for geometric averaging seen in MRI, thus allowing a more complete examination of the affected structures. Lastly, ultrasound is more readily available in most EDs than is MRI, and thus should be considered as an adjunct to the clinical examination and routine radiographic studies.[33–36]

Musculoskeletal ultrasound is most commonly and easily performed with a high-frequency linear transducer. With minimal training, physicians can successfully use the amount of tibial translation to diagnose ACL tears.[37] PCL thickness can easily be assessed in the longitudinal plane and has been shown to have excellent inter-rater reliability and reproducibility after minimal training.[38] Ultrasound has also been used to diagnose PCL injuries in children.[39] The anatomy of the PLC also lends itself to

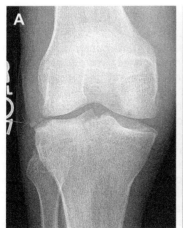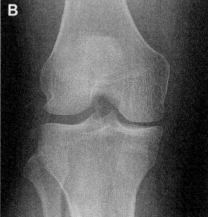

Fig. 2. (*A, B*) AP radiographs showing Segond fractures (note the small avulsed fragment at the lateral tibial plateau). (*Courtesy of* Michael Bond, MD, University of Maryland, College Park, MD.)

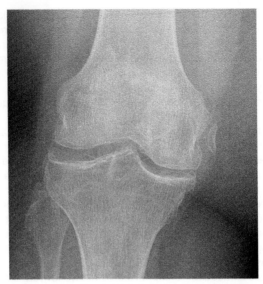

Fig. 3. AP radiograph showing Pellegrini-Stieda lesion (note the large calcification in the MCL distribution). (*Courtesy of* Michael Bond, MD, University of Maryland, College Park, MD.)

ultrasound evaluation and correlates well with MRI.[40] Protocols are also being developed to incorporate ultrasound in the diagnosis of meniscal injuries.[41,42]

Despite the technological advances mentioned earlier, MRI still remains the preferred imaging modality among orthopedic surgeons. The anatomic detail obtained from MRI allows for operative planning. However, it is important to remember that MRI is not 100% sensitive or specific. Meniscal injuries can be particularly difficult to diagnose on MRI.[43,44] When reviewing MRI reports, it is imperative to consider the radiologist's experience as well as the strength of the magnet used because both variables have been shown to have wide inter-rater reliability.[45]

ACL Injuries

Sports participation accounts for most ACL tears.[1,46] Both contact and noncontact tears are common, and the rate of tears is reaching epidemic numbers in some sports.[47–50] The typical mechanism of injury is often a valgus force applied to an extended knee; rotation is commonly involved as well. However, the specific subset of snowboarders typically tear the ACL by a flat landing on a flexed knee with moderate-severe compression.[51] Regardless of the mechanism, patients often hear or feel a pop as the ACL tears. The patient can often ambulate immediately after the disruption; however, this typically becomes more difficult as the resultant effusion develops and enlarges. Moderate effusions are commonly seen within 2 to 3 hours of injury. Routine knee radiographs should be performed to detect the presence of a Segond fracture, although MRI is the diagnostic imaging test of choice for suspected ACL tears.[52] If an MRI is performed, it is important to differentiate between native and reconstructed ACLs because the signs of tears vary between them.[53] It is also imperative that the evaluating physician considers the likelihood of concomitant ligamentous and meniscal injuries. A recent retrospective study showed that an acute ACL tear complicated the diagnosis of lateral meniscal tears, particularly tears of the posterolateral horn.[44] The physical examination finding of joint line tenderness, often believed to heighten suspicion for meniscal tears, is not reliable in patients with concurrent ACL tears.[54] Patients with isolated ACL tears may be safely discharged from the ED in a hinged knee brace (fully unlocked) and crutches. However, early orthopedic referral is needed to ensure the initiation of physical therapy that can maximize preoperative range of motion, particularly extension.

Several ACL reconstruction techniques are commonly used. It is helpful for the emergency physician to be familiar with these techniques, particularly when evaluating acute and chronic postoperative patients, because the complications seen with each vary. Cadaveric grafts typically use the Achilles tendon to reconstruct the torn ligament, whereas autografts are typically taken from the hamstring tendon or the patellar tendon. Currently, patellar tendon grafts are the most commonly performed, but there is no consensus.[55–58] Difficulty kneeling, patellar fracture, and patellar tendon rupture are seen after patellar tendon grafts, whereas hamstring weakness and a slower return to regular activity are seen with hamstring tendon grafts.[59] All may be concerns of postoperative patients presenting to the ED. Postoperative infection is also common, with septic arthritis and tuberculosis being reported.[60–62]

Age more than 50 years was previously considered a relative contraindication to ACL reconstruction, but the increasing activity level of the baby boomers has seen this theory lose validity.[63] Timing of ACL reconstruction in children has also been controversial. Treatment options include delayed reconstruction until skeletal maturity has been achieved or reconstruction as the child is still growing. Current recommendations favor immediate reconstruction, because the rate of postinjury meniscal tears is significantly lower with early intervention.[64,65]

Failure to surgically reestablish knee anatomy after ACL tear can alter the structure of the collateral ligaments, further altering knee mechanics and predisposing the patient to MCL and LCL injuries.[66] Delays in reconstruction can lead to meniscal tears, further contributing to knee instability and premature arthritic changes.[67,68] ACL reconstruction, and particularly the lack of reconstruction, can significantly accelerate the development of knee osteoarthritis.[69] However, it the precise degree to which lack of reconstruction accelerates the progression of osteoarthritis remains to be determined. A recent meta-analysis concluded that previous estimates of postoperative osteoarthritis have overestimated the incidence of disease.[70] Postoperative osteoarthritis may be partially caused by chronic quadriceps weakness, thus the role of physical therapy and return to activity should be reinforced in the ED.[71] Concurrent ACL reconstruction with menisectomy has been shown to result in greater arthritic changes than reconstruction alone.[72] This finding is augmented by a retrospective study showing that up to 61% of medial, and 74% of lateral, meniscal tears healed spontaneously during recovery from ACL reconstruction, raising the question of whether menisectomy should be performed at the time of ACL reconstruction.[73] A meta-analysis furthers the recommendation to avoid menisectomy at the time of ACL reconstruction.[74] A review of knee injuries among National Football League players showed that menisectomy shortens the career (games played, games started, and years in the league) significantly more than ACL reconstruction. The combination of menisectomy with ACL reconstruction shortened all 3 playing parameters more than either procedure in isolation.[75]

As more emergency physicians also practice sports medicine, it is prudent to discuss the possibility of preventing ACL tears. A retrospective study by Rishiraj and colleagues[76] determined that bracing the previously reconstructed knee is helpful in preventing recurrent injuries but there seems to be no benefit to the native knee.

Some investigators advocate jump training, quadriceps/hamstring strengthening, and core strengthening programs as means to prevent ACL tears, particularly noncontact injuries.[77–84]

PCL Injuries

Isolated PCL disruptions are rare, accounting for approximately 7% of all athletic-related knee injuries.[85] Half of these injuries were associated with other ligamentous insults.[85] The most common mechanism for this injury is a posteriorly directed force applied to a flexed knee, either through contact with the dashboard during a motor vehicle crash or through contact with the ground during a fall. Effusions are rare because the PCL is extraarticular.[86] If an effusion is present, this should heighten suspicion for concomitant ligamentous injury and/or knee dislocation. Patients with isolated PCL tears can also be discharged from the ED in a hinged knee brace (fully unlocked) with orthopedic follow-up. Those with suspected multiple ligamentous injuries may require immediate orthopedic consultation, particularly if dislocation or PLC injury is suspected.

Treatment of isolated PCL tears was previously nonoperative but there has been a recent movement toward operative intervention for these cases.[87–90] A variety of graft options are available including patellar tendon, quadriceps tendon, Achilles tendon, and tibial tendon. Both autograft and allografts are commonly used. Similar postoperative complications are seen with these grafts as are found with ACL reconstruction. Chronic PCL deficiency also contributes more significantly than was previously believed to the development of premature osteoarthritis, particularly in the medial compartment.[91] The chronically torn PCL also places increasing stress and stretch on the PLC, further increasing the risk of disruption of this complex as well.[92] Caution must be used when evaluating studies of PCL injury outcome, because a wide range of methods and evaluation scales were used.[93]

PLC Injuries

Patients with suspected PLC (see **Fig. 3**) disruptions merit orthopedic consultation before discharge from the ED. The presence of concomitant ligamentous injuries should not delay orthopedic evaluation because staged surgical interventions are the standard of care when the PLC is disrupted. Recent studies have demonstrated significantly reduced morbidity and higher functioning when repair or reconstruction of the PLC is performed within 10 to 14 days of injury.[94,95] Delayed operative attempts are complicated by tissue degeneration and scarring, making proper identification of structures difficult. Failure to address PLC injuries and the instability that results is the most common cause of postoperative ACL failure.[96,97] Despite a multitude of techniques, there seems to be difficulty in fully restoring PCL integrity in the PCL-PLC–deficient knee.[98] Furthermore, the decision to proceed with repair versus reconstruction is still controversial but, from small studies, it seems that reconstruction has significantly better postoperative stability and improved motion.[99] Further debate is ongoing regarding the optimal reconstruction technique.[88,100–102]

Patients with PLC disruptions are also at risk for peroneal nerve injury.[103] It is imperative that a thorough distal neurovascular examination be performed to rule out this complication. Patients with fibular head avulsions or biceps femoris avulsion were at particularly high risk for peroneal nerve involvement.[103]

LCL Injuries

Isolated LCL injuries are uncommon because of the anatomic position of the ligament in the PLC of the knee.[104] As with injuries to the PLC, these injuries typically result from a varus force applied to the knee regardless of the position of the knee. Both high-and low-energy mechanisms have been reported to cause LCL injuries, with activities as seemingly benign as yoga causing LCL disruptions.[105] Osteoarthrosis has also been linked to increased risk of LCL abnormalities.[106] Examination maneuvers should include thorough assessment of the PLC as well as isolated examination of the LCL. Varus stress radiographs can be used to further enhance the initial evaluation. Laxity greater than 2.7 mm should heighten suspicion for isolated LCL damage, whereas greater than 4 mm is considered to indicate a PLC injury.[107] If an isolated LCL injury is present, patients may be safely discharged with crutches and a hinged knee brace in the fully unlocked position. Orthopedic follow-up should be within 2 to 3 days of injury to ensure timely definitive imaging. Management of the isolated LCL injury remains controversial, with some investigators advocating operative reconstruction using the semitendinosis tendon as a donor graft, and others advocating conservative management.[108] Bushnell and colleagues[104] recently showed that nonoperative management led to a faster return to activity, including a return to an elite level of competition.

MCL Injuries

The MCL is the most commonly injured of the 4 major knee ligaments.[109] Injuries to the MCL typically result from a valgus force applied to the knee, again with the knee either flexed or extended. Unlike injuries to the other major knee ligaments, a spectrum of MCL injuries is possible. Injuries progress from a simple stretch (grade I) to partial tear (grade II) and complete tear (grade III). Grade I and II injuries typically present with laxity relative to the uninjured knee, whereas a grade III injury lacks a firm endpoint during stress testing. In addition to joint laxity, the patient is typically tender over the site of the injury; ecchymosis is common as well. The MCL is extraarticular, thus effusions are rare.

Treatment of MCL injuries, particularly grade I and II injuries, is nonoperative. These patients may also be safely discharged in a hinged knee brace (fully unlocked to allow functional weight bearing as tolerated) and crutches, with orthopedic follow-up.[109] It is imperative that the patient not be sent home with a straight-leg knee immobilizer because this can hinder recovery.[110] The need for rapid referral to physical therapy should be stressed to patients on discharge from the ED. Early mobility exercises and therapeutic ultrasound can significantly accelerate recovery.[111] Management of grade III injuries is slightly more controversial. These injuries were historically treated operatively. Barring the presence of a large associated avulsion fracture, it is now recommended that individuals with grade III tears undergo a trial of nonoperative management.[109,112–114] As with other ligamentous disruptions, a variety of operative techniques may be performed, including primary repair, allografts, and autografts (semitendinous and gracilis tendon harvests).[109]

MCL reconstruction in the concomitantly ACL-deficient knee is not recommended. Multiple studies have shown no difference in overall knee stability when ACL reconstruction has been performed while allowing the MCL to heal nonoperatively.[112–114] The 6- to 8-week delay from time of injury to ACL reconstruction provides adequate time for MCL healing.[113] This finding also highlights the need for immediate physical therapy while awaiting definitive operative intervention. Operative management of MCL injuries with concurrent ACL and PCL injuries is not recommended, although the lower incidence of this injury results in fewer data to fully evaluate outcomes.[112]

One exception to the operative intervention of MCL injuries exists; the patient with Pellegrini-Stieda syndrome. Given the amount of calcification usually seen with this diagnosis, surgical excision of the abnormal growth is often required.[115]

Meniscal Injuries

Meniscal injuries are different from ligamentous disruptions. Because of their anatomic location and their role in shock absorption, the menisci are subjected to significantly more breakdown through normal activities than are the other structures of the knee. Degenerative tears are almost as common as traumatic injuries. An MRI study of asymptomatic patients more than 50 years of age showed rates of meniscal tears ranging from 19% among 50 to 59 year olds and 56% among those more than 70 years old.[116] Patients with meniscal abnormalities typically present with generalized knee pain localizing to either the medial or lateral joint lines. However, joint line tenderness (or lack thereof) is not a reliable finding in patients with chronic ACL deficiency.[54] Effusions may be seen but usually do not develop until at least 4 to 6 hours from the time of the tear. Patients may notice a clicking sensation when walking, as the meniscal fragments slide between the tibia and the femur. Similarly, locking of the knee joint is possible if the fragment does not disengage from between the 2 bones. Neither of these findings is definite because the location and the size of the tear affects the likelihood of developing these abnormalities. The presence of an acute meniscal injury should raise concern for the possibility of a concurrent tibial plateau fracture. This relationship has been highlighted with the increased use of MRI.[117]

Patients with isolated meniscal injuries may be safely discharged from the ED with crutches or a cane as needed. Hinged knee braces may also be used; however, knee immobilization is not indicated.[118] Outpatient orthopedic surgery referral is warranted. Treatment can be conservative (physical therapy) or operative (arthroscopic excision of the fragment). A small percentage of meniscal tears can be repaired, but this is dependant on the anatomic location of the tear. It was initially believed that arthroscopy accelerated the development of knee osteoarthrosis more than conservative therapy. A recent study shows that nonoperatively managed meniscal tears also increase the rate of osteoarthrosis relative to the intact meniscus.[119]

Meniscal abnormalities are often seen in children, with tears and discoid menisci being the most common.[120] In cases of discoid meniscus, the meniscus is typically larger than normal with a more oval morphology compared with the normal C-shaped morphology. Children with discoid menisci can note pain and snapping with ambulation. They may also present with tears because the morphologic changes result in more instability than is seen in the typical meniscus and thus predispose the patient to injury. Pediatric menisci have increased vascularity relative to the adult structure and are thus more amenable to surgical repair rather than excision.[120]

Knee Dislocation

Knee dislocation results from disruption of at least 3 of the 4 major ligaments of the knee. This is one of the true orthopedic emergencies. Two mechanisms of injury are possible; high-velocity trauma and apparently minor trauma in obese patients.[121] A recent study suggested that the low-velocity mechanism may be more common than higher forces.[122] Two classification schemes are commonly encountered in clinical practice. The first describes the final position of the tibia relative to the femur; anterior, posterior, medial, lateral, and rotary dislocations are possible. A newer classification system describing the dislocation according to the resulting ligamentous disruptions has recently been gaining favor.[123]

Patients sustaining knee dislocations present in 2 distinctively different fashions. Given the amount of force required to disrupt most ligaments, the joint capsule is frequently disrupted as well. This prohibits formation of an effusion and often results in spontaneous reduction of the dislocation, thus masking the severity of the injury.[123] If the joint capsule integrity has been maintained, significant deformity is likely on presentation. Ecchymosis may be noted with both presentations. The ED physician must maintain a high index of suspicion for knee dislocation if significant laxity is present because of the need to ensure the integrity of the popliteal artery and the tibial nerve.[124]

If the dislocated knee has not spontaneously reduced, reduction should be performed as quickly as possible. Before performing the reduction, the examiner should ensure that a buttonhole deformity is not present. Simple inspection and an inability to passively range the knee should heighten the suspicion for a buttonhole deformity. With this defect, the medial femoral condyle is embedded in the joint capsule, making closed reduction impossible. The buttonhole deformity has also been reported on MRI.[125] The typical reduction technique is to apply longitudinal traction to the tibia to dislodge the proximal tibia from its resting spot on the femur. Once the tibia is freed from the femur, a force opposite to the direction of the dislocation should be applied to restore normal leg alignment.[124] Care should be taken to ensure that any rotary component is also corrected. Once reduction is achieved, the knee should be placed in a locked hinged knee brace with slight (15°–20°) flexion. External fixators may be used as a temporizing measure in cases of extreme instability.[126,127]

Reduction should ideally be performed within 6 hours of the injury; risk of neurovascular compromise and the development of compartment syndrome increase with prolonged time of dislocation.[124,128] Neurovascular evaluations should be performed both before and after reduction. In addition to manual palpation, the ankle-brachial index (ABI) should be calculated to further evaluate the popliteal artery. Angiography was previously performed following any knee dislocation. Recent studies have shown that this invasive study should be reserved for patients with absent pulses, neurologic deficits, or abnormal ABIs. An ABI less than 0.9 has been shown to have a positive predictive value of 100% for vascular injuries requiring surgical exploration and repair.[129] Current therapeutic recommendations suggest that patients with normal vascular examinations should be admitted for at least 24 hours of observation, with neurovascular checks every 2 to 3 hours.[130] Any change in neurovascular status during the observation period is an indication for immediate angiography.[126] CT angiography has started to replace traditional angiography because the CT-based modality is more readily available than the latter study. Furthermore, Doppler studies are also gaining favor as an integral component of the neurovascular examination.[131–135]

Peroneal nerve injury is sustained with approximately 20% of knee dislocations.[136] Both sensory (deficits over the lateral aspect of the leg, dorsum of the foot, or first web space) and motor deficits (weakness of the extensor hallucis longus, anterior tibialis, and peroneal muscles, producing loss of great toe extension, foot drop, and weakness of ankle eversion, respectively) typically result. In cases of suspected peroneal nerve injury, the affected foot should be splinted in a neutral position to minimize tension on the nerve.

Staged operative intervention on the multiple ligamentous injured knee is now preferred to a single, large-scale repair.[137–139] PCL and PLC injuries are typically repaired within 10 days of the injury.[140] ACL reconstruction is commonly delayed 6 to 8 weeks from the injury, allowing any resultant effusion to resolve and allowing for reestablishment of normal range of motion.[128] The question of repair versus reconstruction discussed earlier in reference to isolated ligamentous injuries also applies to operative planning for the multiple ligamentous injured knee.[126,138]

Patellar Dislocation

Patellar dislocations typically result from a varus force applied to a flexed knee. Dislocations can also occur from the forced contraction of a flexed quadriceps. Patellar dislocation has been reported following aggressive use of the Wii, resulting in the term Wii knee.[141] The lateral patellar retinaculum is significantly stronger than its medial counterpart, making lateral dislocations the more common injury. On arrival at the ED, the knee is typically flexed, with an obvious lateral deformity; effusion and ecchymosis may also be present. Prereduction radiographs (AP, lateral, and sunrise views) are recommended to evaluate for concomitant fractures before the reduction attempt; osteochondral fractures are most commonly seen.[142,143] Sedation may be needed to achieve reduction, which is performed by extending the knee and simultaneously applying a valgus force to the dislocated patella. Once normal alignment is reestablished, the extensor mechanism should be assessed to ensure integrity of the quadriceps and patellar tendons. The extremity should then be placed in a straight-leg knee immobilizer and postreduction films should be performed. Patients with successful reductions may be discharged with the straight-leg knee immobilizer, crutches, and orthopedic follow-up.

The increased use of MRI has highlighted the higher-than-expected rate of injuries associated with patellar dislocation. Meniscal tears, MCL disruptions, and osteochondral fractures have all been significantly associated with dislocations.[144] Classic complications following patellar dislocation include persistent instability, subluxation, repeat dislocation, and accelerated osteoarthrosis. Recent prospective studies comparing operative with nonoperative therapies showed a significant reduction in the redislocation rate in the surgically treated group. However, the rate of return to baseline activity was similar between groups.[145,146] Surgical intervention is commonly recommended; however, timing of the procedure varies. Immediate repair is generally recommended in physically active patients, whereas some surgeons advocate delaying surgical intervention until after a second dislocation.[147] If operative intervention is planned, a variety of techniques may be used to reestablish the medial retinaculum and the medial patellofemoral ligament. The hamstring tendon is commonly used as donor graft.[148,149] As with other knee injuries, surgical repair is still controversial in children, with recent literature advocating intervention before closure of the physes.[150]

Patellar Fracture

Patellar fractures result from the same mechanisms as PCL injuries; fall onto a flexed knee and dashboard injury.[151] Several fracture patterns are possible (transverse, horizontal, avulsion, and stellate), resulting in a variety of presentations. Effusion and ecchymosis are common with all fracture types, but a palpable defect may or may not be detected. Although the neurovascular examination is typically benign, the key physical examination finding is the status of the extensor mechanism. Routine knee radiographs should be performed to further delineate the extent of the injury. Patients with intact extensor mechanisms can be discharged from the ED in a straight-leg knee immobilizer with crutches and orthopedic follow-up. Patients who cannot extend the leg should be seen by orthopedics immediately because internal fixation is often performed within 24 hours of the injury.[152,153]

Quadriceps and Patellar Tendon Rupture

The quadriceps and patellar tendons most commonly rupture because of trauma, particularly forced quadriceps contraction with a flexed knee. Degenerative tears and disruptions secondary to chronic medical conditions (diabetes, Lyme disease)

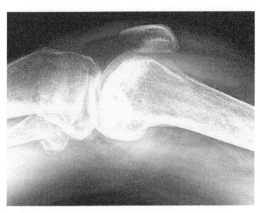

Fig. 4. Lipohemarthrosis.

are also seen but are significantly less common than traumatic mechanisms.[154] There is an age predilection for each injury because patients more than 40 years of age tend to tear the quadriceps tendon, whereas younger patients are more likely to sustain patellar tendon disruptions.[46] Patients typically present with a large knee effusion and moderate pain. Although obvious tendon defects may be appreciable, it is imperative to assess the integrity of the extensor mechanism. The position of the patella on standard lateral knee view may indicate a tendon rupture, with quadriceps tendon

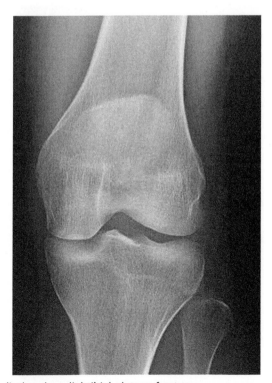

Fig. 5. Minimally displaced medial tibial plateau fracture.

rupture resulting in low-riding patellae, and patellar tendon rupture creating high-riding patellae. A minimally invasive technique to assess quadriceps tendon integrity has been proposed[155] but has yet to gain clinical support. Ultrasound has also been shown to be reliable in diagnosing quadriceps rupture.[156,157] Patellar tendon disruptions were initially believed to be an isolated injury; however, a recent study indicates that this may not be the case, thus highlighting the need for a complete knee examination.[158] Patients with tendon rupture should be placed in a straight-leg knee immobilizer and undergo orthopedic evaluation. Operative fixation within a month of injury has been shown to improve clinical outcome.[159]

Tibial Plateau Fractures

Tibial plateau fractures occur when varus or valgus forces are applied to the knee, typically when the knee is flexed. Both low- and high-velocity mechanisms are seen.[160] Lateral plateau fractures occur more frequently than medial plateau fractures; bicondylar injuries are also possible. Joint line tenderness, ecchymosis, and effusion are commonly seen with all 3 fracture patterns. Crepitance may be present with larger fractures. Initial radiographic evaluation should include the routine knee series as well as cross-table lateral and oblique views. The identification of a lipohemarthrosis (layering of fat, blood, and synovial fluid) on the cross-table lateral view strongly indicates a tibial plateau fracture (**Fig. 4**). The presence of a lipohemarthrosis can be confirmed by arthrocentesis when red blood cells and fat cells are seen on microscopic examination of the fluid.

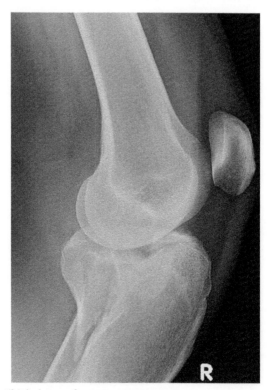

Fig. 6. Bicondylar tibial plateau fracture.

Table 2
Recommended brace and settings for selected injuries

Injury	Brace	Setting	Orthopedic Evaluation
ACL	Hinged brace	Fully unlocked	3–5 d
PCL	Hinged brace	Fully unlocked	3–5 d
MCL	Hinged brace	Fully unlocked	3–5 d
LCL (isolated)	Hinged brace	Fully unlocked	3–5 d
PLC	Hinged brace	Fully unlocked	In ED
Meniscal tear	± Hinged brace	Fully unlocked	3–5 d
Patella dislocation	Knee immobilizer		3–5 d
Patella fracture (extensor intact)	Knee immobilizer		1–3 d
Patella fracture (extensor disrupted)	Knee immobilizer		In ED
Tibial plateau fracture	Knee immobilizer		In ED
Quadriceps/patellar tendon rupture	Knee immobilizer		In ED if bilateral; otherwise 1–3 d

If plain radiographs are indeterminate and there is high clinical suspicion for tibial plateau fracture, CT with narrow window parameters (2 mm) should be performed.[161] CT may also be warranted when plateau fractures are seen on routine radiographs because it is important to determine the exact amount of fracture displacement (**Figs. 5** and **6**). As little as 2 to 3 mm of displacement requires operative therapy to reestablish the weight-bearing surface. Open and arthroscopic techniques as well as external fixators are commonly used.[162,163] Plateau fractures may occur in isolation or may be seen with compartment syndrome, in conjunction with collateral ligament injuries (typically the collateral ligament opposite the fracture), meniscal injuries, or with knee dislocation, again highlighting the need for a thorough examination of the injured knee.[117,164–166] A recent study comparing acute imaging modalities (CT and MRI) has shown that CT misses only 2% of ligamentous injuries associated with tibial plateau fractures, further enhancing the diagnostic value of the study; however, MRI is still recommended for definitive operative planning.[117,167] Given the need for operative intervention with small amounts of fracture depression, orthopedic consultation should be obtained in the ED for all patients with tibial plateau fractures.

SUMMARY

The knee is subjected to a variety of forces throughout the course of regular activity, thus making knee pain a common presentation to the ED. In addition to following basic trauma protocols, thorough neurovascular and musculoskeletal examinations should be performed and supplemented with appropriate imaging. Emergency physicians should also consider recent developments in knee anatomy and function when evaluating the patient with an acutely injured knee. **Table 2** summarizes the types of brace, brace setting, and recommended follow-up for common knee and leg injuries diagnosed in the ED.

REFERENCES

1. Gianotti SM, Marshall SW, Hume PA, et al. Incidence of anterior cruciate ligament injury and other knee ligament injuries: a national population-based study. J Sci Med Sport 2009;12(6):622–7.

2. Hugston JC, Jacobsen KE. Chronic posterolateral rotatory instability of the knee. J Bone Joint Surg Am 1985;67:351.

3. Gollehon DL, Torzilli PA, Warren RF. The role of posterolateral and cruciate ligaments in the stability of the human knee. J Bone Joint Surg Am 1987;69:233–42.

4. Maynard MJ, Deng X, Wickiewicz TL, et al. The popliteofibular ligament: rediscovery of a key element in posterolateral stability. Am J Sports Med 1996;24:311–5.

5. Seebacher JR, Inglis AE, Marshall JL, et al. The structure of the posterolateral corner of the knee. J Bone Joint Surg Am 1982;64:536–41.

6. Watanabe Y, Moriya H, Takahashi K, et al. Functional anatomy of the posterolateral structures of the knee. Arthroscopy 1993;9:57–62.

7. Vinson EN, Major NM, Helms CA. The posterolateral corner of the knee. AJR Am J Roentgenol 2008;190:449–58.

8. Hardaker WT Jr, Garret WE Jr, Bassett FH 3rd. Evaluation of acute traumatic hemarthrosis of the knee joint. South Med J 1990;83(6):640–4.

9. Noyes FR, Bassett RW, Grood ES, et al. Arthroscopy in acute traumatic hemarthrosis of the knee. Incidence of anterior cruciate ligament tears and other injuries. J Bone Joint Surg Am 1980;62(5):687–95.

10. Maffulli N, Binfield PM, King JB, et al. Acute hemarthrosis of the knee in athletes. A prospective study of 106 cases. J Bone Joint Surg Br 1993;75(6):945–9.

11. Smith TO, Daview L, O'Driscoll ML, et al. An evaluation of the clinical tests and outcome measures used to assess patellar instability. Knee 2008;15(4):255–62.

12. Guillodo Y, Rannou N, Dubrana F, et al. Diagnosis of anterior cruciate ligament rupture in an emergency department. J Trauma 2009;65(5):1078–82.

13. Torg JS, Conrad W, Kalen V. Clinical diagnosis of anterior cruciate instability in the athlete. Am J Sports Med 1976;4(2):84–93.

14. Jain DK, Amaravati R, Sharma G. Evaluation of the clinical signs of anterior cruciate ligament and meniscal injuries. Indian J Orthop 2009;43(4):375–8.

15. Benjaminse A, Gokeler A, van der Schans CP. Clinical diagnosis of an anterior cruciate ligament rupture: a meta-analysis. J Orthop Sports Phys Ther 2006;36(5):267–88.

16. Solomon DH, Simel DL, Bates DW, et al. The rational clinical examination. Does this patient have a torn meniscus or ligament of the knee? Value of the physical examination. JAMA 2001;286(13):1610–20.

17. Griffith CJ, LaPrade RF, Johansen S, et al. Medial knee injury: Part 1, static function of the individual components of the main medial knee structures. Am J Sports Med 2009;37(9):1762–70.

18. Wijdicks CA, Griffith CJ, LaPrade RF, et al. Medial knee injury: Part 2, load sharing between the posterior oblique ligament and superficial medial collateral ligament. Am J Sports Med 2009;37(9):1771–6.

19. Hugston JC, Norwood LA. The posterolateral drawer test and external recurvatum test for posterolateral rotatory instability of the knee. Clin Orthop 1980;147:82–7.

20. Konan S, Rayan F, Haddad FS. Do physical diagnostic tests accurately detect meniscal tears? Knee Surg Sports Traumatol Arthrosc 2009;17(7):806–11.

21. Harrison BK, Abell BE, Gibson TW. The Thessaly test for detection of meniscal tears: validation of a new physical examination technique for primary care medicine. Clin J Sport Med 2009;19(1):9–12.

22. Garavaglia G, Lubbeke A, Dubois-Ferriere V, et al. Accuracy of stress radiography techniques in grading isolated and combined posterior knee injuries: a cadaveric study. Am J Sports Med 2007;35(12):2051–6.

23. Garofalo R, Fanelli GC, Cikes A, et al. Stress radiography and posterior pathological laxity of knee: comparison between two different techniques. Knee 2009;16(4):251–5.

24. Bennett DL, George MJ, EL-Khoury GY, et al. Anterior rim tibial plateau fractures and posterolateral knee injury. Emerg Radiol 2004;10(2):76–83.

25. Covey DC. Injuries of the posterolateral corner of the knee. J Bone Joint Surg Am 2001;83(1):106–18.

26. Kaplan PA, Walker CW, Kilcoyne RF, et al. Occult fracture patterns of the knee associated with anterior cruciate ligament tears: assessment with MR imaging. Radiology 1992;183(3):835–8.

27. Nawata K, Teshima R, Suzuki T. Osseous lesions associated with anterior cruciate ligament injuries. Assessment by MRI at various periods after injuries. Arch Orthop Trauma Surg 1993;113(1):1–4.

28. Harish S, O'Donnell P, Connell D, et al. Imaging of the posterolateral corner of the knee. Clin Radiol 2006;61:457–66.

29. Wang JC, Shapiro MS. Pellegrini-Stieda syndrome. Am J Orthop 1995;24(6):493–7.

30. McAnally JL, Southam SL, Mlady GW. New thoughts on the origin of the Pellegrini-Stieda: the association of PCL injury and medial femoral epicondylar periosteal stripping. Skeletal Radiol 2009;38(2):193–8.

31. Tajima G, Nozaki M, Iriuchishima T, et al. Morphology of the tibial insertion of the posterior cruciate ligament. J Bone Joint Surg Am 2009;91(4):859–66.

32. Lorenz S, Elser F, Brucker PU, et al. Radiological evaluation of the anterolateral and posteromedial bundle insertion sites of the posterior cruciate ligament. Knee Surg Sports Traumatol Arthrosc 2009;17(6):683–90.

33. Kaplan PA, Matamoros A, Anderson JC. Sonography of the musculoskeletal system. AJR Am J Roentgenol 1990;155:237–45.

34. Jacobson JA. Musculoskeletal ultrasound and MRI: which do I choose? Semin Musculoskelet Radiol 2005;9(2):135–49.

35. Finlay K, Friendman L. Ultrasonography of the lower extremity. Orthop Clin North Am 2006;37(3):245–75.

36. Blankenbaker DG, De Smet AA. The role of ultrasound in the evaluation of sports injuries of the lower extremities. Clin Sports Med 2006;25(4):867–97.

37. Palm HG, Bergenthal G, Ehry P, et al. Functional ultrasonography in the diagnosis of acute anterior cruciate ligament injuries: a field study. Knee 2009;16(6):441–6.

38. Sorrentino F, Iovane A, Nicosia A, et al. Role of high-resolution ultrasonography without and with real-time spatial compound imaging in evaluating the injured posterior cruciate ligament: preliminary study. Radiol Med 2009;114(2):312–20.

39. Karabay N, Sugun TS, Toros T. Ultrasonographic diagnosis of the posterior cruciate ligament injury in a 4-year old child: a case report. Emerg Radiol 2009;16(5):415–7.

40. Barker RP, Lee JC, Healy JC. Normal sonographic anatomy of the posterolateral corner of the knee. AJR Am J Roentgenol 2009;192:73–9.

41. Shanbhogue AK, Sandhu MS, Singh P, et al. Real time spatial compound ultrasound in the evaluation of meniscal injuries: a comparison study with conventional ultrasound and MRI. Knee 2009;16(3):191–5.

42. Shetty AA, Tindall AJ, James KD, et al. Accuracy of hand-held ultrasound scanning in detecting meniscal tears. J Bone Joint Surg Br 2008;90(8):1045–8.

43. Venkatanarasimha N, Kamath A, Mukherjee K, et al. Potential pitfalls of a double PCL sign. Skeletal Radiol 2009;38(8):735–9.

44. Laundre BJ, Collins MS, Bond JR, et al. MRI accuracy for tears of the posterior horn of the lateral meniscus in patients with acute anterior cruciate ligament injury and the clinical relevance of missed tears. AJR Am J Roentgenol 2009; 193(2):515–23.

45. Krampla W, Roesel M, Svoboda K, et al. MRI of the knee: how do field strength and radiologist's experience influence diagnostic accuracy and interobserver correlation in assessing chondral and meniscal lesions and the integrity of the anterior cruciate ligament? Eur Radiol 2009;19(6): 1519–28.

46. Clayton RA, Court-Brown CM. The epidemiology of musculoskeletal tendinous and ligamentous injuries. Injury 2008;39(12):1338–44.

47. Agel J, Arendt EA, Bershadsky B. Anterior cruciate ligament injury in National Collegiate Athletic Association basketball and soccer: a 13 year review. Am J Sports Med 2005;33(4):524–30.

48. Ireland ML. Anterior cruciate ligament injury in female athletes: epidemiology. J Athl Train 1999;34(2):150–4.

49. Mihata LC, Beutler AI, Boden BP. Comparing the incidence of anterior cruciate ligament injury in collegiate lacrosse, soccer, and basketball players: Implications for anterior cruciate ligament mechanism and prevention. Am J Sports Med 2006;34(6):893–4.

50. Arendt EA, Agel J, Dick R. Anterior cruciate ligament injury patterns among collegiate men and women. J Athl Train 1999;34(2):86–92.

51. Davies H, Tietjens B, Van Sterkenburg M, et al. Anterior cruciate ligament injuries in snowboarders: a quadriceps-induced injury. Knee Surg Sports Traumatol Arthrosc 2009;17(9):1048–51.

52. Behairy NH, Dorgham MA, Khaled SA. Accuracy of routine magnetic resonance imaging in meniscal and ligamentous injuries of the knee: comparison with arthroscopy. Int Orthop 2009;33(4):961–7.

53. Kheder EM, Abd El-Bagi ME, El-Hosan MH. Anterior cruciate ligament graft tear. Primary and secondary magnetic resonance signs. Saudi Med J 2009;30(4): 465–71.

54. Shelbourne KD, Benner RW. Correlation of joint line tenderness and meniscus pathology in patients with subacute and chronic anterior cruciate ligament injuries. J Knee Surg 2009;22(3):187–90.

55. Duquin TR, Wind WM, Fineberg MS, et al. Current trends in anterior cruciate ligament reconstruction. J Knee Surg 2009;22(1):7–12.

56. Andersson D, Samuelsson K, Karlsson J. Treatment of anterior cruciate ligament injuries with special reference to surgical technique and rehabilitation: an assessment of randomized controlled trials. Arthroscopy 2009;25(6): 653–85.

57. Cohen SB, Yucha DT, Ciccotti MC, et al. Factors affecting patient selection of graft type in anterior cruciate ligament reconstruction. Arthroscopy 2009; 25(9):1006–10.

58. Sun K, Tian SQ, Zhang JH, et al. Anterior cruciate ligament reconstruction with bone-patellar tendon-bone autograft versus allograft. Arthroscopy 2009;25(7): 750–9.

59. Piva SR, Clinds JD, Klucinec BM, et al. Patella fracture during rehabilitation after bone-patellar tendon-bone anterior cruciate ligament reconstruction: 2 case reports. J Orthop Sports Phys Ther 2009;39(4):278–86.

60. Mouzopoulos G, Fotopoulos VC, Tzurbakis M. Septic knee arthritis following ACL reconstruction: a systematic review. Knee Surg Sports Traumatol Arthrosc 2009;17(9):1033–42.
61. Wang C, Ao Y, Wang J, et al. Septic arthritis after arthroscopic anterior cruciate ligament reconstruction: a retrospective analysis of incidence, presentation, treatment, and cause. Arthroscopy 2009;25(3):243–9.
62. Nag HL, Negoi DS, Nataraj AR, et al. Tubercular infection after arthroscopic anterior cruciate ligament reconstruction. Arthroscopy 2009;25(2):131–6.
63. Trojani C, Sane JC, Coste JS, et al. Four-strand hamstring tendon autograft for ACL reconstruction in patients aged 50 years or older. Orthop Traumatol Surg Res 2009;95(1):22–7.
64. Cohen M, Ferretti M, Quarteiro M, et al. Transphyseal anterior cruciate ligament reconstruction in patients with open physes. Arthroscopy 2009;25(8):831–8.
65. Henry J, Chotel F, Chouteau J, et al. Rupture of the anterior cruciate ligament in children: early reconstruction with open physes or delayed reconstruction to skeletal maturity? Knee Surg Sports Traumatol Arthrosc 2009;17(7):748–55.
66. Van de Velde SK, DeFrate LE, Gill TJ, et al. The effect of anterior cruciate ligament deficiency on the in vivo elongation of the medial and lateral collateral ligaments. Am J Sports Med 2007;35(2):294–300.
67. Tayton E, Verma R, Higgins B, et al. A correlation of time with meniscal tears in anterior cruciate ligament deficiency: stratifying the risk of surgical delay. Knee Surg Sports Traumatol Arthrosc 2009;17(1):30–4.
68. Yoo JC, Ahn JH, Lee SH, et al. Increasing incidence of medial meniscal tears in nonoperatively treated anterior cruciate ligament insufficiency patients documented by serial magnetic resonance imaging studies. Am J Sports Med 2009;37(8):1478–83.
69. Louboutin H, Debarge R, Richou J, et al. Osteoarthritis in patients with anterior cruciate ligament rupture: a review of risk factors. Knee 2009;16(4):239–44.
70. Oiestad BE, Engebretsen L, Storheim K, et al. Knee osteoarthritis after anterior cruciate ligament injury: a systematic review. Am J Sports Med 2009;37(7):1434–43.
71. Palmieri-Smith RM, Thomas AC. A neuromuscular mechanism of posttraumatic osteoarthritis associated with ACL injury. Exerc Sport Sci Rev 2009;37(3):147–53.
72. Ichiba A, Kishimoto I. Effects of articular cartilage and meniscus injuries at the time of surgery on osteoarthritic changes after anterior cruciate ligament reconstruction in patients under 40 years old. Arch Orthop Trauma Surg 2009;129(3):409–15.
73. Pujol N, Beaufils P. Healing results of meniscal tears left in situ during anterior cruciate ligament reconstruction: a review of clinical studies. Knee Surg Sports Traumatol Arthrosc 2009;17(4):396–401.
74. Beaufils P, Hulet C, Dhenain M, et al. Clinical practice guidelines for the management of meniscal lesions and isolated lesions of the anterior cruciate ligament of the knee in adults. Orthop Traumatol Surg Res 2009;95(6):437–42.
75. Brophy RH, Gill CS, Lyman S, et al. Effect of anterior cruciate ligament reconstruction and meniscectomy and length of career in National Football League athletes: a case control study. Am J Sports Med 2009;37(11):2102–7.
76. Rishiraj N, Taunton JE, Lloyd-Smith R, et al. The potential role of prophylactic/functional knee bracing in preventing knee ligament injury. Sports Med 2009;39(11):937–60.

77. Alentorn-Geli E, Myer GD, Silvers HJ, et al. Prevention of non-contact anterior cruciate ligament injuries in soccer players. Part 1: mechanisms of injury and underlying risk factors. Knee Surg Sports Traumatol Arthrosc 2009; 17(7):705–29.
78. Alentorn-Geli E, Myer GD, Silvers HJ, et al. Prevention of non-contact anterior cruciate ligament injuries in soccer players. Part 2: a review of prevention programs aimed to modify risk factors and to reduce injury rates. Knee Surg Sports Traumatol Arthrosc 2009;17(8):859–79.
79. Boling MC, Padua DA, Marshall SW, et al. A prospective investigation of biomechanical risk factors for patellofemoral pain syndrome: the joint undertaking to monitor and prevent ACL injury (JUMP-ACL) cohort. Am J Sports Med 2009; 37(11):2108–16.
80. Brophy RH, Chiaia TA, Maschi R, et al. The core and hip in soccer athletes compared by gender. Int J Sports Med 2009;30(9):663–7.
81. Iversen MD, Friden C. Pilot study of female high school basketball players' anterior cruciate ligament injury knowledge, attitudes, and practices. Scand J Med Sci Sports 2009;29(4):595–602.
82. Lim BO, Lee YS, Kim JG, et al. Effects of sports injury prevention training on the biomechanical risk factors of anterior cruciate ligament injury in high school female basketball players. Am J Sports Med 2009;37(9):1728–34.
83. McLean SG, Samorezov JE. Fatigue-induced ACL injury risk stems from a degradation in central control. Med Sci Sports Exerc 2009;41(8):1661–72.
84. Wells L, Dyke JA, Albaugh J, et al. Adolescent anterior cruciate ligament reconstruction: a retrospective analysis of quadriceps strength recovery and return to full activity after surgery. J Pediatr Orthop 2009;29(5):486–9.
85. Hugston JC, Andrews JR, Cross MJ, et al. Classification of knee ligament instabilities. Part II. The lateral compartment. J Bone Joint Surg Am 1976;58(2): 173–9.
86. Ramos LA, de Carvalho RT, Cohen M, et al. Anatomic relation between the posterior cruciate ligament and the joint capsule. Arthroscopy 2008;24(12): 1367–72.
87. Hermans S, Corten K, Bellemans J. Long-term results of isolated anterolateral bundle reconstructions of the posterior cruciate ligament: a 6- to 12-year follow-up study. Am J Sports Med 2009;37(8):1499–507.
88. Kim SJ, Kim TE, Jo SB, et al. Comparison of the clinical results of three posterior cruciate ligament reconstruction techniques. J Bone Joint Surg Am 2009;91(9): 2543–9.
89. Matava MJ, Ellis E, Gruber B. Surgical treatment of posterior cruciate ligament tears: an evolving technique. J Am Acad Orthop Surg 2009;17(7):435–46.
90. McAllister DR, Miller MD, Sekiya JK, et al. Posterior cruciate ligament biomechanics and options for surgical treatment. Instr Course Lect 2009;58:377–88.
91. Van de Velde SK, Bingham JT, Gill TJ, et al. Analysis of tibiofemoral cartilage deformation in the posterior cruciate ligament-deficient knee. J Bone Joint Surg Am 2009;91(9):167–75.
92. Kozanek M, Fu EC, Van de Velde SK, et al. Posterolateral structures of the knee in posterior cruciate ligament deficiency. Am J Sports Med 2009;37(3):534–41.
93. Watsend AM, Osestad TM, Jakobsen RB, et al. Clinical studies on posterior cruciate ligament tears have weak design. Knee Surg Sports Traumatol Arthrosc 2009;17(2):140–9.

94. Cooper JM, McAndrews PT, LaPrade RF. Posterolateral corner injuries of the knee: anatomy, diagnosis, and treatment. Sports Med Arthrosc 2006;14(4): 213–20.
95. Malone AA, Dowd GSE, Saifuddin A. Injuries of the posterior cruciate ligament and posterolateral corner of the knee. Injury 2006;37:485–501.
96. Chen FS, Rokito AS, Pitman ML. Acute and chronic posterolateral rotatory instability of the knee. J Am Acad Orthop Surg 2000;8:97–110.
97. O'Brien SJ, Warren RF, Pavlov H, et al. Reconstruction of the chronically insufficient anterior cruciate ligament with the central third of the patellar ligament. J Bone Joint Surg Am 1991;73:278–86.
98. Apsingi S, Nguyen T, Bull AM, et al. A comparison of modified Larson and 'anatomic' posterolateral corner reconstructions in knees with combined PCL and posterolateral corner deficiency. Knee Surg Sports Traumatol Arthrosc 2009;17(3):305–12.
99. Stannard JP, Brown SL, Farris RC, et al. The posterolateral corner of the knee: repair versus reconstruction. Am J Sports Med 2005;33(6):881–8.
100. Markolf KL, Graves BR, Sigward SM, et al. How well do anatomical reconstructions of the posterolateral corner restore varus stability to the posterior cruciate ligament-reconstructed knee? Am J Sports Med 2007;35(7):1117–22.
101. Shi SY, Ying XZ, Zheng Q, et al. Isometric reconstruction of the posterolateral corner of the knee. Acta Orthop Belg 2009;75(4):504–11.
102. Stannard JP, Brown SL, Robinson JT, et al. Reconstruction of the posterolateral corner of the knee. Arthroscopy 2005;21(9):1051–9.
103. Botomley N, Williams A, Birch R, et al. Displacement of the common peroneal nerve in posterolateral corner injuries of the knee. J Bone Joint Surg Br 2005; 87(9):1225–6.
104. Bushnell BD, Bitting SS, Crain JM, et al. Treatment of magnetic resonance imaging-documented isolated grade III lateral collateral ligament injuries in National Football League athletes. Am J Sports Med 2010;38(1):86–91.
105. Patel SC, Parker DA. Isolated rupture of the lateral collateral ligament during yoga practice: a case report. J Orthop Surg 2008;16(3):378–80.
106. Chen YH, Carrino JA, Raman SP, et al. Atraumatic lateral collateral ligament complex signal abnormalities by magnetic resonance imaging in patients with osteoarthrosis of the knee. J Comput Assist Tomogr 2008;32(6):982–6.
107. LaPrade RF, Heikes C, Bakker AJ, et al. The reproducibility and repeatability of varus stress radiographs in the assessment of isolated fibular collateral ligament and grade-III posterolateral knee injuries. An in vitro biomechanical study. J Bone Joint Surg Am 2008;90(10):2069–76.
108. Coobs BR, LaPrade RF, Griffith CJ, et al. Biomechanical analysis of an isolated fibular (lateral) collateral ligament reconstruction using an autogenous semitendinous graft. Am J Sports Med 2007;35(9):521–7.
109. Miyamoto RG, Bosco JA, Sherman OH. Treatment of medial collateral ligament injuries. J Am Acad Orthop Surg 2009;17:152–61.
110. Thornton GM, Johnson JC, Maser RV, et al. Strength of medial structures of the knee joint are decreased by isolated injury to the medial collateral ligament and subsequent joint immobilization. J Orthop Res 2005;23:1191–8.
111. Sparrow KJ, Finucand SD, Owen JR, et al. The effects of low-intensity ultrasound on medial collateral ligament healing in the rabbit model. Am J Sports Med 2005;33:1048–56.

112. Kovachevich R, Shah JP, Arens AM, et al. Operative management of the medial collateral ligament in the multi-ligament injured knee: an evidence-based systematic review. Knee Surg Sports Traumatol Arthrosc 2009;17(7):823–9.

113. Noyes FR, Barber-Westin SD. The treatment of acute combined ruptures of the anterior cruciate and medial ligaments of the knee. Am J Sports Med 1995;23: 380–9.

114. Petersen W, Laprell H. Combined injuries of the medial collateral ligament and the anterior cruciate ligament. Early ACL reconstruction versus late ACL reconstruction. Arch Orthop Trauma Surg 1999;119(5-6):258–62.

115. Theivendran K, Lever CJ, Hart WJ. Good result after surgical treatment of Pellegrini-Stieda syndrome. Knee Surg Sports Traumatol Arthrosc 2009; 17(10):1231–3.

116. Englund M, Guermazi A, Gale D, et al. Incidental meniscal findings on knee MRI in middle-aged and elderly persons. N Engl J Med 2008;359(11):1108–15.

117. Mustonen AOT, Koivikko MP, Lindhal J, et al. MRI of acute meniscal injury associated with tibial plateau fractures: prevalence, type, and location. AJR Am J Roentgenol 2008;191:1002–9.

118. Singhal M, Patel J, Johnson D. Knee: medial ligament injuries. In: DeLee JC, Drez D Jr, Miller MD, editors. DeLee: DeLee and Drez's orthopaedic sports medicine. 3rd edition. Philadelphia (PA): Saunders; 2009.

119. Englund M, Guermazi A, Roemer FW, et al. Meniscal tear in knees without surgery and the development of radiographic osteoarthritis among middle-aged and elderly persons: the multicenter oseteoarthritis study. Arthritis Rheum 2009;60(3):831–9.

120. Kramer DE, Micheli FJ. Meniscal tears and discoid meniscus in children: diagnosis and treatment. J Am Acad Orthop Surg 2009;17(11):698–707.

121. Peltola EK, Lindahl J, Hietaranta H, et al. Knee dislocation in overweight patients. AJR Am J Roentgenol 2009;192:101–6.

122. Bui KL, Ilaslan H, Parker RD, et al. Knee dislocations: a magnetic resonance imaging study correlated with clinical and operative findings. Skeletal Radiol 2008;37(7):653–61.

123. Robertson A, Nutton RW, Keating JF. Dislocation of the knee. J Bone Joint Surg Br 2006;88:706–11.

124. Seroyer ST, Musahl V, Harner CD. Management of the acute knee dislocation: the Pittsburgh experience. Injury 2008;39:710–8.

125. Harb A, Lincold D, Michaelson J. The MR dimple sign in irreducible posterolateral knee dislocations. Skeletal Radiol 2009;38(11):1111–4.

126. Levy BA, Fanelli GC, Whelan DB, et al. Controversies in the treatment of knee dislocations and multiligament reconstruction. J Am Acad Orthop Surg 2009; 17(4):197–206.

127. Zaffagnini S, Iacono F, LoPresti M, et al. A new hinged dynamic distractor for immediate mobilization after knee dislocations: technical note. Arch Orthop Trauma Surg 2008;128(11):1233–7.

128. Medvecky MJ, Zazulak BT, Hewett TE. A multidisciplinary approach to the evaluation, reconstruction and rehabilitation of the multi-ligament injured athlete. Sports Med 2007;37(2):169–87.

129. Mills WJ, Barei DP, McNair P. The value of the ankle-brachial index for diagnosing arterial injury after knee dislocation: a prospective study. J Trauma 2004;56:1261–5.

130. Johnson ME, Foster L, DeLee JC. Neurologic and vascular injuries associated with knee ligament injuries. Am J Sports Med 2008;36(12):2448–62.

131. Abou-Sayed H, Berger DL. Blunt lower-extremity trauma and popliteal artery injuries: revisiting the case for selective arteriography. Arch Surg 2002;137(5):585–9.

132. Chapman J, Pallin D. Popliteal air following penetrating trauma. Am J Emerg Med 2006;24:638.

133. Miller-Thomas MM, West OC, Cohen AM. Diagnosing traumatic arterial injury in the extremities with CT angiography: pearls and pitfalls. Radiographics 2005;25(Suppl 1):S133.

134. Nicandri GT, Chamberlain AM, Wahl CJ. Practical management of knee dislocations: a selective angiography protocol to detect limb-threatening vascular injuries. Clin J Sport Med 2009;19(2):125–9.

135. Peng PD. CT angiography effectively evaluates extremity vascular trauma. Am Surg 2008;74:103.

136. Niall DM, Nutton RW, Keating JF. Palsy of the common peroneal nerve after traumatic dislocation of the knee. J Bone Joint Surg Br 2005;87:664–7.

137. Bin SI, Nam TS. Surgical outcome of 2-stage management of multiple knee ligament injuries after knee dislocation. Arthroscopy 2007;23(10):1066–72.

138. Fanelli GC, Edson CJ, Reinheimer KN. Evaluation and treatment of the multiligament-injured knee. Instr Course Lect 2009;58:389–95.

139. Ibrahim SA, Ahmad FH, Salah M, et al. Surgical management of traumatic knee dislocation. Arthroscopy 2008;24(2):178–87.

140. Levy BA, Dajani KA, Whelan DB, et al. Decision making in the multiligament-injured knee: an evidence-based systematic review. Arthroscopy 2009;25(4):430–8.

141. Robinson RJ, Barron DA, Grainger AJ, et al. Wii knee. Emerg Radiol 2008;15(4):255–7.

142. Stefancin JJ, Parker RD. First-time traumatic patellar dislocation: a systematic review. Clin Orthop Relat Res 2007;455:93–101.

143. Felus J, Kowalczyk B, Lejman T. Sonographic evaluation of the injuries after traumatic patellar dislocations in adolescents. J Pediatr Orthop 2008;28(4):397–402.

144. Guerrero P, Li X, Patel K, et al. Medial patellofemoral ligament injury patterns and associated pathology in lateral patella dislocation: an MRI study. Sports Med Arthrosc Rehabil Ther Technol 2009;1(1):17.

145. Camanho GL, Viegas Ade C, Bitar AC, et al. Conservative versus surgical treatment for repair of the medial patellofemoral ligament in acute dislocations of the patella. Arthroscopy 2009;25(6):620–5.

146. Sillanpaa PJ, Mattila VM, Maenpaa H, et al. Treatment with and without initial stabilizing surgery for primary traumatic patellar dislocation. A prospective randomized study. J Bone Joint Surg Am 2009;91:263–73.

147. Colvin AC, West RV. Patellar instability. J Bone Joint Surg Am 2008;90:2751–62.

148. Panagopoulos A, van Niekerk L, Triantafillopoulos IK. MPFL reconstruction for recurrent patella dislocation: a new surgical technique and review of the literature. Int J Sports Med 2008;29(5):359–65.

149. Ronga M, Oliva F, Longo UG, et al. Isolated medial patellofemoral ligament reconstruction for recurrent patellar dislocation. Am J Sports Med 2009;37(9):1735–42.

150. Nietosvaara Y, Paukku R, Palmu S, et al. Acute patellar dislocation in children and adolescents. Surgical technique. J Bone Joint Surg Am 2009;91(Suppl 2):139–45.

151. Atkinson PJ, Haut RC. Injuries produced by blunt trauma to the human patellofemoral joint vary with flexion angle of the knee. J Orthop Res 2001;19:827–33.

152. Pritchett JW. Nonoperative treatment of widely displaced patella fracture. Am J Knee Surg 1997;10:145–7.
153. Brostroum A. Fracture of the patella: a study of 422 patellar fractures. Acta Orthop Scand Suppl 1972;143:1.
154. Pandya NK, Zgonis M, Ahn J, et al. Patellar tendon rupture as a manifestation of Lyme disease. Am J Orthop 2008;37(9):e167–70.
155. Jolles BM, Garofalo R, Gillain L, et al. New clinical test in diagnosing quadriceps tendon rupture. Ann R Coll Surg Engl 2007;89:259–61.
156. Heyde CE, Mahlfeld K, Stahel PF, et al. Ultrasonography as a reliable diagnostic tool in old quadriceps tendon ruptures: a prospective multicentre study. Knee Surg Sports Traumatol Arthrosc 2005;13(7):564–8.
157. LaRocco BG, Zlupko G, Sierzenski P. Ultrasound diagnosis of quadriceps tendon rupture. J Emerg Med 2008;35(3):293–5.
158. McKinney B, Cherney S, Penna J. Intra-articular knee injuries in patients with knee extensor mechanism ruptures. Knee Surg Sports Traumatol Arthrosc 2008;16(7):633–8.
159. Ramseier LE, Werner CML, Heinzelmann M. Quadriceps and patellar tendon rupture. Injury 2006;37:516–9.
160. Berkson EM, Virkus WW. High-energy tibial plateau fractures. J Am Acad Orthop Surg 2006;14(1):20–31.
161. McEnery KW, Wilson AJ, Pilgram TK, et al. Fractures of the tibial plateau: value of spiral CT coronal plane reconstruction for detecting displacement in vitro. Am J Roentgenol 1994;163:1177–84.
162. Duan XJ, Yang L, Guo L, et al. Arthroscopically assisted treatment for Schatzker type I-V tibial plateau fractures. Chin J Traumatol 2008;11(5):288–92.
163. Papagelopoulos PJ, Partsinevelos AA, Themistocelous GS, et al. Complications after tibia plateau fracture surgery. Injury 2006;17:475–84.
164. Badhe S, Baiju D, Elliot R, et al. The 'silent' compartment syndrome. Injury 2009;40(2):1879.
165. Stark E, Stucken C, Trainer G, et al. Compartment syndrome in Schatzker type VI plateau fractures and medial condylar fracture-dislocations treated with temporary external fixation. J Orthop Trauma 2009;23(7):502–6.
166. Abdel-Hamid MZ, Chang CH, Chan YS, et al. Arthroscopic evaluation of soft tissue injuries in tibial plateau fractures: retrospective analysis of 98 cases. Arthroscopy 2006;22(6):669–75.
167. Mui LW, Engelsohn E, Umans H. Comparison of CT and MRI in patients with tibial plateau fracture: can CT findings predict ligament tear or meniscal injury? Skeletal Radiol 2007;36(2):145–51.

Leg, Ankle, and Foot Injuries

Dennis P. Hanlon, MD*

KEYWORDS

• Ankle • Calcaneus • Talus • Lisfranc

Injuries to the leg, ankle, and foot are common in patients seeking emergency care. In many cases, the emergency provider (EP) can provide initial care and have the patient follow up as an outpatient. In some cases, emergent orthopedic consultation is required. The EP must be aware of the anatomy, common injuries, important injuries, and potential complications associated with these injuries.

TIBIAL AND FIBULA SHAFT FRACTURES

Tibial fractures are the most common long-bone fracture. These injuries vary from minimally displaced fractures to acutely limb-threatening injuries because of vascular, neurologic, and extensive soft tissue involvement. The tibia has little protection on the anterior surface because the skin and subcutaneous tissue are thin (**Fig. 1**). As a result, it is the most common long bone to have an open fracture.[1]

As with most paired bones, a displaced fracture of the tibial shaft is associated with a fibula fracture 75% to 85% of the time (**Fig. 2**).[2] Isolated fibula fractures are caused by direct trauma and usually are less serious than tibial fractures. Proximal fibula fractures may be associated with a peroneal nerve injury.

Tibial and fibula shaft fractures are associated with multiple complications including osteomyelitis, delayed or nonunion, reflex sympathetic dystrophy, deep vein thrombosis, and compartment syndrome.[3] The lower leg is divided into 4 major compartments by the fascia. Excessive pressure within any compartment produces ischemic pain and nerve damage unless treated expediently. Pain out of proportion to injury is a classic finding of compartment syndrome; however, this can be difficult to judge with an underlying distracting tibial and/or fibula fracture. Increased pain with passive stretching of the affected muscles and decreased sensation in the affected nerve distribution are reliable findings suggestive of compartment syndrome.[4]

The most commonly used method for classifying open fractures is the Gustilo classification. In this system, grade 1 open fractures have skin lesions of less than 1 cm and a clean, simple bone fracture with minimal comminution. Grade 2 open fractures

Operations, Allegheny General Hospital, 320 East North Avenue, Pittsburgh, PA 15212, USA
* 200 Windermere Ct, McMurray, PA 15317.
E-mail address: dhanlon@wpahs.org

Emerg Med Clin N Am 28 (2010) 885–905
doi:10.1016/j.emc.2010.09.001   emed.theclinics.com

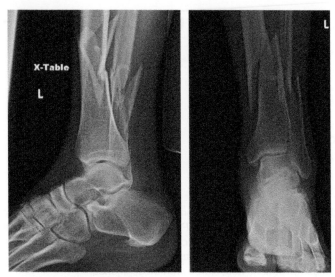

Fig. 1. Anteroposterior (AP) and lateral views of an open pen, comminuted tibia, and fibula fracture. The lateral view shows the scant soft tissue protection of these bones.

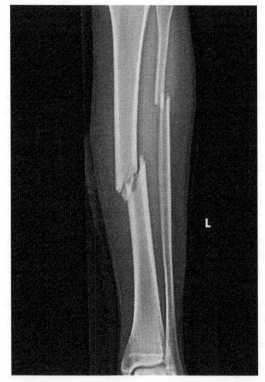

Fig. 2. Moderately displaced tibia and fibula fracture.

have skin lesions greater than 1 cm, no extensive soft tissue damage, and minimal crush injury with moderate comminution. Grade 3 open fractures have extensive skin damage with muscle and neurovascular involvement, comminution of fracture, and instability. Grade 3 fractures are further subdivided into 3a (severe comminution or segmental fractures), 3b (periosteal bone stripping, severe comminution, and contamination), and 3c (arterial damage). Amputation is rare for grade 1 and 2 open fractures, but it is necessary in more than 20% of grade 3c fractures.[5]

Tibial shaft fractures are usually easily diagnosed. These fractures are the result of a high-energy mechanism, and patients must be evaluated thoroughly to exclude other injuries. Orthopedic consultation is required for most tibial and fibula shaft fractures. Urgent operative debridement is required for open fractures. While waiting for operative intervention, the leg should be splinted, sterile dressings should be applied to the overlying wounds, tetanus immunization updated if needed, and prophylactic intravenous antibiotics should be administered. Closed tibial and fibula shaft fractures, particularly if displaced, are at risk for compartment syndrome and may warrant admission for observation and subsequent operative intervention. In a recent study, diaphyseal tibia fractures had an 8% rate of compartment syndrome.[6] Isolated fibular fractures rarely develop complications and can be managed with protected weight bearing. Closed tibial and fibula shaft fractures are splinted in a long leg splint with the knee at 10° to 20° of flexion.[2]

ANKLE SPRAINS

The evaluation of ankle injuries is a daily occurrence in the practice of emergency medicine. Ankle sprains make up most of these injuries. In addition, ankle sprains are the most common injury in sports, accounting for 15% to 20% of sports-related injuries.[7,8] There are 3 main varieties of ankle sprains. The lateral sprain or inversion sprain is the most common. An isolated medial sprain or eversion sprain is uncommon because of the strength of the deltoid ligament. The medial malleolus will usually fracture before the deltoid ligament tears.[9] The high or syndesmotic ankle sprain has received much attention recently from sports medicine specialists. These syndesmotic sprains take longer to heal and may require surgery.[10] All types of ankle sprains are graded on the level of severity. In grade 1 injuries, only stretching of the involved ligaments has occurred. Grade 2 injuries have partial tears of the involved ligaments; grade 3 injuries have complete tears or ruptures of involved ligaments. Although the management of the different types of sprains has substantial overlap, there are some differences in findings and prognosis.[8,9] The history, physical exam, and radiographic imaging must consider injuries that may mimic ankle sprains (**Table 1**).

The lateral sprain is the most common sprain, accounting for 85% of such injuries because of the anatomic design of the ankle.[11] The distal articulation of the tibia and fibula creates the ankle mortise. It is primarily a hinge-type joint allowing approximately 20° of dorsiflexion and 30 to 50° of plantar flexion. The ankle also has 25° of eversion and inversion that occurs at the subtalar joint. The ankle mortise is widest anteriorly so the joint is least stable with the foot plantar flexed. With the strength difference between the deltoid ligament medially and the lateral ligamentous complex, inversion injuries occur much more commonly than eversion injuries. The anterior talofibular ligament is the most commonly injured ligament.[12] It runs from the front of the lateral malleolus to the anterolateral aspect of the talus. With further inversion stress, the calcaneofibular ligament is injured. This ligament runs from the tip of the lateral malleolus to the lateral aspect of the calcaneus. The posterior talofibular ligament is the strongest of the 3

Table 1
Ankle sprain mimics

Entity	Mechanism	Key to Avoiding Misdiagnosis
Avulsion fractures lateral malleolus	Same mechanism as sprain	Close scrutiny of radiographs (see **Fig. 4**)
Proximal fifth metatarsal fractures	Vertical or medially directed force applied to a plantar flexed foot	Point tenderness base of fifth metatarsal
Lisfranc fractures	Axial load on a plantar flexed foot	Ecchymosis on the plantar aspect of the midfoot
Achilles tendon ruptures	Sudden acceleration or forced dorsiflexion	Weak plantar flexion; positive Thompson test
Talar avulsion fractures	Inversion mechanism	Dorsal tenderness (see **Fig. 5**)
Navicular avulsion fractures	Inversion mechanism	Bifurcate ligament
Rupture of peroneal tendons	Forced dorsiflexion; snapping sensation posterolateral ankle	Weakness of eversion

lateral ligaments. It is almost horizontal in its orientation and runs from the fossa in the inner aspect of the lateral malleolus to the posterior tubercle of the talus.

The physical examination of a lateral ankle sprain will reveal tenderness and swelling of the lateral ankle. The anterior drawer test may reveal a more significant injury, a grade 3 sprain. To perform this test, with the patient sitting and the ankle in 10° to 15° of plantar flexion, cup the heel with one hand and provide counter traction to the tibia with the other while attempting to translate the fibula from anterior to posterior. Increased movement and pain indicates a positive test.[9] Compare with the uninjured side because a 2-mm difference may be significant.[9,12] In addition, a dimple may appear just anterior to the lateral malleolus. Finally, there may be the sensation of no definite endpoint compared with the other side. The talar tilt test is performed by applying slight adduction and eversion stress to the midfoot. If both the anterior talofibular ligament and fibulocalcaneal ligament are ruptured, there will be movement of the talus within the mortise.[9]

The medial sprain or eversion sprain is uncommon because of the strength of the deltoid ligament. The superficial component of the deltoid ligament connects the medial malleolus to the medial calcaneus, sustentaculum tali centrally, anteriorly to the tarsal navicular. The deep component of the deltoid ligament connects to the neck, body, and posterior portion of talus. There will be tenderness, swelling, and ecchymosis to the medial aspect of the ankle. In the external rotation stress test, an external rotation force is applied to a dorsiflexed ankle. If painful, the test is positive.[9,13] In particular, the proximal fibula must always be examined with any medial ankle injury to evaluate for a possible Maissoneuve fracture.

The high or syndesmotic ankle sprain is an injury to the ligaments of the distal tibiofibular syndesmosis. These ligaments include the anterior inferior tibiofibular ligament, posterior inferior tibiofibular ligament, the inferior transverse ligament, and the interosseous ligament. These sprains account for 10% to 20% of all ankle sprains, with an increased incidence in certain sports such as skiing and hockey.[13] The most common mechanism of injury is external rotation. Usually the foot is planted on the ground with internal rotation of the leg and body with respect to the foot.[10] The patient will complain of pain anteriorly between the distal tibia and fibula at the level of the ankle joint. There will usually be difficulty bearing weight.[14]

The physical examination of a syndesmotic ankle sprain will reveal a tender, swollen ankle. The squeeze test is performed by compressing the proximal tibia and fibula. It is positive if this maneuver produces pain at the ankle.[9,13] Another test to detect syndesmosis injuries is the crossed-leg test. While sitting, the patient rests the midtibia of the affected leg on the knee of the unaffected leg. A downward force is applied to the medial side of the knee. If pain is produced in the area of syndesmosis, the test is positive.[15] Tenderness length, the distance that tenderness extends proximal to the ankle joint, correlates with the degree of injury and return to sports.[16]

The indications for diagnostic imaging are discussed later. A standard ankle series includes anteroposterior (AP), oblique, and lateral views. With plain radiographs, a widened medial clear space will be noted on the mortise view. The medial clear space, which extends from the lateral border of the medial malleolus to the medial border of the talus, should not exceed 2 to 3 mm. A widened medial clear space implies a deltoid ligament rupture, syndesmosis disruption, or both (**Fig. 3**).[17] A decrease in the amount of tibiofibular overlap, usually greater than 2 mm on the mortise view and greater than 6 mm on the AP view, suggests an injury to the syndesmosis. This finding may also be seen with a deltoid ligament rupture. A syndesmotic injury may also be radiographically unapparent.[14] Stress films are not useful acutely, but may be beneficial for the orthopedist in follow-up.

The initial treatment of ankle sprains incorporates the well-known RICE therapy (rest, ice, compression, and immobilization). The different types of sprains will have some modification of this therapy based on severity and type of sprain. The treatment of severe lateral ankle sprains is conservative, with either a posterior splint or an Aircast brace (DonJoy Inc, Vista, CA, USA) with initial non-weight bearing.[18–20] Boyce and colleagues[20] showed improved ankle function at 10 days and 1 month after injury

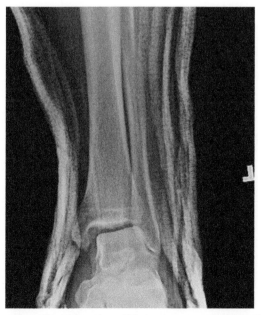

Fig. 3. Disrupted mortise with widened medial clear space and a talar tilt.

using an Aircast versus an elastic bandage. With first-time ankle sprains, a combination of elastic wrap and Air-stirrup brace (DonJoy Inc, Vista, CA, USA) allowed injured patients a faster return to preinjury status.[21] In athletes, some authorities advocate surgical repair of isolated medial sprains.[10] A suspected syndesmotic injury should be splinted, non–weight bearing, and have early orthopedic referral. Syndesmotic ankle sprains without diastasis can be managed conservatively.[14] Acute, unstable syndesmosis injuries should be repaired surgically).[10,16]

The complications of ankle sprains include prolonged pain, recurrence, and chronic laxity. Almost one-third of athletes will have a recurrent ankle sprain within 1 year.[22] One-third to one-half of patients will still have some symptoms at 3 years.[22] In addition to these complications, syndesmotic ankle sprains are prone to the formation of heterotropic ossification within the interosseous membrane.[16]

ANKLE FRACTURES

The Ottawa ankle rules were developed because of the low yield of routine ankle radiographs in the assessment of ankle injuries. These rules decrease the number of films by up to 30% without missing clinically significant fractures.[23,24] The Ottawa ankle rules state that an ankle series is indicated in the following circumstances: (1) tenderness along the distal 6 cm of the posterior tibia or the tip of the medial malleolus, (2) tenderness along the distal 6 cm of the posterior fibula or the tip of the lateral malleolus, and (3) the inability to bear weight for 4 steps, immediately and in the emergency department (ED). Similarly, the Ottawa foot rules state that a foot series is indicated in the following circumstances: (1) tenderness at the base of the fifth metatarsal, (2) tenderness at the navicular bone, and (3) the inability to bear weight for 4 steps, immediately and in the ED.[23]

There are 2 fracture classification schemes that are commonly used. The Danis-Weber classification scheme is based on the location of the fibular fracture, which determines the need for operative intervention because it reveals the status of the

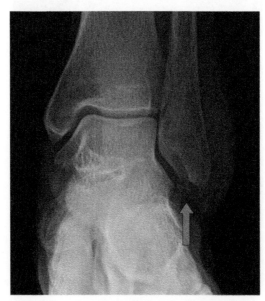

Fig. 4. Avulsion fracture of lateral malleolus with soft tissue swelling.

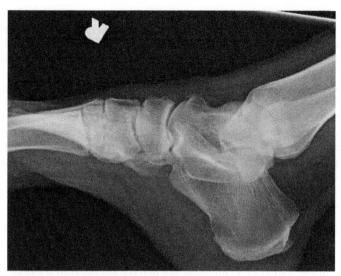

Fig. 5. Talar and tarsal navicular avulsion fractures.

syndesmosis. The other major system is the Lauge-Hansen classification, which is based on mechanism of injury. The Danis-Weber classification scheme is more useful to EPs, with its anatomic basis and correlation with the need for surgery.[9,25] In Weber type A injuries, the fibula fracture occurs distal to the mortise. These fractures are stable and managed conservatively with immobilization. In Weber type B injuries, the fibula fracture occurs at the level of the mortise. Generally, these fractures are unstable and require operative repair (**Fig. 6**). A truly isolated fibula fracture at the level of the plafond would be the exception, and this injury could be managed conservatively. In Weber type C injuries, the fibula fracture occurs above the level of the mortise.

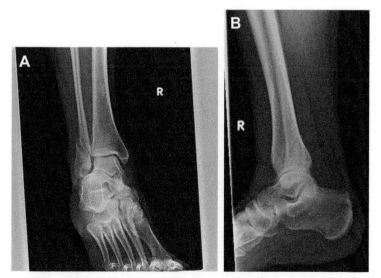

Fig. 6. (*A*) AP and (*B*) lateral views of Weber B fracture: oblique fibula fracture at level of the plafond.

These fractures are unstable and require operative repair because of disruption of the syndesmosis. The initial management includes immobilization, non–weight-bearing status, pain control, and early orthopedic referral. Some patients will be admitted because of swelling, pain control, comorbidities, or plans for early operative intervention.

If there are fractures or ligament ruptures on both sides of the ankle, the resulting injury will be unstable. Because of the instability of these ankle fractures, these injuries are often fracture-dislocations of the ankle. If there is an obvious fracture-dislocation with any evidence of vascular compromise, the ankle should be reduced emergently (**Fig. 7**). Do not wait for radiographs unless they are immediately available. There are several important specific fractures of the ankle including pilon fractures, Maissoneuve fractures, and triplane fractures, which are discussed later.

PILON FRACTURES

Pilon fractures are intraarticular fractures of the distal tibia extending into the metaphysis. These fractures are also referred to as plafond fractures and account for 7% of tibial fractures.[6] In French, the term pilon means pestle, which correlates with the mechanism of this injury. Pilon fractures are usually the result of a high-energy axial load force such as a fall from heights or a front-end motor vehicle collision. These fractures are often associated with other lower extremity injuries, pelvic fractures, and lumbar spine injuries.[26] These fractures have been reported with a low-energy mechanism such as skiing.

These injuries are not usually a diagnostic problem. Pilon fractures have obvious deformities and often associated soft tissue injury. Plain radiographs are diagnostic (**Fig. 8**). Computed tomography (CT) scan may help evaluate the degree of comminution to help in operative planning, but it is not required emergently in the acute setting.

Although the diagnosis may be easy, the management can be difficult. These fractures have a high rate of nonunion and wound infections, and are particularly challenging to manage with extensive soft tissue injury.[26] There are worse outcomes in patients who are diabetic,[27] and outcomes are generally poor after nonoperative treatment. Surgery is indicated for open fractures, displaced fractures, rotational

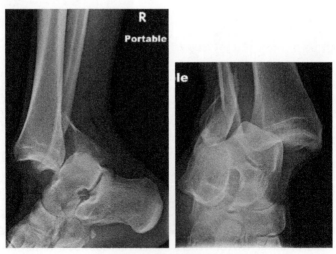

Fig. 7. AP and lateral views of unstable ankle fracture-dislocation.

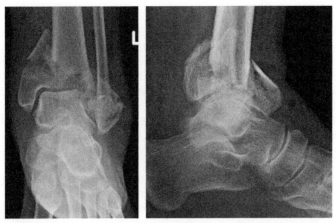

Fig. 8. AP and lateral views of a typical pilon fracture: comminuted and intraarticular. Also, note the extensive soft tissue air.

deformity, and articular fragments with a step-off greater than 2 mm.[26] These injuries need to be carefully assessed and observed for vascular compromise compartment syndrome.[6]

MAISSONEUVE FRACTURE

This fracture is caused by an external rotational force applied to the ankle. The Maissoneuve fracture consists of a proximal fibula fracture, syndesmosis disruption, and either a deltoid ligament rupture or medial malleolus fracture. Any medial ankle injury requires the careful evaluation of the proximal fibula.

Ankle radiographs will show a widened medial clear space if the deltoid ligament is ruptured or a transverse medial malleolus fracture is present (**Fig. 9**). The tibiofibular overlap may also be decreased, but the proximal fibula fracture will be missed without a radiograph of the entire tibia and fibula bones.

The initial treatment includes posterior splinting, non–weight bearing, and early orthopedic follow-up. Definitive treatment is open reduction and internal fixation (ORIF).

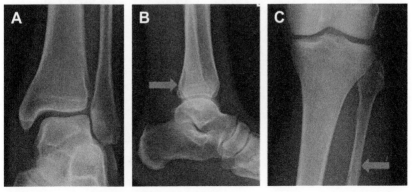

Fig. 9. (*A*) AP and (*B*) lateral view of the ankle showing widened medial clear space consistent with rupture of deltoid ligament. The arrow points to an associated posterior malleolus fracture. (*C*) A subtle proximal fibula fracture.

TRIPLANE FRACTURES

This multiplanar fracture has a transverse component (growth plate), a sagittal component (epiphysis), and a coronal component (distal tibial metaphysis). It occurs during adolescence before complete closure of the distal tibial physis. The asymmetric closure of the distal tibia growth plate allows this type of fracture to occur with an eversion stress. This force moves along the nonfused lateral aspect of the distal tibia growth plate until it meets the fused area and is transmitted into the epiphysis and metaphysis. It accounts for 5% to 10% of pediatric intraarticular fractures.[28,29]

The physical examination shows the typical findings of a fracture with exquisite tenderness, swelling, and the inability to bear weight. A deformity may be present depending on the degree of displacement.

Plain radiography usually reveals the fracture, (**Fig. 10**) although the findings may be subtle. The distal tibial metaphysis, the coronal component, is most readily identified on the lateral view.[29] Approximately half of triplane fractures have an associated fibula fracture.[30] CT provides invaluable preoperative information and better detail, including important information of the congruity of the articular surface (**Fig. 11**).[31]

The initial treatment will be immobilization in a posterior splint and non–weight bearing. Definitive treatment generally requires operative intervention unless the fracture is nondisplaced. Orthopedists may attempt closed reduction of a triplane fracture, but it is only successful 30% to 50% of the time.[30] Whether a closed reduction should be attempted routinely before surgery in displaced triplane fracture is controversial.[29,31]

ACHILLES TENDON RUPTURE

Achilles tendon rupture is a common injury to recreational athletes that is missed up to 25% of the time on initial visits.[32] Most patients are asymptomatic before

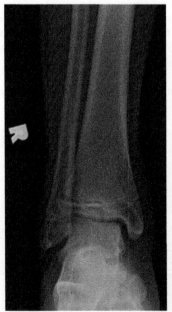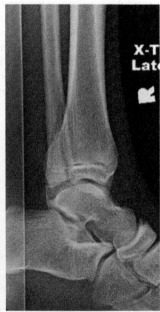

Fig. 10. AP and lateral views of a triplane fracture of the distal tibia. Widening of the lateral portion of the distal tibia physis. A vertical lucency extends through the middle of the epiphysis. Subtle fracture lines extend into the metaphysis.

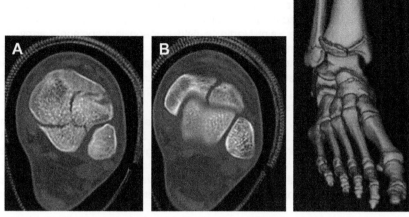

Fig. 11. (A, B) CT shows the extent of the fracture of the distal tibial metaphysis. (C) CT reconstruction of a triplane fracture.

rupture, without symptoms of Achilles tendonitis. Classically, patients feel a pop while accelerating, decelerating, or jumping. Although this injury is initially painful, the pain may be minimal or spontaneously resolved by the time of presentation. Most ruptures occur 2 to 6 cm above the insertion on the calcaneus.[32,33] There is an increased incidence with gout, lupus, chronic renal failure, rheumatoid arthritis, fluoroquinolone use, and chronic corticosteroid use.[33] The incidence of Achilles tendon rupture has increased as people have become more active in middle age and later.[34]

An accurate, focused physical examination is essential because the diagnosis is primarily clinical. A palpable defect may be present 2 to 6 cm above the calcaneus; however, this defect may be obscured by edema or hemorrhage.[35] The patient may have some plantar flexion from the actions of the flexor digitorum, flexor hallucis longus, tibialis posterior, peroneus longus, and peroneus brevis. There may be increased dorsiflexion on passive range of motion if not limited by pain or swelling. A positive Thompson test confirms the suspected diagnosis.[9] This test is performed, with the patient prone and the knee flexed to 90°, by squeezing the calf muscles just distal to its maximum width. With an intact Achilles tendon, the foot will plantar flex. If the Achilles tendon is ruptured, then there will be no plantar flexion.

Diagnostic imaging is unnecessary unless there is concern for an associated fracture or the diagnosis is unclear. Radiographs will be negative or have some subtle soft tissue findings. Ultrasound can diagnose complete and partial tears, but it is operator dependent. Magnetic resonance imaging (MRI) is accurate even for partial tears, but it is usually not necessary in the ED. Most Achilles tendon ruptures are complete.

The ED treatment is to splint in plantar flexion with no weight bearing and provide early orthopedic referral. The optimal definitive treatment is controversial. Surgical repair has a decreased risk of recurrent rupture and allows a faster return to sports or activities.[36] Conservative management eliminates surgical complications including wound infections, but the rate of recurrent rupture ranges from 8% to 39%.[35] Percutaneous surgical techniques decrease the surgical complication rate without an increase in the rate of rerupture compared with open methods.[37]

LISFRANC FRACTURE/SPRAIN

Lisfranc injuries represent a spectrum of midfoot injuries from frank fracture-disloca-tions to sprains of the tarsometatarsal joint. This joint is known as the Lisfranc joint after Jacques Lisfranc de Saint-Martin, a field surgeon in Napoleon's army. This surgeon developed an amputation technique at the tarsometatarsal joint to avoid infection and frostbite. Although fracture-dislocations are uncommon injuries, sprains to this joint are being increasingly recognized, particularly among athletes.[38,39] Twenty percent of these rare, complex injuries are missed.[40] The miss rate is even higher with subtle injuries in neuropathic diabetics.[41]

Motor vehicle collisions, falls, and athletic events are the most common mecha-nisms for Lisfranc injuries. Equestrian riders who get a foot caught in a stirrup after falling from the horse may injure this joint. Higher-energy mechanisms generally cause fracture-dislocations, whereas lower-energy mechanisms may cause only ligamen-tous injuries. In athletes, the mechanism often involves an axial load on a plantar-flexed foot.[42] Rotational force to a plantar-flexed foot may also produce a Lisfranc injury.

The Lisfranc joint is the articulation between the midfoot and forefoot. This tarsome-tatarsal joint relies on both bony and ligamentous support for its stability. The middle cuneiform–second metatarsal articulation is recessed providing additional stability to the Lisfranc joint and the transverse arch of the foot.[43] The solitary Lisfranc ligament runs from the plantar lateral aspect of the medial cuneiform to the plantar medial aspect of the second metatarsal. Injury to this ligament results in loss of the longitu-dinal and transverse arch.[44] The intermetatarsal ligaments connect all the metatarsals, but there are no intermetatarsal ligaments between the first and second metatarsals. The dorsal intermetatarsal ligaments are weaker than the plantar ligaments, resulting in an increased incidence of dorsal dislocations.

The physical examination may reveal tenderness at the Lisfranc joint, and swelling and ecchymosis on the plantar aspect of the midfoot.[45] This is not specific for Lisfranc injury, but it warrants further investigation.[45] Intense swelling may mask a deformity.[40] This swelling may be significantly out of proportion to a negative radiograph. Passive movement of the individual heads of the metatarsals produces pain at the tarsometa-tarsal joint. Passive pronation with adduction of the forefoot with the hindfoot stabi-lized will elicit pain and may reveal instability.[40] These stress tests are difficult and unreliable in the unanesthetized patient.

Diagnostic imaging of these injuries includes the standard radiographic series of the foot with an AP, lateral, and oblique view. On the AP view of a normal foot, the lateral border of the medial cuneiform should align with the lateral border of the first meta-tarsal, and the medial border of the base of the second metatarsal should line up with the medial border of the middle cuneiform. The second tarsometatarsal joint should be 1 cm proximal to the first tarsometatarsal joint and 0.5 cm proximal to the third tarsometatarsal joint. On the oblique view, the lateral border of the lateral cuneiform should align with the lateral border of the third metatarsal, and the medial border of the fourth metatarsal should line up with the medial border of the cuboid. On the lateral view, the superior border of the first metatarsal base should align with the superior border of the medial cuneiform. Diastasis greater than 2 mm between the first and second metatarsal suggests a Lisfranc injury and is consistent with a third degree sprain.[42] The fleck sign, referring to an avulsion from the second metatarsal base or medial cuneiform, may be the only sign of a Lisfranc injury.[42] Standard radio-graph series appear normal in up to 50% of cases. Even significant injuries can reduce spontaneously, making the diagnosis of Lisfranc injuries difficult (**Fig. 12**).

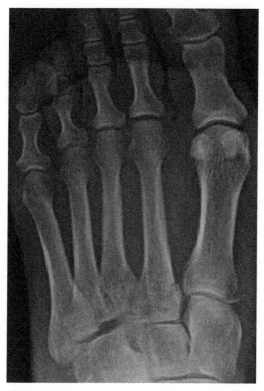

Fig. 12. Lisfranc fracture.

Weight-bearing AP and lateral views may help with the diagnosis but are not needed in the ED. These views may be technically difficult acutely because of significant pain. Advanced imaging including CT, bone scans, and MRI can greatly assist accurate diagnosis, but these tests are not indicated in the ED. CT provides excellent bony detail and may identify small avulsion fractures or detect misalignment that suggests Lisfranc injury. MRI can identify individual ligament ruptures and predict midfoot instability.[43]

The emergency management of Lisfranc injuries depends on the severity of the injury. Fracture-dislocations with significant swelling need to be observed for compartment syndrome and require orthopedic consultation. Displaced Lisfranc injuries require ORIF because most closed reductions cannot be maintained with casting alone. Nondisplaced Lisfranc injuries can be managed with a posterior splint and early orthopedic follow-up. These nondisplaced Lisfranc injuries usually require a short leg cast for 6 weeks with weight-bearing views of the foot at 4 to 6 weeks. Lisfranc injuries with less than 2 mm of diastasis on weight-bearing radiographs can be managed conservatively.[39] The best predictor of outcome is stable anatomic alignment.[46] There is a high incidence of posttraumatic arthritis with Lisfranc injuries. All patients with pain in the area of the Lisfranc joint should receive prompt referral to an orthopedist to avoid missing subtle injuries.

PROXIMAL FIFTH METATARSAL FRACTURES

The proximal fifth metatarsal is the most common site of midfoot fractures.[47,48] The clinical presentation of fractures involving the proximal fifth metatarsal is similar to that of ankle sprains, often resulting in an inaccurate diagnosis if a cursory examination is performed at the initial presentation. Any patient with an inversion injury, or ankle sprain, must have the base of the fifth metatarsal palpated and filmed if tender. There are 2 basic types of proximal fifth metatarsal fractures: the avulsion fracture of the fifth metatarsal tuberosity and fracture of the proximal diaphyseal metatarsal shaft, a true Jones fracture.[2,6] The Jones fracture of the fifth metatarsal occurs at least 1.5 cm distal to the metatarsal styloid in the area of the metaphyseal-diaphyseal junction and may be unimpressive radiographically (**Fig. 13**). These 2 fractures vary considerably in treatment, prognosis, and complications. A third type of proximal fifth metatarsal fracture is the proximal diaphyseal stress fracture.[49,50] From an emergency medicine viewpoint, this fracture can be considered in the same manner as a true Jones fracture.[49]

Historically, the mechanism of injury can be similar for these 2 fractures. An inversion of the foot while the ankle is plantar flexed may produce an avulsion fracture of the fifth metatarsal tuberosity. Jones fractures result from a vertical or medially directed force applied to a plantar flexed foot.[50] Acute onset of pain at the base of the fifth metatarsal with difficulty bearing weight will occur. The physical examination will reveal bony tenderness at the base of the fifth metatarsal. Passive inversion and resisted eversion cause pain. Also, compression of the metatarsal heads will produce pain at the base of the fifth metatarsal.

Radiographically, the avulsion fracture of the fifth metatarsal tuberosity will generally be transverse and proximal to the distal cuboid (**Fig. 14**). An apophysis near the base of the fifth metatarsal may be mistaken for an avulsion fracture. Apophyses of early adolescence are oriented parallel to the bone rather than transverse or oblique.

The treatment of nondisplaced avulsion fractures is symptomatic. It includes a walking boot or hard-soled shoe with weight bearing as tolerated. This conservative treatment should continue until symptoms subside, usually within 4 to 6 weeks. Displaced avulsion fractures greater than 2 mm, or articular surface step-off with the cuboid or involving more than one-third of the cubometatarsal articulation surface, require orthopedic referral and subsequent surgical treatment.[51]

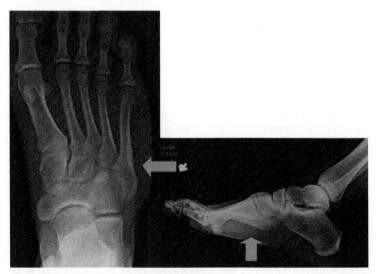

Fig. 13. AP and lateral views of a Jones fracture.

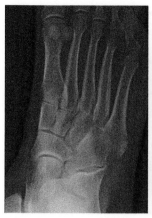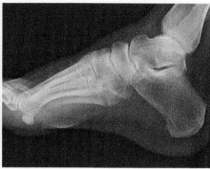

Fig. 14. AP and lateral views of an avulsion fracture of the fifth metatarsal tuberosity.

The early treatment of Jones fractures involves posterior splinting with non–weight bearing and early orthopedic follow-up. ORIF is the preferred treatment of athletes and active patients.[52,53] Prolonged immobilization may be required if conservative treatment is used. These fractures have a high rate of nonunion, delayed union, and recurrence when managed conservatively.[53] Proximal fifth metatarsal diaphyseal stress fractures heal even more poorly.[50]

CALCANEAL FRACTURES

Calcaneal fractures are associated with a high-energy, axial load mechanism.[54] In 30% of cases, another lower extremity fracture is associated with a calcaneal fracture, and compression fractures of the lumbar spine occur in 10% to 15% of cases.[54] In addition to being the largest tarsal bone, it is the most frequently fractured tarsal bone. These fractures are bilateral in 7% of cases. Approximately 25% to 30% of cases are extra-articular, so the subtalar joint (talocalcaneal joint) is involved in most cases.[55,56] The patient will be unable to bear weight.

The physical examination must include a search for associated injuries. In addition, the heel will be swollen, tender, and ecchymotic. The heel will be markedly tender with gentle cupping of the examiner's hand. Mondor sign is a midplantar ecchymosis seen with calcaneal fractures.[57]

Although diagnostic of the fracture, the standard foot series does not always reveal the full extent of subtalar joint involvement, which is important for treatment decisions (**Fig. 15**). Evaluating the Bohler angle may help diagnose a fracture with compression. On the lateral view of the foot, a line drawn from the posterior tuberosity of the calcaneus to the apex of the posterior facet forms a 20° to 40° angle with a line drawn from the apex of the posterior facet to the apex of the anterior process.[9,17] A calcaneal fracture must be suspected if this angle is less than 20° or greater than 40°. An axial view (Harris view) can be used to view the subtalar joint and calcaneal tuberosity if standard radiographs do not reveal a suspected fracture (**Fig. 16**). CT has greatly improved the ability to accurately evaluate complex fractures including the extent of subtalar joint involvement (**Fig. 17**).

There is no consensus on optimal management. A substantial subset of these fractures does poorly regardless of management.[58] A 15-year study of displaced, intraarticular calcaneal fractures failed to show any difference in clinical outcomes between

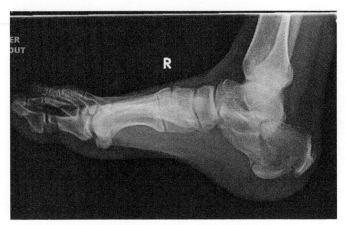

Fig. 15. Lateral foot radiograph showing a calcaneal fracture.

operative and conservative treatment.[58] Early complications include fracture blisters and compartment syndrome. Late complications include subtalar arthritis, chronic pain, wound infection, and sural neuritis.[43] The goal of surgical management is to restore the height and length of the calcaneus, realign the posterior facet of the subtalar joint, and restore the mechanical axis of the hindfoot. Displaced calcaneal fractures require orthopedic consultation. Extra-articular fractures are treated conservatively with a few exceptions. These exceptions include displaced fractures

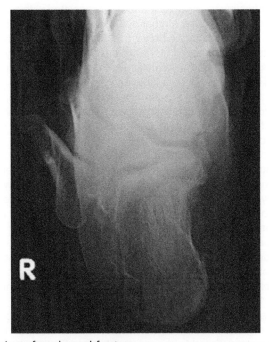

Fig. 16. An axial view of a calcaneal fracture.

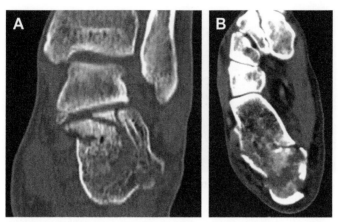

Fig. 17. (*A*) CT shows an intraarticular fracture with subtalar involvement. (*B*) CT shows the comminuted calcaneal fracture.

of the sustentaculum tali, posterior fractures, and some calcaneal body fractures.[58] With a fracture of the sustentaculum tali, the flexor hallucis longus tendon may be interposed with nonoperative management of displaced fractures.[6,58]

TALAR FRACTURES

The talus is the second largest tarsal bone and the second most commonly fractured tarsal bone.[6] Its fractures are typically divided into major and minor fractures. Major talar fractures include fractures to the body, head, or neck of the talus.[6] Fifty percent of major talar injuries are talar neck fractures.[6] Patients with major talar fractures typically describe a high-energy hyperdorsiflexion of the ankle joint as the mechanism of injury, such as motor vehicle crashes or falls from a height. Minor talar fractures include avulsion fractures of the lateral, medial, and posterior processes as well as those from the superior neck and head. These injuries are caused by sudden forces applied to an inverted, dorsiflexed foot.[59] The presentation is that of lateral ankle pain after an inversion mechanism. A fracture of the lateral process of the talus has become a common snowboarding injury.[60,61]

There are no unique findings on physical examination. There may be loss of the hindfoot contour, swelling, tenderness, and ecchymosis. The foot and ankle must be assessed for any open wounds, ischemic skin changes, and neurovascular integrity. Radiographically, most major talar fractures will be shown on standard ankle and foot radiographs (**Fig. 18**). Many minor talar fractures may be occult on plain radiography and require a CT for visualization if these injuries are suspected.[62]

The initial management of minor talar fractures is posterior splinting, non–weight bearing, and orthopedic follow-up. Major talar fractures will usually require ORIF unless precise anatomic alignment is present.[63] Any significantly displaced major talar fracture will require an early closed reduction attempt to decrease the risk of avascular necrosis.[63] Urgent orthopedic consultation is recommended for all major talar fractures.[2]

Complications of major talar fractures include avascular necrosis, skin necrosis, posttraumatic arthritis, malunion, and nonunion. These fractures have a high risk of avascular necrosis because of the tenuous blood supply of the talus.[61,62]

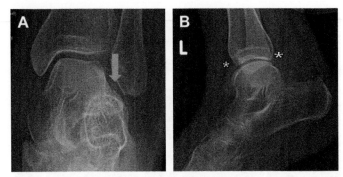

Fig. 18. (*A*) A subtle talar avulsion fracture. (*B*) Lateral view shows ankle effusion (*asterisks*).

SUMMARY

The EP must be aware of the anatomy of the leg, ankle, and foot. The varied presentation of common injuries must be recognized, as well as the unique presentations of uncommon injuries. The astute EP must rely on a focused history and a precise examination to avoid the pitfalls and missed injuries from an over-reliance on radiographic studies. Potential complications associated with these injuries must be anticipated and avoided if possible.

REFERENCES

1. Lyn E, Pallin D, Antosia RE. Knee and lower leg. In: Marx JA, Hockberger RS, Walls RM, et al, editors. Rosen's emergency medicine. Philadelphia: Mosby Elsevier; 2006. p. 770–807.
2. Powers J, Boenau I. Common fractures of the knee and lower leg. Emerg Med 2005;37:46–53.
3. Cannada LK, Anglen JO, Archdeacon MT, et al. Avoiding complications in tibial fractures. J Bone Joint Surg Am 2008;90:1760–8.
4. Hoover TJ, Siefert JA. Soft tissue complications of orthopedic emergencies. Emerg Med Clin North Am 2000;18:115–39.
5. Brinker MR, Bailey DE Jr. Fracture healing in tibia fractures with an associated vascular injury. J Trauma 1997;42:11–9.
6. Park S, Ahn J, Gee AO, et al. Compartment syndrome in tibial fractures. J Orthop Trauma 2009;23:514–8.
7. Fong DT, Man CY, Yung PS, et al. Sports-related injuries attending an accident and emergency department. Injury 2008;39:1222–7.
8. Ivins D. Acute ankle sprain: an update. Am Fam Physician 2006;74:1714–20.
9. Ho K, Abu-Laban RB. Ankle and foot. In: Marx JA, Hockberger RS, Walls RM, et al, editors. Rosen's emergency medicine. Philadelphia: Mosby Elsevier; 2006. p. 808–41.
10. Press CM, Gupta A, Hutchinson MR. Management of ankle syndesmosis injuries in the athlete. Curr Sports Med Rep 2009;8:228–33.
11. Liu SH, Williams JJ. Lateral ankle sprains and instability problems. Clin Sports Med 1994;13:793–809.
12. Haller PR. Leg injuries. In: Tintinalli JE, Kelen GD, Stapczynski JS, editors. Emergency medicine: a comprehensive study guide. New York: McGraw-Hill; 2004. p. 1734–6.

13. Lin CF, Gross MT, Weinhold P. Ankle syndesmosis injuries: anatomy, biomechanics, mechanism of injury, and clinical guidelines for diagnosis and intervention. J Orthop Sports Phys Ther 2006;36:372–84.

14. Nussbaum ED, Hossea TM, Sieler SD, et al. Prospective evaluation of syndesmotic ankle sprains without diastasis. Am J Sports Med 2001;29:31–4.

15. Kiter E, Bozkurt M. The crossed-leg test for examination of ankle syndesmotic injuries. Foot Ankle Int 2005;26:187–8.

16. Zalavras C, Thordarson D. Ankle syndesmotic injury. J Am Acad Orthop Surg 2007;15:330–9.

17. Williamson B, Schwartz DT. The ankle and leg. In: Schwartz DT, Reisdorff E, editors. Emergency radiology. New York: McGraw-Hill; 2000. p. 157–84.

18. Cooke MW, Marsh JL, Clark M, et al. Treatment of severe ankle sprain: a pragmatic randomized controlled trial comparing the clinical effectiveness and cost-effectiveness of three types of mechanical ankle support with tubular bandage. The CAST Trial. Health Technol Assess 2009;13:111–21.

19. Lamb SE, Marsh J, Hutton J, et al. Mechanical supports for acute, severe ankle sprain: a pragmatic, multicentre, randomized controlled trial. Lancet 2008;373: 575–81.

20. Boyce SH, Quigley MA, Campbell S. Management of ankle sprains: a randomized controlled trial of the treatment of inversion injuries using an elastic support bandage or an Aircast ankle brace. Br J Sports Med 2005;39:91–6.

21. Beynnon BD, Renstrom PA, Haugh, et al. A prospective, randomized clinical investigation of the treatment of first-time ankle sprains. Am J Sports Med 2006;34:1401–12.

22. van Rijn RM, van Os AG, Bernsen RM, et al. What is the clinical course of acute ankle sprains? A systematic literature review. Am J Med 2008;121(4): 324–31.

23. Stiell IG, Greenberg GH, McKnight RD, et al. Decision rules for the use of radiography in acute ankle injuries. Refinement and prospective validation. JAMA 1993; 269:1127–32.

24. Bachman LM, Kolb E, Koller MT, et al. Accuracy of Ottawa ankle rules to exclude fractures of the ankle and mid-foot: a systematic review. BMJ 2003; 326:417–22.

25. Stiell IG, Michael JA. Ankle injuries. In: Tintinalli JE, Kelen GD, Stapczynski JS, editors. Emergency medicine: a comprehensive study guide. New York: McGraw-Hill; 2004. p. 1736–41.

26. Tarkin IS, Clare MP, Marcantonio A, et al. An update on the management of high-energy pilon fractures. Injury 2008;39:142–54.

27. Kline AJ, Gruen GS, Pape HC, et al. Early complications following the operative treatment of pilon fractures with and without diabetes. Foot Ankle Int 2009;30: 1042–7.

28. Hermus JP, Driessen MJ, Mulder H, et al. The triplane variant of the tibial apophyseal fracture: a case report and a review of the literature. J Pediatr Orthop B 2003;12:406–8.

29. El-Karef E, Sadek HI, Narin DS, et al. Triplane fracture of the distal tibia. Injury 2000;31:729–36.

30. Jones S, Phillips N, Ali F. Triplane fractures of the distal tibia requiring open reduction and internal fixation. Pre-operative planning using computed tomography. Injury 2003;34:293–8.

31. Kim JR, Song KH, Song KJ, et al. Treatment outcomes of triplane and Tillaux fractures of the ankle in adolescence. Clin Orthop Surg 2010;2:34–8.

32. Ufberg J, Harrigan RA, Cruz T, et al. Orthopedic pitfalls in the ED: Achilles tendon rupture. Am J Emerg Med 2004;22:596–600.
33. Hanlon DP. Bilateral Achilles tendon rupture: an unusual occurrence. J Emerg Med 1992;10:559–61.
34. Sabb TG, Kadakia AR. Non-surgical management of Achilles ruptures. Foot Ankle Clin 2009;14:675–84.
35. Landvater SJ, Renstrom P. Complete Achilles tendon rupture. Clin Sports Med 1992;11:741–58.
36. Mazzone MF, McCue T. Common conditions of the Achilles tendon. Am Fam Physician 2002;65:1805–10.
37. Deangelis JP, Wilson KM, Cox CL, et al. Achilles tendon rupture in athletes. J Surg Orthop Adv 2009;18:115–21.
38. Lattermann C, Goldstein JL, Wukich DK, et al. Practical management of Lisfranc injuries in athletes. Clin J Sport Med 2007;17:311–5.
39. Nunley JA, Vertullo CJ. Classification, investigation, and management of midfoot sprains. Am J Sports Med 2002;30:871–8.
40. Perron AD, Brady WJ, Keats TE. Orthopedic pitfalls in the ED: Lisfranc fracture-dislocation. Am J Emerg Med 2001;19:71–5.
41. Sherief TI, Mucci B, Greiss M. Lisfranc injury: how frequently does it get missed? And how can we improve? Injury 2007;38:856–60.
42. Curtis MJ, Meyerson M, Szura B. Tarsometatarsal joint injuries in the athlete. Am J Sports Med 1993;21:497–502.
43. Raiken SM, Elias I, Dheer S, et al. Prediction of midfoot instability in the subtle Lisfranc injury. Comparison of MRI with intraoperative findings. J Bone Joint Surg Am 2008;91:892–9.
44. Kaar S, Femino J, Morag Y. Lisfranc joint displacement following sequential ligament sectioning. J Bone Joint Surg Am 2007;89:2225–32.
45. Ross G, Cronin R, Hausenblas J. Plantar ecchymosis sign: a clinical aid to diagnosis of occult Lisfranc tarsometatarsal injuries. J Orthop Trauma 1996;10:119–22.
46. Philbin T, Rosenberg G, Sferra JJ. Complications of missed or untreated Lisfranc injuries. Foot Ankle Clin 2003;8:61–71.
47. Fetzer GB, Wright RW. Metatarsal shaft fractures and fractures of the proximal fifth metatarsal. Clin Sports Med 2006;25:139–50.
48. Shuen WM, Boulton C, Batt ME, et al. Metatarsal fractures and sports. Surgeon 2009;7:86–8.
49. Den Hartog BD. Fracture of the proximal fifth metatarsal. J Am Acad Orthop Surg 2009;17:458–64.
50. Hatch RL, Alsobrook JA, Clugston JR. Diagnosis and management of metatarsal fractures. Am Fam Physician 2007;76:817–26.
51. Lawrence SJ, Botte MJ. Jones' fractures and related fractures of the proximal fifth metatarsal. Foot Ankle 1993;14:358–65.
52. Wedmore IS, Charette J. Emergency department evaluation and treatment of ankle and foot injuries. Emerg Med Clin North Am 1994;18:85–113.
53. Mologne TS, Lundeen JM, Clapper MF, et al. Early screw fixation versus casting in the treatment of acute Jones fractures. Am J Sports Med 2005;33:970–5.
54. Germann CA, Perron AD, Miller MD, et al. Orthopedic pitfalls in the ED: calcaneal fractures. Am J Emerg Med 2004;22:607–11.
55. Swanson SA, Clare MP, Sanders RW. Management of intra-articular fractures of the calcaneus. Foot Ankle Clin 2008;13:659–78.
56. Bajammal S, Tornetta P, Sanders D, et al. Displaced intra-articular calcaneal fractures. J Orthop Trauma 2005;19:360–4.

57. Richman JD, Barre PS. The plantar ecchymosis sign in fractures of the calcaneus. Clin Orthop 1986;207:122–5.
58. Ibrahim T, Rowsell M, Rennie W, et al. Displaced intra-articular calcaneal fractures: 15-year follow-up of a randomized controlled trial of conservative versus operative treatment. Injury 2007;38:848–55.
59. McCrory P, Bladin C. Fractures of the lateral process of the talus: a clinical review. Clin Sports Med 1996;6:124–8.
60. Chan GM, Yoshido D. Fracture of the lateral process of the talus associated with snow boarding. Ann Emerg Med 2003;41:854–6.
61. Kirkpatrick DP, Hunter RE, Janes PC, et al. The snowboarder's foot and ankle. Am J Sports Med 1998;26:271–7.
62. Vallier HA, Nork SE, Barei DP, et al. Talar neck fractures: results and outcomes. J Bone Joint Surg Am 2004;86:1616–24.
63. Elgafy H, Ebraheim NA, Tile M, et al. Fractures of the talus: experience of two level 1 trauma centers. Foot Ankle Int 2000;21:1023–9.

Pediatric Orthopedic Emergencies

Rose M. Chasm, MD[a,b,*], Sharon A. Swencki, MD[a]

KEYWORDS

- Pediatric • Orthopedics • Emergency department • Fracture
- Child abuse • Limp

Many well-seasoned emergency physicians often find it challenging to assess and treat pediatric patients regardless of the complaint. Because of anatomic and physiologic differences, pediatric patients experience orthopedic injuries that are both unique and specific to this subset of the population. Emergency physicians must be aware of these nuances to properly diagnose and treat these injuries.

Among children who come to emergency departments (EDs) with an acute traumatic injury, almost 20% will have a fracture.[1] Not surprisingly, boys sustain fractures more commonly than girls during childhood, at a rate of 42% and 27%, respectively.[1,2]

PEDIATRIC BONE ANATOMY

Before any discussion of specific pediatric orthopedic injuries, the major anatomic regions of growing bone must be reviewed briefly (**Fig. 1**). The epiphysis is the rounded end of a long bone at its joint with adjacent bone. It is a secondary ossification center and is separated from the rest of the bone by the cartilaginous epiphyseal plate, or growth plate. This anatomy is important to note because ossification centers and the subsequent closure of the epiphyseal plate become visible on radiograph films at various times, making fracture identification difficult. The shaft or the main midsection of a long bone, otherwise known as the *diaphysis*, is composed of cortical bone. It contains both bone marrow and adipose tissue.

Although obtaining comparison radiographs is not a defined requirement in all pediatric patients, they may be especially helpful for children whose epiphyseal plate has not completely ossified. Most pediatric long bones have ossified by the end of puberty.

---

[a] Department of Emergency Medicine, University of Maryland School of Medicine, 110 South Paca Street, 6th Floor, Suite 200, Baltimore, MD 21201, USA
[b] Combined Emergency Medicine/Pediatrics Residency, University of Maryland Medical Center, 110 South Paca Street, 6th Floor, Suite 200, Baltimore, MD 21201, USA
* Corresponding author. Department of Emergency Medicine, University of Maryland School of Medicine, 110 South Paca Street, 6th Floor, Suite 200, Baltimore, MD 21201.
E-mail address: rchas001@umaryland.edu

Emerg Med Clin N Am 28 (2010) 907–926
doi:10.1016/j.emc.2010.06.003
0733-8627/10/$ – see front matter © 2010 Elsevier Inc. All rights reserved.

emed.theclinics.com

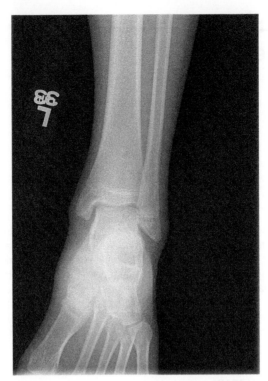

Fig. 1. Radiograph indicating major anatomic regions of pediatric growing bone.

PEDIATRIC FRACTURE TYPES

The periosteum of growing immature pediatric bone is strong but more pliable than completely matured adult bone, often leading to bowing injuries rather than the typical fractures that typically occur in adults. A compressive force in a child may result in a buckle or torus fracture rather than the impacted fractures experienced by adult patients. This type of injury is most commonly seen in distal forearm injuries (**Fig. 2**). Greenstick fractures occur as a result of force applied to the side of a long bone. Only one side of the cortex is disrupted, whereas the other is merely bent (**Fig. 3**). Infants may experience complete bowing of the bone without any interruption of the cortex, leading to a plastic deformation.

Growth plate injuries constitute nearly 20% of all pediatric skeletal injuries.[1] Damage to the physis may disrupt bone growth and lead to limb length discrepancies at that site anywhere from 1% to 10% of the time.[3] Although the degree of growth disturbance is not predictable, the most common growth disturbance is premature partial arrest of linear growth. The Salter-Harris classification stratifies physeal injuries according to the risk of growth disturbance (**Fig. 4**).[4]

The most common physeal fracture, which is seen in half of all growth plate injuries, is a Salter-Harris type II fracture, which involves both the metaphysis and the growth plate. In general, Salter-Harris type I and II fractures have a low risk of growth disturbance. However, the relative risk increases from Salter-Harris type I to V. Other factors, such as severity of injury, which includes the degree of displacement or comminution; patient age; and the particular physis injured are also important.[5] Because

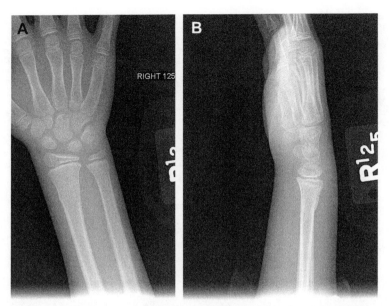

Fig. 2. (*A*, *B*) Radiograph of buckle/torus fracture of distal radius. Note the discrete swelling or interruption of the cortex seen on both views, but seen best on the lateral film (*B*).

nondisplaced Salter-Harris type I and II fractures usually heal well with few complications, emergency physicians may confidently immobilize these injuries in the acute setting, allowing for outpatient follow-up with an orthopedic specialist or the primary pediatrician on a nonurgent basis within a month after injury.[6] Children with nondisplaced Salter-Harris type III, IV, or V fractures should be referred to an orthopedic specialist for urgent definitive care no more than 3 to 5 days after the injury.[6]

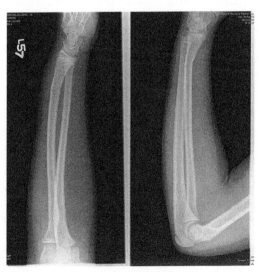

Fig. 3. Radiograph of greenstick fracture of distal radius. Note only one side of the cortex is disrupted whereas the other is merely bent with no cortical interruption.

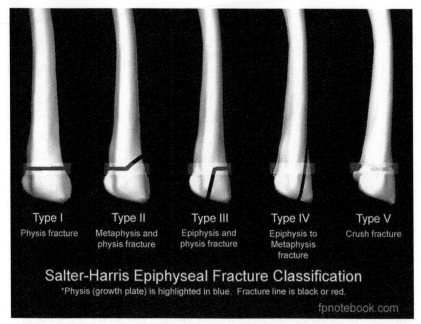

Fig. 4. Diagram of Salter-Harris classification. (*From* Family Practice Notebook.com. Available at: http://www.fpnotebook.com/_media/OrthoFractureSalterHarris.jpg. Accessed August 7, 2010; with permission.)

Differentiating Salter-Harris type I and type V fractures can be problematic, because both involve only the growth plate and may be difficult to identify on plain film. Thus, many authors recommend treating any injury with pain at the physis as a presumed fracture, and recommend early follow-up. Splinting techniques are comparable to those used in adults. Children often require shorter periods of immobilization because pediatric fractures usually heal faster, which is beneficial to patients but problematic for clinicians because they have less time to detect and reduce malpositioned fragments. Children rarely experience stiffness or decreased range of motion after fractures, and therefore repeat visits for pain or need for physical therapy is rare.

Distal Radial Fracture

By far, the most common fracture site in pediatric patients is the distal radius, occurring in two-thirds of children treated for fractures in the ED.[1,7] Because of the increase in certain recreational activities, such as snow- and skateboarding, the incidence of these fractures has increased nearly 40% over the past 3 decades.[8] Most distal radial metaphyseal fractures occur during adolescence, when bone growth velocity peaks, leading to relative bone porosity, and when children engage in activities that put them at risk for injury. The most common mechanism of injury is a fall on an outstretched hand.

Torus fractures are usually nondisplaced and may be very difficult to diagnose on radiographs because the findings may be subtle. These fractures are best seen on the lateral view (see **Fig. 2**). Reduction is unnecessary unless angulation is greater than 15°. These fractures may be placed in a short arm volar splint, and patients should be seen by an orthopedic surgeon within 5 days for conversion to a short arm cast. Patients are typically in a cast for 2 to 4 weeks. Use of a short arm volar splint for the entire length of treatment is an acceptable alternative, obviating the need for urgent follow-up while providing comfort and protection from reinjury.[9–11]

Children with greenstick and complete fractures should be referred to an orthopedic surgeon within 3 to 5 days after injury, because they are at risk of displacement or reangulation associated with growth during healing. Nondisplaced greenstick fractures (see **Fig. 3**) can be treated emergently with a volar short arm splint unless more than 15° of angulation is present. Angulated fractures should emergently undergo closed reduction and immobilization in a long arm splint, with orthopedic follow-up within 3 days.

Distal radial fractures rarely occur in isolation; therefore, radiographs must be reviewed thoroughly for associated ulnar styloid and distal ulnar fractures. Dedicated radiographs of the surrounding joints, including the wrist and elbow, should be obtained to exclude the presence of associated scaphoid and supracondylar fractures, respectively. In addition, nerve injury should be excluded if significant swelling or fracture angulation is present. A complete median and ulnar nerve examination is necessary.

As stated, physeal fractures can be difficult to diagnose. One reliable sign of an occult fracture is the presence of the pronator fat pad along the volar aspect of the distal radius, which can be seen on the lateral view (**Fig. 5**).[12]

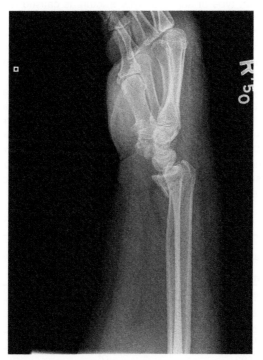

Fig. 5. Radiograph showing a pronator fat pad secondary to distal radius fracture in an adult, but would have a comparable appearance in a child.

Elbow Fracture

Among all pediatric fractures, 10% involve the elbow. These fractures are often complex and challenging to diagnose, and should be managed by an orthopedist because they have the potential for secondary neurovascular injury. More than half of all pediatric elbow fractures are supracondylar, because this is the weakest part of the elbow joint.[13] The younger the child, the more difficult the fracture may be to diagnose, because the elbow has six ossification centers that ossify at various ages from 1 to 11 years. Comparison views and additional oblique views can assist in the diagnosis.[14,15] Although it is unnecessary to memorize the exact ages at which these ossification centers appear or fuse, it is clinically important to know that they appear in a specific sequence. There are two commonly taught mnemonics for this sequence of appearance (**Table 1**). The first is C-R-I-T-O-E (capitellum, radial head, internal or medial epicondyle, trochlea, olecranon, and external or lateral epicondyle). The other is "Come Read My Tale Of Love."

Vital landmarks on radiographs can help diagnose occult fractures. The anterior humeral line is a parallel line that is drawn along the anterior edge of the humerus, and should bisect the middle of the capitellum (**Fig. 6**). Another important landmark is the radiocapitellar line, which should course through the axis of the radius and point directly to the capitellum, regardless of which radiographic view is obtained (**Fig. 7**). Any disruption of the anterior humeral line or the radiocapitellar line indicates a displaced fracture.

One final indication of an occult fracture is the posterior fat pad sign, which is seen on the lateral radiograph.[16] Although the presence of an anterior fat pad or the absence of a posterior fat pad does not rule out an occult fracture, a posterior fat pad is always pathologic, indicating an occult fracture (**Fig. 8**).[16]

The most common type of supracondylar fracture is caused by a fall on an outstretched hand, wherein the outstretched arm is hyperextended and drives the olecranon into the supracondylar portion of the humerus. Displacement is common. Bone fragments retained within the confined space of the elbow, and concomitant swelling, can lead to vascular and neurologic compromise. Thus, a complete neurovascular examination is important to perform.

Compartment syndrome of the distal forearm is another potential complication of a supracondylar fracture. If the patient is experiencing increased pain and has a tense forearm accompanied by paresthesia or increased pain with passive extension of the digits or wrist, compartment syndrome should be considered. Delays in diagnosis can result in Volkmann's ischemic contracture, which results in severe muscle fibrosis and neuropathy, leaving the extremity functionless with few treatment options.[17]

Because of these complications and the fact that most supracondylar fractures are displaced, patients with this fracture should be referred emergently to an orthopedist

Table 1
Sequence of appearance or fusion of ossification centers in the elbow

	Growth Center		Ossification Age
C	Capitellum	Come	1 year
R	Radial head	Read	3 years
I	Internal/Medial epicondyle	My (Medial)	5 years
T	Trochlea	Tale	7 years
O	Olecranon	Of	9 years
E	External/Lateral epicondyle	Love (Lateral)	11 years

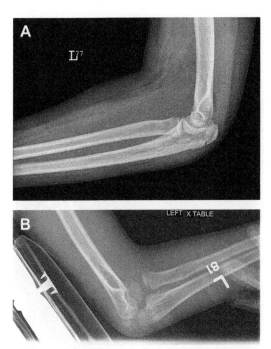

Fig. 6. (A, B) Radiograph depicting an anterior humeral line violation in a supracondylar fracture. The anterior humeral line is the parallel line drawn along the anterior edge of the humerus, and should bisect the middle of the capitellum in a normal radiograph.

for surgical intervention. While awaiting transfer, the extremity should be immobilized in a long arm splint, with the forearm placed in a neutral position and the elbow at 90°. Care should be taken to not apply the splint too tightly, because progression of swelling could result in iatrogenic compartment syndrome.

Nursemaid's Elbow

Radial head subluxation, or nursemaid's elbow, is a common pediatric injury seen in infants as young as 6 months up to older preteen children, but most commonly in children between ages 1 and 3 years. The classic history of injury is a sudden longitudinal traction on the extended arm with the wrist in pronation, as occurs when an uncooperative child is lifted up from the wrist by someone who is taller. This mechanism tears the attachment of the annular ligament to the neck of the radius, with the detached portion becoming trapped between the subluxed radial head and the capitellum.[17] Children are brought to the ED when they refuse to use that arm and hold it in a flexed and pronated position. Traditional teaching to reduce the subluxation has been to perform firm supination of the forearm, with the other hand supporting the elbow in 90° of flexion until a click is heard.

Since 1990, however, several studies have proposed that hyperpronation rather than supination with flexion of the elbow has better success rates and is less painful.[18–20] A Cochrane review of those studies, published in mid-2009, concluded that evidence from those small low-quality trials was too limited to change current practice, and recommended that a randomized prospective trial would be beneficial.[21] Shortly thereafter, Bek and colleagues[21] published a randomized clinical trial of 66 patients,

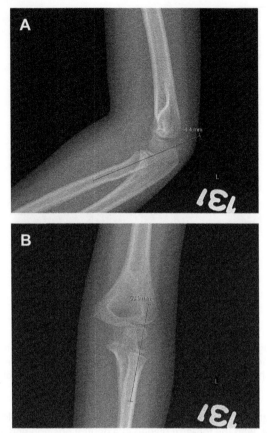

Fig. 7. (*A, B*) Radiograph depicting a radiocapitellar line violation in a supracondylar fracture. The radiocapitellar line courses through the axis of the radius and normally should point directly to the capitellum, regardless of which radiographic view is obtained.

which showed first-time success rates of reduction of 94% with hyperpronation compared with 69% with supination, and second-attempt success rates of 100% with hyperpronation and 91% with supination. Dislocations that could not be relocated with supination were successfully reduced on the first attempt with the hyperpronation method. The authors did not definitively report a difference in pain between the groups.[22]

Ankle Injuries

Before publication of the Ottawa Ankle Rules (OAR), most patients with ankle injuries underwent imaging to rule out fractures. Only 15% of these images were positive for fractures. What initially began as a small single-site trial in Ottawa Hospital by a team of urgent care doctors was expanded to a multicenter study. The results of that study were developed into what is now the generally accepted guideline to determine when radiographs are needed to rule out ankle fractures. These results have a sensitivity of nearly 100% for predicting the presence of a fracture, and reduced the need for radiographs by approximately 35%.[23] The OAR state that radiographs are required

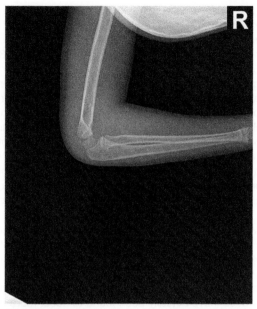

Fig. 8. Radiograph showing posterior fat pad that is pathologic of an elbow fracture.

when the patient has bony pain in the malleolar zone and any one of the following:[24–26]

- Bone tenderness along the distal 6 cm of the posterior edge of the tibia or tip of the medial malleolus
- Bone tenderness along the distal 6 cm of the posterior edge of the fibula or tip of the lateral malleolus
- An inability to bear weight for four steps, both immediately and in the ED.

Although generally accepted for the adult population, the OAR only recently have garnered support for use in children older than 6 years.[26–29] Applying the OAR to younger children is difficult, because they often refuse to ambulate out of fear or lack of cooperation rather than a true inability to bear weight because of a fracture.[27–30]

Gravel and colleagues[30] published a prospective head-to-head comparison of the OAR, Low-Risk Exam, and Malleolar Zone Algorithm, which were all designed to minimize the number of radiographs performed on children after ankle injury. The conclusion was that the OAR identified all children with clinically important fractures, whereas the Low-Risk Exam and Malleolar Zone Algorithm had sensitivities of 87% and 94%, respectively. Based on these findings, the OAR is the most reliable guideline in both adults and children.

CHILD ABUSE

Child abuse often results in orthopedic injuries. Therefore, clinicians must be vigilant to consider abuse (nonaccidental trauma) in the differential diagnosis of any child presenting to the ED with a fracture. A recent study from The Children's Hospital of Philadelphia (CHOP) comparing orthopedic injuries caused by accidental and nonaccidental trauma in children younger than 4 years found that children experiencing nonaccidental trauma were more likely to be younger (11.7 vs 22.1 months), with no gender predominance among the victims.[31] Of all fractures resulting from child abuse, 80% occur in children younger than 18-months,[32] whereas 85% of accidental fractures occur in children older then 5 years.[32]

When assessing whether a fracture occurred accidentally or nonaccidentally, the developmental stage of the child is important to consider. Rib fractures at any age are indicative of nonaccidental trauma,[31,33] and children presenting with multiple fractures are more likely to have experienced abuse.[33] Although no one long bone fracture is indicative of abuse, the study from CHOP found that tibia/fibula, humerus, and femur fractures in patients younger than 18 months are more likely the result of nonaccidental trauma, whereas humerus and femur fractures in children older than 18 months are more likely the result of accidental trauma.[31] Nonaccidental and accidental trauma cannot be easily differentiated in tibia/fibula fractures in children older than 18 months.[31]

A systematic review of literature on fractures and child abuse recently published in the British Medical Journal found that a femoral shaft fracture in a nonambulatory child is highly suspicious for abuse, as are mid-shaft humerus fractures in children younger than 15 months.[33] On the contrary, a supercondylar fracture is likely the result of accidental trauma, especially in older children.[33] Skull fractures, although often thought to be an indicator of abuse, have actually been found to occur more often in accidental trauma.[31,33]

Long bone diaphysis (shaft) fractures are the most common types of fractures seen in abuse, but are not diagnostic of nonaccidental trauma.[34] However, metaphyseal–epiphyseal fractures (**Fig. 9**) can be considered diagnostic of abuse in children

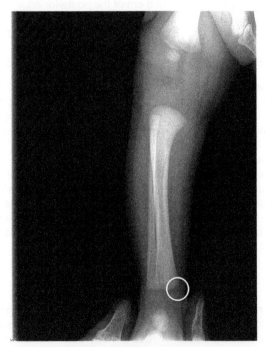

Fig. 9. Radiograph showing distal tibial metaphysis fracture in an infant.

younger than 5 years, and may be seen almost exclusively in infants.[34,35] These fractures, sometimes referred to as bucket-handle or corner fractures, occur when indirect sheering forces are applied to the infant's limb in a pulling or twisting motion, causing avulsion of the immature periosteum at the metaphysis.[34,36]

When nonaccidental trauma is suspected, it must be reported to the proper governmental authorities, as mandated by law nationwide.[37] In these cases, a thorough physical examination focusing on other signs of nonaccidental injury, and detailed documentation are necessary.[37] The clinician should also be prepared to provide testimony or a sworn statement on the child's behalf should legal action result.[37]

THE CHILD WITH A LIMP

Another common cause of concern is the child presenting to the emergency department with a limp or refusal to ambulate. A Scottish study found the incidence of children presenting to the ED with a limp to be 1.8 per 1000 visits.[38] This group had a slight male predominance (male:female ratio of 1.7:1) and a median age of 4.35 years.[38] This presentation poses a challenge to clinicians, because the differential diagnosis of the child with the limp is broad (**Box 1**). Most children with a limp have a benign, self-limiting condition, but the presence of a limp may herald the existence of a severe, life-threatening condition, such as osteosarcoma and leukemia.[39] In these latter cases, a delay in diagnosis can lead to significant morbidity and mortality.

Most patients can be managed entirely in the ED.[38] The onus for the emergency physician is determining which children have a presentation necessitating further workup with laboratory and radiologic studies.

History

History should be obtained from both the caretaker and the patient. If there is any reason to suspect abuse, the patient should be interviewed separately from the parent. Onset and duration of the limp and the presence of pain or trauma are important aspects of the history. Older children can be prompted to localize the pain to one area; however, the presence of referred pain from an adjacent joint must be considered. The young child may be unable to localize the pain, and may simply refuse to walk. If the young child prefers to crawl, pathology of the foot is a more likely diagnosis.[40]

A thorough review of systems is especially important in children presenting with a limp; fever, weight loss, malaise, and respiratory symptoms may be important clues in diagnosis. These concomitant symptoms should suggest a more serious cause of the limp, such as infection, a rheumatologic condition, or malignancy. Timing of the pain may also be a clue to its cause. Rheumatologic conditions more often cause pain that is worse in the morning.[40] A family history of rheumatologic conditions or neuromuscular diseases should be ascertained, because these disease entities are often inherited.

The age of the child at presentation may offer clues to the cause of the gait disturbance. A breakdown of differential diagnoses common for different age groups are provided in **Box 2**.

Physical Examination

Walking requires the integration of nearly all of the body's biomechanical systems. Gait can be affected by a disturbance in the neurologic system, including upper and lower motor neurons or motor end plates, and the musculoskeletal system, including muscles, bones, joints, and ligaments. Pain, weakness, or structural abnormalities of the spine, pelvis, or lower extremity can all affect gait.

Box 1
Differential diagnosis of limp

Trauma

Fractures

Sprains/strains

Contusion

Child abuse

Overuse syndromes

Inflammatory disease

Juvenile rheumatoid arthritis

Systemic lupus erythematosus

Rheumatic fever

Transient synovitis

Congenital abnormality

Developmental dysplasia of the hip

Limb length discrepancy

Sickle cell disease

Cerebral palsy

Orthopedic abnormality

Legg-Calvé-Perthes disease

Slipped capital femoral epiphysis

Infection

Septic arthritis

Osteomyelitis

Diskitis

Soft tissue infection

Neoplasm

Osteosarcoma

Ewing's sarcoma

Lymphoma

Leukemia

The normal gait is a fluid movement consisting of a swing and stance phase. Distinguishing between specific patterns of gait abnormalities can help pinpoint the cause of the limp. The most common gait disturbance is the antalgic gait, which is caused by pain. In the antalgic gait, the stance phase is shortened in an effort to prevent pain in the affected limb. Trendelenburg gait is seen with pathology of the hip. This gait is characterized by a shift in the torso over the affected leg during the stance phase. Steppage gait indicates the inability to dorsiflex the foot. The patient will flex at the hip and knee to allow for the foot to clear the ground. Equinus or toe-walking may indicate limb-length discrepancy, either real or perceived. Knee

---

Box 2
Common diagnoses by age

Age 1–3 years

Septic hip

Developmental dysplasia of the hip

Leg-length discrepancy

Fractures

Age 4–10 years

Legg-Calvé-Perthes disease (idiopathic osteonecrosis of the femoral head)

Juvenile rheumatoid arthritis

Toxic synovitis

Neoplasm

Age 11 years–adult

Overuse syndromes

Avascular necrosis

Slipped capital femoral epiphysis

Gonococcal septic arthritis

Sprains/fracture

All ages

Trauma

Child abuse

Septic arthritis

Osteomyelitis

Neoplasm

Leukemia

Neuromuscular disorders

---

pain or quadriceps weakness may cause the child to keep the leg stiff, causing a vaulting gait.[39,41,42]

The most important part of the physical examination is the observation of the patient walking with and without shoes. Examination of the patient should focus on thoroughly observing their gait—the stance and swing phase of both limbs. During this part of the examination, the child should have as little clothing on as possible from waist down to allow thorough inspection of the lower extremities.[42] Having the child hop and walk on heels and toes can reveal coordination problems and less-obvious or isolated muscle weakness.[42] Abdominal and genital examinations should also be included to rule out diagnoses such as appendicitis or testicular torsion.[42]

Position of comfort should be observed. Tenderness, deformity, erythema, swelling, and range of motion (ROM) should be tested in both of the lower extremities and the lower spine. The child's footwear should be inspected for wear patterns and external causes of gait disturbance, such as foreign body in the shoe.

Laboratory Studies

The decision to obtain laboratory studies in these patients is based on history and physical examination findings. If infection, inflammation, or malignancy are considered as the cause of the limp, a complete blood count with differential, erythrocyte sedimentation rate (ESR), and C-reactive protein (CRP) should be obtained. More specialized laboratory studies, such as Lyme titer and rheumatoid factor, can be obtained as warranted.

Joint fluid is the gold standard for diagnosing septic arthritis, and must be obtained if infection is suspected. This fluid should be sent for Gram stain, culture, and cell count. Blood and bone cultures should be obtained in cases of suspected infections, such as osteomyelitis.

Imaging Studies

Plain radiographs of the affected joint are generally the first diagnostic test and are indicated in almost all cases.[43] Radiographs of the joint above and below the affected or painful joint should be considered because of the possibility of referred pain. One study noted that up to 10% of children with positive hip radiographs had no complaints of hip pain.[38] Although some authors have suggested that toddlers, who are nonverbal, may benefit from being screened with radiograph films of the lower extremities from hip to foot,[44,45] others have found that this may not be warranted in the well-appearing child.[46] Imaging of the unaffected extremity for comparison should always be considered. Patients with complaints of back pain, neurologic deficits, or tenderness or deformity of the back should undergo imaging of the spine. Plain radiographs may be the only imaging modality needed for most patients. Frog-leg lateral views should be ordered for patients with a hip disorder, because singe-view anteroposterior pelvis films may miss significant pathology.

Ultrasound is the preferred imaging modality for detecting effusion of the hip.[47] Bedside ultrasound has been embraced by emergency physicians as a tool to aid in rapid diagnosis in the ED. With its increasing availability, bedside ultrasound can be used as a screening tool to detect effusion, and then as an aid to guide arthrocentesis of the hip.[48,49] To perform this examination, the linear transducer should be used while the patient lies supine. The probe should be placed obliquely parallel to the long axis of the femoral neck and the distance measured between the femoral neck and the posterior surface of the iliopsoas muscle.[48] A measurement of more than 5 mm[50,51] or a difference of 2 mm from the unaffected hip[50–52] indicates a joint effusion.

Bone scintigraphy may be needed when history, physical examination, and radiologic studies fail to localize the cause of the limp in children with persistent symptoms. This imaging modality can help identify stress fracture, occult fracture, metastases, tumors, and infection.[53,54] Although radionucleotide bone scans are unlikely to be an available diagnostic tool for emergency physicians, some experts have suggested that this modality should be used much earlier in the diagnosis of children with a limp.[42] Disease entities such as osteomyelitis may be evident on a bone scintigraphy scan days before abnormalities are seen on plain radiographs, and bone scintigraphy is 25% to 50% more sensitive than radiography in detecting fractures.[53]

The role of CT in the limping child is limited given the high dose of radiation and the efficacy of other imaging modalities.[54] MRI is useful for detecting stress fractures, osteonecrosis, osteomyelitis, myositis, and other abnormalities of surrounding tissue.[42,54]

Synopsis

When evaluating children presenting with a limp, emergency physicians should focus on controlling the pain, attempt to pinpoint the cause of the limp, initiate therapy for any identified cause, and arrange for appropriate disposition and follow-up.[41] In the well-appearing child with a limp, no systemic symptoms, and no concerning history or physical examination, a minimal workup consisting of plain radiographs with observation and reevaluation in a few days has been suggested.[40]

Table 2 summarizes differential diagnoses and their correlating history, physical examination, proposed workup, and disposition for pediatric patients with a limp.

Pitfalls

One pitfall in diagnosing the cause of a limp in a child is attributing the limp to "growing pains." "Growing pains" is a diagnosis of exclusion and should be made only if the patient has bilateral leg pain only in the evening or at night; the child should not have a limp, pain, or symptoms during the day.[40,55] To support the diagnosis of growing pains, the child must have a completely normal physical examination (ie, no limp). Diagnostic imaging and laboratory testing are probably not warranted. These children should not have any systemic symptoms, localizing signs, joint involvement, or limitation of activity.[55] Therefore, children presenting with a limp cannot be experiencing growing pains.

Another pitfall is the diagnosis of "groin pull" in preteens or teenagers who present with hip or groin pain. This diagnosis is rare in adolescents. During the examination, a slipped capital femoral epiphysis (SCFE) must be excluded.[56] Anteroposterior and frog-leg lateral radiographs should be obtained. One technique to diagnose SCFE is to obtain an anteroposterior radiograph of the pelvis and draw Klein's line, a line that, when drawn parallel to the superior edge of the femoral neck, should intersect the epiphysis of the femoral head. If the line does not intersect the epiphysis, SCFE is diagnosed. However, recent evidence calls into question whether this is a reliable method of diagnosis, finding a low sensitivity of Klein's line, especially in mild cases.[57] The study by Green and colleagues[57] proposes a modification of Klein's line, comparing the epiphyseal width lateral to Klein's line, which should differ by less than 2 mm between hips (**Fig. 10**). If the measured width between sides is more than 2 mm, the side with the smallest width would be diagnosed as a SCFE.[57]

The diagnosis of a malignancy in a child is troubling and an important "can't miss" situation for emergency physicians. A study from the DuPont Institute in Delaware found that 11.6% of children diagnosed with leukemia at their institution presented with a limp.[58] These children had an antalgic gait and were experiencing hip or knee pain. Most patients had mild fever and lymphadenopathy, and hepatosplenomegaly was common.[58] Laboratory findings included elevated ESR, anemia, thrombocytopenia, and increased lymphocytes and blast cells on the peripheral blood smear.[58]

One of the most common diagnostic dilemmas in children presenting with a limp is the distinction between transient synovitis and septic arthritis of the hip. Kocher and colleagues[59] described a clinical prediction rule in the differentiation of septic arthritis versus transient synovitis of the hip. These criteria include a white blood cell (WBC) count greater than 12,000 cells/mm^3, ESR greater than 40 mm/h, presence of fever, and the inability to bear weight.[59] More recently, a study found fever to be the best predictor of septic arthritis, along with elevated CRP, elevated ESR, refusal to weight bear, and an elevation of the WBC count.[60]

Table 2
Differential diagnoses, examination findings, and management for children with a limp

Differential	History	Physical Examination	Laboratory	Imaging	Disposition/Follow-up
Traumatic	Injury	Deformity, localized pain, decreased ROM, swelling	None	Plain films, bone scan	Orthopedics/primary care follow-up
Inflammatory disease	Long-term pain, pain in multiple joints, family history, recent illness (transient synovitis)	Warmth or erythema in one or more joints	CBC, ESR, CRP, joint aspirate	Plain films, ultrasound	Rheumatology/primary care follow-up
Congenital abnormality	Since birth	Deformity, leg-length discrepancy, decreased ROM	None	Plain films	Orthopedics/primary care follow-up
Orthopedic abnormality	Painless limp, knee, hip or thigh pain, appropriate age, obesity	Limited ROM, asymmetric ROM, painful ROM	None	Plain films	Orthopedics consult for disposition
Infection	Fever, chills, pain, erythema	Warmth, erythema	CBC, ESR, CRP, joint aspirate	Plain films, MRI, bone scan	Admission with orthopedic consult
Neoplasm	Pain, irritable hip or knee, fever, constitutional symptoms	Lymphadenopathy, hepatosplenomegaly, mass	CBC, ESR, CRP, alkaline phosphatase, calcium, electrolytes	Plain films, MRI, CT, bone scan, staging	Hematology/oncology consult for disposition

Abbreviations: CBC, complete blood count with differential; CRP, C-reactive protein; ESR, erythrocyte sedimentation rate; ROM, range of motion.
Adapted from Leet AL, Skaggs DL. Evaluation of the acutely limping child. Am Fam Physician 2000;61:1011–8; with permission.

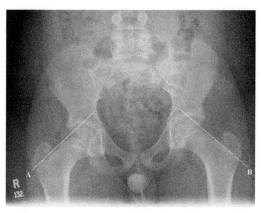

Fig. 10. (A) Mildly displaced SCFE. (B) Normal hip. In this case, Klein's Line intersects the femoral epiphysis on both sides, however by applying Green's modification—comparing the length of femoral epiphysis lateral to Klein's Line—a subtle SCFE is diagnosed.

SUMMARY

The ED evaluation of children with orthopedic complaints is complicated by their unique conditions (eg, radial head dislocation, limp) and the difference in how they must be treated for conditions that affect children and adults. Emergency physicians must be aware of these differences to ensure proper timely diagnosis and management, which can reduce the risk of long-term disability.

An understanding of fractures unique to growing bone, such as buckle/torus and greenstick types, will provoke clinicians to have a keener eye when reviewing pediatric radiographs. The Salter-Harris classification provides a proven, generally accepted stratification of injury to describe and properly disposition pediatric fractures. Emergency physicians must also recognize a distal radial fracture, because it is the most common pediatric fracture, and the many complications of the supracondylar fracture. Although this article dedicates great attention to the differences in orthopedic injuries sustained by adults and children, some similarities exist. Expanding evidence shows that the various guidelines to determine the probability of ankle fractures and need for radiographs in adults may also be used in children.

Children presenting to the ED with a limp or refusal to bear weight can pose a significant challenge for emergency physicians. The differential diagnosis is wide and, although most children will have a benign course, life-threatening causes can present in a similar fashion. Therefore, emergency physicians must be comfortable with the workup of this complaint and be aware of factors in the child's history and physical examination that should lead to a thorough search for a more serious cause of the patient's symptoms.

REFERENCES

1. Wilkins KE. The incidence of fractures in children. In: Rockwood CA, Wilkins KE, Beaty JH, editors. 4th edition, Fractures in children, vol. 3. Philadelphia: Lippincott-Raven; 1996. p. 3–17.
2. Landin LA. Fracture patterns in children: analysis of 8,682 fractures with special reference to incidence, etiology and secular changes in a Swedish urban population 1950–1979. Acta Orthop Scand 1983;54:1–109.

3. Growth plate fractures. Your orthopaedic connection, American Academy of Orthopaedic Surgeons, May 2009. Available at: http://orthoinfo.aaos.org/topic.cfm?topic=A00040. Accessed February 15, 2010.
4. Salter RB, Harris WR. Injuries involving the epiphyseal plate. J Bone Joint Surg Am 1963;45:587.
5. Peterson CA, Peterson HA. Analysis of the incidence of injuries to the epiphyseal growth plate. J Trauma 1972;12:275–81.
6. Eiff MP, Hatch RL. Boning up on common pediatric fractures. Contemp Pediatr 2003. [Online].
7. Khosla S, Melton LJ, Dekutoski MB, et al. Incidence of childhood distal forearm fractures over 30 years: a population based study. JAMA 2003;290:1479–85.
8. Solan MC, Rees R, Daly K. Current management of torus fractures of the distal radius. Injury 2002;33:503–5.
9. Sherbino J. How do I treat pediatric wrist fractures? Ann Emerg Med 2009;54(4):541–2.
10. Randsborg PH, Sivertsen EA. Distal radius fractures in children: substantial difference in stability between buckle and greenstick fractures. Acta Orthop 2009;80(5):585–9.
11. Musharafieh RS, Macari G. Salter-Harris I fractures of the distal radius misdiagnosed as wrist sprain. J Emerg Med 2000;19:265–70.
12. Townsend DJ, Bassett GS. Common elbow fractures in children. Am Fam Physician 1996;53:2031–41.
13. Chacon D, Kissoon N, Brown T, et al. Use of comparison radiographs in the diagnosis of traumatic injuries of the elbow. Ann Emerg Med 1992;21:895–9.
14. Kissoon N, Galpin R, Gayle M, et al. Evaluation of the role of comparison radiographs in the diagnosis of traumatic elbow injuries. J Pediatr Orthop 1995;15:449–53.
15. Skaggs DL, Mirzayan R. The posterior fat pad sign in association with occult fracture of the elbow in children. J Bone Joint Surg Am 1999;81:1429–33.
16. Wheeless CR III. Wheeless' textbook of orthopedics. Division of Orthopedics, Duke University Medical Center, Durham (NC), last updated January 3, 2010. Available at: http://www.wheelessonline.com. Accessed February 12, 2010.
17. Green DA, Linares MY, Garcia Pena BM, et al. Randomized comparison of pain perception during radial head subluxation reduction using supination-flexion or forced pronation. Pediatr Emerg Care 2006;22(4):235–8.
18. Macias CG, Bothner J, Wiebe R. A comparison of supination/flexion to hyperpronation in the reduction of radial head subluxations. Pediatrics 1998;102(1):e10.
19. Schunk JE. Radial head subluxation: epidemiology and treatment of 87 episodes. Ann Emerg Med 1990;19(9):1019–23.
20. Krul M, van der Wouden JC, van Suijlekom-Smit LW, et al. Manipulative interventions for reducing pulled elbow in young children. Cochrane Database Syst Rev 2009;4:CD007759.
21. Bek D, Yildiz C, Kose O, et al. Pronation versus supination maneuvers for the reduction of 'pulled elbow': a randomized clinical trial. Eur J Emerg Med 2009;16(3):135–8.
22. Stiell IG, Greenberg GH, McKnight RD, et al. A study to develop clinical decision rules for the use of radiography in acute ankle injuries. Ann Emerg Med 1992;21(4):384–90.
23. Stiell IG, McKnight RD, Greenberg GH, et al. Implementation of the Ottawa ankle rules. JAMA 1994;271(11):827–32.

24. Bachmann LM, Kolb E, Koller MT, et al. Accuracy of Ottawa ankle rules to exclude fractures of the ankle and mid-foot: systematic review. BMJ 2003; 326(7386):417.
25. Stiell I, Wells G, Laupacis A, et al. Multicentre trial to introduce the Ottawa ankle rules for use of radiography in acute ankle injuries. Multicentre Ankle Rule Study Group. BMJ 1995;311(7005):594–7.
26. Clark KD, Tanner S. Evaluation of the Ottawa ankle rules in children. Pediatr Emerg Care 2003;19(2):73–8.
27. Brehaut JC, Stiell IG, Visentin L, et al. Clinical decision rules "in the real world": how a widely disseminated rule is used in everyday practice. Acad Emerg Med 2005;12:948–56.
28. Dowling S, Spooner CH, Liang Y, et al. Accuracy of Ottawa ankle rules to exclude fractures of the ankle and midfoot in children: a meta-analysis. Acad Emerg Med 2009;16(4):277–87.
29. Myers A, Canty K, Nelson T. Are the Ottawa ankle rules helpful in ruling out the need for x ray examination in children? Arch Dis Child 2005;90:1309–11.
30. Gravel J, Hedrei P, Grimard G, et al. Prospective validation and head-to-head comparison of 3 ankle rules in a pediatric population. Ann Emerg Med 2009; 54(4):534–40.
31. Pandya NK, Baldwin K, Wolfgruber H, et al. Child abuse and orthopaedic injury patterns: analysis at a level I pediatric trauma center. J Pediatr Orthop 2009; 29(6):618–25.
32. Worlock P, Stower M, Barbor P. Patterns of fractures in accidental and non-accidental injury in children: a comparative study. Br Med J (Clin Res Ed) 1986;293(6539):100–2.
33. Kemp AM, Dunstan F, Harrison S, et al. Patterns of skeletal fractures in child abuse: systematic review. BMJ 2008;337:a1518. DOI: 10.1136/bmj.a1518.
34. Merten DF, Radkowski MA, Leonidas JC. The abused child: a radiological reappraisal. Radiology 1983;146(2):377–81.
35. Caffey J. Some traumatic lesions in growing bones other than fractures and dislocations: clinical and radiological features: the Mackenzie Davidson Memorial Lecture. Br J Radiol 1957;30(353):225–38.
36. Kleinman PK. Diagnostic imaging in infant abuse. AJR Am J Roentgenol 1990; 155(4):703–12.
37. Kellogg ND, American Academy of Pediatrics Committee on Child Abuse and Neglect. Evaluation of suspected child physical abuse. Pediatrics 2007;119(6): 1232–41.
38. Fischer SU, Beattie TF. The limping child: epidemiology, assessment and outcome. J Bone Joint Surg Br 1999;81(6):1029–34.
39. Sawyer JR, Kapoor M. The limping child: a systemic approach to diagnosis. Am Fam Physician 2009;79(3):215–24.
40. Leet AL, Skaggs DL. Evaluation of the acutely limping child. Am Fam Physician 2000;61(4):1011–8.
41. Lin BW, Schraga ED, Stevens KJ. Pediatrics, limp. Medscape, updated October 2, 2009. Available at: http://emedicine.medscape.com. Accessed November 20, 2009.
42. De Boeck H, Vorlat. Limping in childhood. Acta Orthop Belg 2003;69(4):301–10.
43. Barkin RM, Barkin SZ, Barkin AZ. The limping child. J Emerg Med 2000;18(3): 331–9.
44. Illingworth CM. 128 Limping children with no fracture, sprain, or obvious cause. Clin Pediatr (Phila) 1978;17(2):139–42.

45. Oudjhane K, Newman B, Oh KS, et al. Occult fractures in preschool children. J Trauma 1988;28(6):858–60.
46. Blatt SD, Rosenthal BM, Barnhart DC. Diagnostic utility of lower extremity radiographs of young children with gait disturbance. Pediatrics 1991;87(2):138–40.
47. Wright N. Diagnostic imaging of the hip in the limping child. J Accid Emerg Med 2000;17:46–9. Best Evidence Topic Reports.
48. Tsung JW, Blaivas M. Emergency department diagnosis of pediatric hip effusion and guided arthrocentesis using point-of-care ultrasound. J Emerg Med 2008; 35(4):393–9.
49. Shavit I, Eidelman M, Galbraith R. Sonography of the hip joint by the emergency physician: its role in the evaluation of children presenting with acute limp. Pediatr Emerg Care 2006;22(8):570–3.
50. Valley VT, Stahmer SA. Targeted musculoarticular sonography in the detection of joint effusions. Acad Emerg Med 2001;8(4):361–7.
51. Chhem RK, Cardinal E, editors. Guidelines and gamuts in musculoskeletal ultrasound. New York: Wiley-Liss; 1999. p. 141.
52. Zieger MM, Dörr U, Schulz RD. Ultrasonography of hip joint effusions. Skeletal Radiol 1987;16(8):607–11.
53. Linebarger JS, Roy ML. Focus on diagnosis: common nuclear medicine studies in pediatrics. Pediatr Rev 2007;28(11):415–7.
54. Fordham L, Gundermann R, Blatt ER. ACR appropriateness criteria. Limping child, Ages 0–5 years. American College of Radiology, last reviewed in 2007. Available at: http://www.acr.org. Accessed November 20, 2009.
55. Asadi-Pooya AA, Bordbar MR. Are laboratory tests necessary in making the diagnosis of limb pains typical for growing pains in children? Pediatr Int 2007;49(6): 833–5.
56. Gholve PA, Cameron DB, Mills MB. Slipped capital femoral epiphysis update. Curr Opin Pediatr 2009;21:39–45.
57. Green DW, Mogekwu N, Scher DM, et al. A modification of Klein's Line to improve sensitivity of the anterior-posterior radiograph in slipped capital femoral epiphysis. J Pediatr Orthop 2009;29(5):449–53.
58. Tuten HR, Gabos PG, Kumar SJ, et al. The limping child: a manifestation of acute leukemia. J Pediatr Orthop 1998;18(5):625–9.
59. Kocher MS, Mandiga R, Zurakowski D, et al. Validation of a clinical prediction rule for the differentiation between septic arthritis and transient synovitis of the hip in children. J Bone Joint Surg Am 2004;86(8):1629–35.
60. Caird MS, Flynn JM, Leung YL, et al. Factors distinguishing septic arthritis from transient synovitis of the hip in children. A prospective study. J Bone Joint Surg Am 2006;88(6):1251–7.

Emergency Orthogeriatrics: Concepts and Therapeutic Alternatives

Christopher R. Carpenter, MD, MSc[a],*, Michael E. Stern, MD[b]

KEYWORDS

- Orthogeriatric care • Therapeutic alternatives
- Care models • Osteoporosis

Geriatric adult emergency department (ED) visits increased by 34% between 1993 and 2003, a trend that will double annual volumes among those aged 65 to 74 years from 6.4 million to 11.7 million by 2013.[1] The fastest growing segment of the population is the old-old (>85 years) who also happen to be using the ED at the highest rate.[2] Geriatric patients already consume more ED time and resources than younger populations[3] and orthopedic injuries represent a substantial proportion of their emergency care issues. After age 50 years, the lifetime risks for fractures in women are hip 17.5%, vertebrate 16%, and Colles 16%. In men aged 50 years and older, the lifetime risks of fracture are hip 6%, vertebrate 5%, and Colles 2.5%.[4] In the United States, the National Hospital Ambulatory Care Survey reported 21 million injury-related ED visits among adults more than 65 years of age from 2000 to 2004, including 22% with fractures.[5] Geriatric trauma is not unique to North American emergency medicine. In the United Kingdom, injuries represent 33% of older adult complaints presenting to EDs.[2] Currently, more than 250,000 hip fractures present to EDs in the United States each year, but this number is projected to double by 2040.[6] Despite the evolving epidemiologic imperative in the Institute of Medicine report, *Hospital-Based Emergency Care: At the Breaking Point*, geriatric issues that will shape twenty-first century acute care were widely underemphasized.[7,8]

Aging is associated with a variety of physiologic changes that affect emergency orthopedic care.[9,10] Hormonal changes and malnutrition result in osteoporosis, which

---

[a] Division of Emergency Medicine, Barnes Jewish Hospital, Washington University in St Louis, Campus Box 8072, 660 South Euclid Avenue, St Louis, MO 63110, USA
[b] Department of Emergency Medicine, New York-Presbyterian Hospital, Weill Cornell Medical College, 525 East 68th Street, New York, NY 10021, USA
* Corresponding author.
E-mail address: carpenterc@wusm.wustl.edu

Emerg Med Clin N Am 28 (2010) 927–949
doi:10.1016/j.emc.2010.06.005
0733-8627/10/$ – see front matter © 2010 Elsevier Inc. All rights reserved.

increases the likelihood and severity of fractures and concomitantly affects orthopedic surgical management.[4,11–14] In distinction, frailty is poorly defined and difficult to quantify but prevalent and associated with suboptimal recovery.[15] Furthermore, diminished gastrointestinal (GI) absorption of medications and impaired renal function impede effective pain management.[16] Functionally, balance and gait problems diminish independence and increase the risk of falls; 27% of community-dwelling older adults suffer a fall each year.[17]

Therapeutically, older adult orthopedic injury management offers unique challenges. In patients with hip fracture, preoperative delirium is reported in 34% to 92% of cases.[18] Not surprisingly, delirium is independently associated with poor functional recovery.[19,20] Previously undiagnosed dementia, usually unrecognized by ED physicians,[21] can be present in 40% of patients.[22,23] Dementia is an independent risk factor for delirium.[24] In addition, cognitive dysfunction can impede timely analgesia,[25] impair full informed consent, and delay prompt diagnosis.[9] Delayed diagnosis and surgical management can adversely affect fracture recovery and increase mortality.[26]

Unfortunately, the traditional emergency care model is not geriatric friendly.[27] For example, standing level falls are a leading cause of older adult fractures and traumatic mortality,[28] but patients who have fallen rarely receive guideline-directed care in today's ED.[29,30] For prevention, previously described fall risk factors lack ED validation so identifying high-risk subsets can be challenging.[17,31] Although one trial reported success with an ED-initiated multidisciplinary intervention to prevent falls,[32] others have not reported reduced fall rates or fall injuries with different models.[33,34] In addition, emergency medicine clinical decision rules for orthopedic injuries often lack validation in older patients.[35,36] This review summarize some of the unique therapeutic options and models in caring for geriatric ED patients with skeletal injuries.

GERIATRIC PHYSIOLOGY

Physiologic changes associated with aging are universal and affect every organ system, generally resulting in a decline in functional reserve capacity. However, these expected changes do not represent disease processes.[37,38] An age-related loss of both reserve and the ability to maintain homeostatic mechanisms, especially under conditions of physiologic stress, results in an increased risk of injury and disease. The resulting trauma or illness is often a complex and synergistic interplay between coexisting disease and the normal processes of aging.[39] Falls in the elderly and the traumatic orthopedic injuries that result are one example.

The musculoskeletal system undergoes several important changes with aging. As a percentage of total body weight, lean body mass decreases, whereas total body fat increases. Loss of muscle mass resulting from a decrease in the number of muscle fibers causes a reduction in muscle strength. After the age of 60 years, muscle strength decreases by approximately 33%, contributing to difficulty in maintaining balance and predisposing the elderly to subsequent falls.[40] Other intrinsic factors related to aging compound the risks of falls and injury, including impaired coordination, peripheral neuromuscular dysfunction, and deficits in vision, equilibrium, gait, proprioception, and cognition.[31,41,42] Physical activity can improve or slow the progression of some of these age-related deficits and therefore has been found to reduce the risk of falling.[34,43–46] Exercise has been shown to increase muscle strength, with specific resistance training actually increasing muscle mass and improving neural coordination and strength.[47–49]

The loss of skeletal bone mass and density in the elderly is another important physiologic change associated with the risk of orthopedic injury (**Fig. 1**). Bone loss

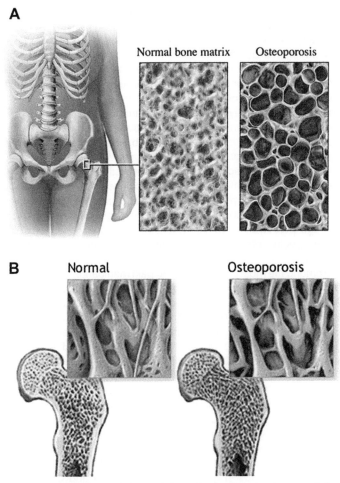

Fig. 1. (*A, B*) Osteoporosis. This artistic rendition of normal and osteoporotic bone demonstrates the striking difference in bone density and bone microstructure. (*From* Nucleus Medical Media, Inc, Kennesaw, Georgia; with permission; MedlinePlus Medical Encyclopedia. Available at: http://www.nlm.nih.gov/medlineplus/ency/imagepages/17156.htm. Accessed June 18, 2010.)

occurs at different rates for women (greatly accelerated during the postmenopausal period) and men, but by age 60 years they have equal rates of bone loss, with increased loss of total bone mass for both at age 80 years. In addition, there are age-related changes to bone quality. This decline in bone integrity combined with the loss of bone mass and changes in its distribution all result in loss of bone strength.[14] Skeletal fragility occurs as the bones become more vulnerable to the mechanical forces of trauma, causing injuries to elderly patients to occur with less transmitted kinetic energy compared with younger populations.

GERIATRIC PHARMACOLOGY

Poor pain management in the elderly is unfortunately a common problem.[50–52] Several barriers to timely and effective analgesia exist, including inadequate knowledge about pain assessment and management, failure to assess for pain, physician misperception that pain is a natural and expected consequence of aging, concerns about the use of analgesics in patients with cognitive dysfunction or other comorbid illnesses, or in postoperative patients a dogma that pain should be expected after surgery.[53–55] Oligoanalgesia, the undertreatment of pain, has many deleterious consequences including[56–58] delirium,[59,60] or other impaired cognitive function,[61,62] decreased functional independence,[54,63] depression,[64,65] poorer clinical outcomes,[60] as well as increased hospital length of stay, health care use and overall costs.[66,67] The American Pain Society, the American Geriatrics Society, and the Agency for Health Care Policy and Research (AHCPR) have created evidence-based clinical practice and quality assurance pain management guidelines for clinicians.[16]

Effective and safe pain management in the older adult must incorporate knowledge of age-related changes that affect both pharmacokinetics and pharmacodynamics: drug absorption, distribution, metabolism, excretion, and the physiologic response to drugs.[68] The 3 most commonly used geriatric analgesics are nonsteroidal antiinflammatory drugs (NSAIDs), acetaminophen, and narcotic analgesics.[16,69,70] Each drug class has specific pharmacologic considerations in the geriatric orthopedic patient.

NSAIDs are among the most commonly used pain medications in the elderly because they provide effective rapid and sustained relief for mild to moderate pain, and they can decrease the swelling and tenderness associated with both acute and postoperative inflammation.[70] However, NSAIDs are associated with significant adverse effects, especially GI and renal toxicity, which are particularly prevalent in the elderly. An age-related decrease in gastric bicarbonate secretion, blood flow, and mucosal function, as well as delayed gastric emptying time, all contribute to a loss of stomach protection and an increased risk of gastritis, ulcer formation, and GI bleeding.[68] Bleeding complications from NSAIDs also occur in the esophagus, duodenum, and small and large intestine.[71] Misoprostol, an oral cytoprotective prostaglandin E1 analogue, acts by replacing GI mucosal prostaglandins that have been reduced by NSAIDs. Cotherapy for NSAIDs with misoprostol has been shown to decrease the incidence of adverse GI events such as perforations and bleeds by 40%.[16,72]

An age-related decline in renal blood flow, functional renal mass, and tubular efficiency causes a decrease in glomerular filtration rate and creatinine clearance, thus affecting drug elimination by the kidneys.[71] Therefore, the elderly depend more on prostacyclin-mediated renal afferent arteriolar vasodilatation to maintain glomerular blood flow. Because NSAIDs impair this compensatory mechanism, a further decrease in renal elimination of drugs occurs.[71] Because creatinine production decreases with a decline in lean body mass that parallels the reduction in creatinine clearance associated with aging, serum creatinine levels are not a reliable marker of renal function in the elderly. Creatinine clearance is a more reliable marker of renal function. As a result of this renal dysfunction, increased drug serum levels and subsequent clinical toxicity can result.[68,71] NSAIDs can also directly cause papillary necrosis and interstitial nephritis.[73] In addition, because NSAIDs are highly lipid soluble with extensive protein binding, they are distributed widely in increased adipose stores of the elderly. Malnourished elderly patients with reduced plasma protein levels also have increased levels of unbound (active) drug.

Antihypertensive medications the activity of which is mediated via renal prostaglandins (such as β-blockers and angiotensin-converting agents) may well be inhibited by NSAIDs, causing hyperkalemia, fluid retention, hypertension, and frank heart failure.[71] Cyclooxygenase-2 (COX-2) inhibitors have an improved GI safety profile with approximately the same analgesic efficacy compared with conventional NSAIDs.[74,75]

However, they show no decrease in the risk of renal complications and appear to increase the risk of cardiovascular thrombotic events in patients not taking aspirin.[76]

Based on available data, it is not yet possible to accurately quantify the risk of NSAID use in the elderly, in terms of number needed to harm (NNH) for renal injury and gastropathy, along with the number needed to treat (NNT) for effective analgesia. To date, NSAIDs as a class of medication have not been deemed inappropriate for use in the elderly population because of inadequate evidence, with 2 specific exceptions. Indomethacin has been labeled as inappropriate because of toxicity to the central nervous system (CNS), as well as phenylbutazone because of its risk of bone marrow suppression.[77] Current guidelines call for judicious use of NSAIDs with low doses and short-term therapy, as well as close monitoring of renal and gastrointestinal function, blood pressure, and fluid status during and immediately after therapy in all elderly patients.[78]

Acetaminophen (alone and in combination with other medications) is the most widely used analgesic in the world and is often used to treat mild to moderate pain in the elderly. Yet, its safe use must incorporate dosage and length-of-therapy adjustments for older adults. Acetaminophen hepatic metabolism in aging adults is multifactorial and can be affected by physiologic changes of aging, lifestyle, genotype, comorbidities, as well as interactions with other medications. As a result, acetaminophen metabolism may be reduced by 50% in this population.[71] Decreased hepatic blood flow and an age-related decline in functional hepatocyte number and enzyme activity affects first-pass metabolism and the clearance of certain drugs. Aging also alters the nonsynthetic hepatic biotransformation reactions (eg, oxidative) more readily than synthetic enzymatic reactions (eg, conjugation). In an acute overdose (usually unintentional) or when the maximum daily dose is exceeded over a prolonged period, metabolism by conjugation becomes saturated, and excess acetaminophen undergoes oxidative metabolism by the CYP enzymes to a reactive metabolite, N-acetyl-p-benzoquinone-imine (NAPQI) leading to liver necrosis. Therefore, traditionally therapeutic doses (4 g/24 h) and long-term high-dose (>2 g/24 h) acetaminophen use in older adults can result in liver and even renal injury, as a result of similar enzymatic reactions occurring in extrahepatic organs.[79–81] In addition, because acetaminophen has a maximum dose beyond which it has no additional analgesic efficacy (ceiling effect), it has limited use for the moderate to severe pain that often accompanies an orthopedic injury.[16]

Evidence suggests that physicians' biases and knowledge deficits are the main culprits for improperly managing pain in the elderly.[55] Misconceptions occur most commonly with treatment using opioid analgesics. In addition, older patients themselves have misperceptions about addiction and drug abuse that can contribute to the barrier to proper/improved pain management. Intentional nonadherence (deciding to discontinue or change the dose of a drug) and unintentional nonadherence (misreading the label or forgetting a dose) are common with elderly patients.[82] Yet, studies of cancer, medical, and burn patients suggest that the medical treatment of pain with opioids rarely leads to drug abuse or iatrogenic opioid addiction.[16]

Opioid analgesics are central to proper pain management in elderly patients with orthopedic injuries.[83] However, individual agents (synthetic vs nonsynthetic) have different pharmacokinetic and pharmacodynamic profiles, and knowledge of these differences is imperative to provide safe and effective analgesia. Morphine (a nonsynthetic opiate) is the most commonly used.[16] It relieves all types of pain with no ceiling effect. Steady state can be achieved within 1 day as a result of an effective half-life (parent drug and its metabolites) of 3 to 4 hours.[16] Morphine is eliminated in the liver via conjugation and therefore is not greatly affected by hepatic changes associated with aging. However, its metabolites are excreted by the kidneys. These age-related renal changes and altered pharmacokinetics cause a prolonged half-life, therefore, a reduction in morphine dose or a lengthened time interval between dosing should be used in elderly patients.[84] Standing doses of narcotic analgesics should be avoided in older patients with dehydration, acute renal failure, or oliguria pre- or postoperatively.[16] Instead, as-needed administration of the opiate should be initiated, as this has the added benefit of requiring the physician to reassess the patient's pain requirements and general condition on a regular basis.

Although morphine may be administered via virtually every conceivable route, site-specific bioavailability exists. Transdermal and transmucosal routes have the lowest bioavailability. Because of alterations in the clearance of opioids, because of the effect that an age-related decrease in hepatic blood flow has on rapid first-pass hepatic metabolism, higher oral or rectal doses of morphine compared with subcutaneous or intravenous administration may not be required for the same analgesic effect.[16,71] When using an equianalgesic dosing table for opioid analgesics, this potential age-related change in pharmacokinetics should be taken into consideration.[85]

Understanding the side effects of opioids and how to manage them is an important aspect of their effective usage. The most common adverse effects are constipation, nausea, vomiting, and sedation; dizziness, hallucinations, confusion, and respiratory depression occur less frequently.[16] All of these side effects are treatable, and some are mitigated by the development of tolerance over time.[16] Sedation and mild confusion are predictable side effects of opioid dose escalation, but care must be taken to distinguish these symptoms from delirium, which confers significant morbidity and mortality. However, delirium has been shown to occur more commonly as a result of the undertreatment of pain rather than as an adverse effect of opioids.[59,60]

The updated Beer guidelines clearly state that certain analgesics should be avoided in the elderly, including pentazocine, propoxyphene, and meperidine.[77] Pentazocine, a mixed opiate agonist/antagonist, increases the risk of seizures as well as other effects on the CNS compared with other analgesics. Propoxyphene has doubtful efficacy in the elderly and can potentiate the anticoagulant effect of warfarin.[71,86] In addition, it has an active metabolite, norpropoxyphene, with a long half-life that increases the risk of CNS toxicity.[87] Meperidine lowers the seizure threshold, has poor analgesic efficacy, causes sedation, and has cardiotoxicity, especially in patients with renal insufficiency or hepatic dysfunction, caused by an active metabolite, normeperidine, with a long half-life.[71,77]

ACUTE FRACTURE ANALGESIC ALTERNATIVES

Aging physiology with concomitant comorbid illnesses including occult cognitive dysfunction and labile blood pressure all complicate acute fracture pain reduction in older adults. In addition, traditional narcotic analgesia can cause delirium and increase the risk of falls. Specific management strategies may augment or replace narcotic analgesia in geriatric orthopedic injury therapy for the 3 most common fractures (hip, vertebral, Colles).[88] For example, in osteoporotic vertebral compression fractures, 5 randomized trials with 246 subjects have demonstrated significantly improved pain control at 1 week with salmon calcitonin (daily doses of 100 IU IM or 200 IU intranasal or 200 IU suppository) with reduced concomitant analgesic use.[89]

The femoral nerve provides much of the sensory innervation to the femur. Fracture pain originates from the sensitive periosteum and quadriceps muscle spasm. In addition to appropriate splinting, acute ED analgesia for hip and distal femur fracture is most commonly intravenous systemic narcotic agents (hydromorphone, morphine). Femoral nerve blocks (**Fig. 2**) reduce pre- and postoperative hip fracture pain.[90]

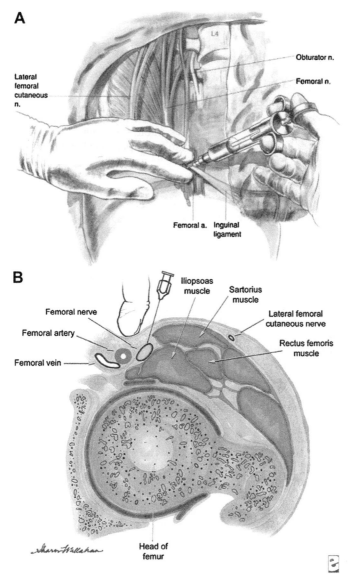

Fig. 2. (*A, B*) Femoral nerve block. A femoral nerve block can be easily performed in the ED by using anatomic landmarks (ie, palpation of the femoral artery) or by using ultrasound guidance to localize the femoral artery and the high-signal femoral nerve that lies lateral to the artery. (*A: From* Brown DL, Clifford JA, Wild J. Atlas of regional anesthesia 2006. p. 113–21, Fig. 13-4. Available at: http://polanest.webd.pl/pliki/varia/books/AtRegAn/micro189.lib3.hawaii.edu_ 3a2127/das/book/body/0/1353/i4-u1.0-b1-4160-2239-2..50017-5–f4.fig.htm. Accessed June 18, 2010; with permission; *B: Reprinted from* eMedicine.com, 2009. Available at: http:// emedicine.medscape.com/article/1143675-overview. Accessed June 18, 2010; with permission.)

McGlone and colleagues[91] assessed femoral nerve blocks performed by house staff and ED physicians for femoral shaft fractures using lignocaine (mean onset 8.7 minutes, mean duration 3.8 hours) or bupivacaine (mean onset 9.3 minutes, mean duration 11.5 hours) with sufficient analgesia to permit comfortable manipulation of the injured extremity within 15 minutes of injection in most cases. A similar population of geriatric adults with femoral neck fractures randomized to systemic analgesia alone or femoral nerve block performed by an orthopedic surgeon using 0.3 mL/kg of 0.25% bupivacaine demonstrated significantly improved pain scores at 15 minutes and 2 hours in the nerve block patients.[92] Others have reported similar successes without any adverse events related to nerve blocks.[93,94] The 3-in-1 femoral nerve block infiltrates the femoral nerve sheath then tracks cranially and laterally anesthetizing the femoral and obdurator nerves, lumbar plexus, and lateral cutaneous nerves. In one randomized controlled trial of femoral neck fracture victims, trained ED physicians using the 3-in-1 block provided patients with faster pain relief (2.8 hours vs 5.8 hours) with significantly less morphine.[95]

Although early femoral nerve block investigations used house staff, ED, or orthopedic physicians to administer the anesthetic locally without imaging or extra equipment, anesthesiologists today use a nerve stimulator to identify the nerve before instilling the medication.[96,97] No study has demonstrated that the nerve stimulator-based or anesthesiology-based approach is superior to femoral nerve blocks performed by ED physicians. However, compared with the fascial pop technique, ultrasound-guided femoral nerve blocks provide faster analgesia and permit identification of the adjacent vascular structures.[98,99] Nurse-based femoral nerve block teams have also been described.[100]

For femoral nerve blocks (see **Fig. 2**), bupivacaine (0.5%) is the analgesic of choice based on duration of action, greater degree of motor blockade, and accumulating trial evidence. The dose is 0.3 mL/kg to a maximum volume of 20 mL to maximize analgesia without significantly increasing the risk of cardiotoxicity.[95] With the patient in the supine position, a 7- to 9-MHz linear array ultrasound probe in the transverse orientation is used to identify the femoral artery and high-signal area lateral to the artery where the nerve lies.[99,101] Under ultrasound visualization, a 22-guage short beveled needle is inserted at a 45° angle and advanced to the iliopectinal fascia in the immediate proximity of the nerve. After aspirating to ensure that a vessel has not been penetrated, 0.5% bupivicaine (0.3 mg/kg up to 20 mg) is administered with deposition directly visualized sonographically. The 3-in-1 femoral nerve block involves distal compression following administration of the local anesthetic, which then tracks cranially and laterally anesthetizing the femoral and obdurator nerves, lumbar plexus, and lateral cutaneous nerves.[99]

Colles fracture-related pain can be managed with a systemic analgesia, a hematoma block, or a Bier block. To place a hematoma block, one aspirates directly over the fracture hematoma before injecting 5 to 15 mL of 1% lidocaine.[102] Hematoma blocks do not require periprocedural fasting, but they offer inferior analgesia compared with a Bier block.[103,104] The risks of hematoma blocks include the introduction of an infectious agent at the fracture site so injection should never occur through nonsterile skin or in an open fracture.[102,105] In addition, lidocaine hematoma blocks have been associated with delirium and seizures.[106]

OSTEOPOROSIS

Osteoporosis is the most common metabolic bone disorder, affecting 200 million people worldwide and more than 10 million people in the United States. Those at risk for developing the disease total another 18 million in the United States alone.[14,107] The lifetime risk of osteoporotic fractures in a 50-year-old white woman has been estimated to be 30% to 40% in the United States, including a 15% to 18% risk for hip fractures.[108] Yet, because osteoporosis is a clinically silent disease, often only manifesting with a fracture after a fall, it is under-recognized and undertreated.[14] However, as physician awareness increases, appropriate medical management is improving.[109]

Causes of osteoporosis are multifactorial. Several factors influence the development of osteoporosis, including age, gender, race, lifestyle, body weight, and peak bone mass, which occurs during the fourth decade. Primary osteoporosis can be divided into type I (postmenopausal) osteoporosis and type II (age-related) osteoporosis. Type I osteoporosis is linked to menopause as a result of estrogen deficiency. In women, accelerated bone loss occurs in the perimenopausal period, with roughly 3% to 5% per year lost during the first decade after menopause onset.[9,110] Subsequently, the loss of bone mass and density proceeds at a rate of 1% per year for women. Type I osteoporotic fractures occur in bones with higher trabecular content: vertebrae, pelvis, distal radius, and proximal femur. Type II osteoporosis affects both genders older than 70 years of age and is characterized by less rapid bone loss (0.5%–3% per year). Hip fractures predominate in this group. Type II osteoporosis is attributable to increases in parathyroid hormone levels, and decreased circulating vitamin D, growth hormone, and insulinlike growth factors.[9] Secondary causes include medications, endocrine disorders, chronic renal disease, hematopoietic disorders, immobilization, inflammatory arthropathy, nutrition, gastrointestinal disorders, liver disease, and connective tissue disorders.[14] For men in particular, specific factors such as alcohol abuse, glucocorticoid excess, and hypogonadism contribute to 50% of their osteoporosis.[111]

Osteoporosis is characterized by significant bone loss as a result of a simultaneous reduction in bone mass and deterioration of bone microstructure (see **Fig. 1**), leading to increased bone fragility and a subsequent increased risk of fracture. The World Health Organization defines osteoporosis as a T-score of greater than 2.5 standard deviations less than the mean of young healthy individuals at their peak bone mass.[112] This bone mineral density (BMD) measurement is obtained using a dual energy X-ray absorptiometry (DEXA) scan. Increased fracture risk has been shown to be correlated with a low BMD.[113] Additional laboratory studies must be performed in the work-up of osteoporosis: levels of calcium, 25-hydroxy vitamin D, parathyroid, bone alkaline phosphatase, urinary calcium and creatinine, thyroid-stimulating hormone, complete blood count, serum and urine protein electrophoresis, and liver function tests.[14]

To prevent the devastating sequelae of osteoporosis, appropriate treatment, both pharmacologic and nonpharmacologic, must be initiated after diagnosis. Pharmacologic treatment includes calcium, vitamin D, bisphosphonates, calcitonin, estrogen, and selective estrogen receptor modulators (SERMs). Osteoporosis management extends beyond pills, capsules, and pharmaceutical prescriptions. Although recent trials have cast doubt on their efficacy, minimally invasive treatment options for spinal compression fractures (vertebroplasty and kyphoplasty) continue to be studied.[114–116] Other nonpharmaceutical treatments such as hip protectors, posture training supports, as well as balance and exercise training programs should be used as complements to optimize the outcomes for patients with osteoporosis.[14]

Treatment with a daily requirement of 1200 to 1500 mg of calcium is recommended and is better absorbed in the citrate form, as it dissolves at all pH levels. A daily dose of vitamin D (400–800 IU) is recommended in addition to the calcium, with even higher dosing for elderly patients with little sun exposure. In elderly women, the administration of both calcium and vitamin D has been shown to prevent hip and other nonvertebral fractures.[117] In a follow-up study, intention-to-treat analysis showed a 36-month benefit in terms of reduction in both types of fractures, with decreased probability (odds ratios of 0.72 and 0.73, respectively).[118]

The most potent drugs in the prevention and treatment of osteoporosis are the bisphosphonates, which strongly bind to the hydroxyapatite of bone and inhibit osteoclast activity. Alendronate and risedronate are widely used and decrease the fracture rate for both the spine and hip. The oral route can cause GI side effects, especially for prone, hospitalized patients, therefore remaining upright for at least 30 minutes after administration is recommended.[14] In type I osteoporosis, the Fracture Intervention Trial (FIT) demonstrated that alendronate increased BMD and decreased the risk of vertebral and hip fractures.[119,120] In addition, alendronate has been shown to be efficacious for men and patients on steroids. The length of bisphosphonate treatment remains unclear, but usually ends after 5 years because of a plateau in bone mass measurements and the potential risk of microfracture accumulation.[14]

In a 5-year randomized, double-blind, placebo-controlled study, nasal calcitonin was shown to increase BMD and decrease the risk of vertebral fractures by 33% in women. Calcitonin also acted as an effective analgesia for bony pain secondary to fracture.[121] However, calcitonin has not been shown to provide any protection against hip fractures.[122,123] Estrogen has been used widely in postmenopausal women as hormone replacement therapy (HRT) to alleviate symptoms. Although estrogen has been shown to decrease the incidence of hip and spine fractures by 35%, it is not recommended for treatment of osteoporosis because of its potential health risks (increased risk of breast cancer and thrombotic events).[14] Raloxifene, a SERM, may increase BMD, but is not as effective as bisphosphonates at treating osteoporosis, and it confers a risk of venous thromboembolism and causes hot flashes.[124]

Parathyroid hormone (PTH) has shown promise in treating osteoporosis. PTH works by increasing BMD, bone resorption, and formation, and enhancing bone architecture and integrity.[125] Several studies have shown that PTH reduces the risk of fracture by increasing the connectivity of bone,[126] thickening trabeculae,[127] increasing cortical thickness, and inhibiting osteocyte apoptosis.[128] However, compared with bisphosphonates, PTH takes 3 to 6 months longer to provide fracture protection, and more recent studies indicate that its place in treatment algorithms is still unclear.[14]

Nonpharmacologic treatment methods are an important part of the comprehensive multidisciplinary approach in the treatment of osteoporosis. Some trials have shown that polypropylene hip protectors (**Fig. 3**) reduce hip fractures[129] and improve self-efficacy in frail older adults, defined as the belief in their own ability to avoid falling. However, other trials have failed to demonstrate a benefit so further research is currently underway.[130–133] The major drawback of hip protectors is noncompliance.[134] Posture training supports are lightweight orthoses, worn backpack style, that have been shown to provide symptomatic relief and increase extensor muscle strength in patients with thoracic kyphosis, as well as reduce vertebral fractures in estrogen-deficient women.[135,136] Tai chi chuan, a Chinese martial art form that involves slow-motion routines, has been shown to improve balance and is associated with a 47.5% reduction in risk of falls.[137] Several studies have shown that continued exercise training can increase BMD, yet it has not been shown to reduce fracture rates.[14]

CARE MODELS

Fracture management can be variable as shown by research demonstrating that age and geography may affect orthopedic management decisions.[138] A timely assessment of older adult fracture victim's preexisting functional status and support network is essential to guide effective acute orthopedic management.[139] Dementia may impede or inhibit appropriate rehabilitation, whereas medical comorbidities may significantly alter the risk-to-benefit ratio for operative intervention. Most research suggests that

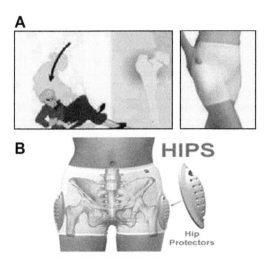

Fig. 3. (A, B) Hip protectors. Several trials have shown that polypropylene hip protectors reduce hip fracture, although low compliance rates impede widespread use. (*From* Kiel D. Hip protectors. Slide presentation at the Surgeon General's Workshop on Osteoporosis and Bone Health. Washington, DC; 12–13 December 2002. Available at: http://www. surgeongeneral.gov/library/bonehealth/chapter_6.html. Accessed June 18, 2010; with permission). (*From* e-pill, LLC, Wellesley, MA. Available at: http://www.hipprotectors.com. Accessed June 18, 2010; with permisssion.)

for hip fractures, an operative delay beyond 48 hours increases mortality, although older patients with fracture merit careful assessment of surgical risk.[140,141] Complications of delayed definitive care and prolonged immobility include pressure ulcers, thromboembolism, and pneumonia. Therefore, prompt preoperative recognition of surgical and nonsurgical injuries along with relevant geriatric syndromes requires a team approach involving orthopedics, anesthesiology, geriatrics, physiotherapy, and dieticians in conjunction with emergency medicine.[142] In addition, in the postoperative period following a hip fracture multidisciplinary rehabilitation has demonstrated a trend toward improved functional outcomes with lower caregiver burdens.[143]

Amatuzzi and colleagues[144] noted a sustained in-hospital mortality decrease (5% to 1.4%) in elderly patients with hip fracture for 4 years in Brazil after initiating an orthogeriatric group practice including educational outreach programs and routine joint orthopedic and geriatric evaluation of all ED patients with fractures. Their model also includes weekly meetings to discuss inpatient progress and outpatient therapy issues. Comprehensive geriatric interventions involving uniform older adult orthopedic patient assessment by a geriatrician, rehabilitation specialist, and social worker reduced in-hospital mortality and 3-month functional outcomes, but did not affect 6- or 12-month outcomes.[145] Similar management models have been described elsewhere (**Fig. 4**).[146,147] A decade's experience with a hip fracture clinical pathway at the New York University Hospital for Joint Diseases was associated with significant decreases in acute hospital length of stay, in-hospital mortality (5.3% vs 1.5%), and 1-year mortality (14.1% vs 8.8%).[148] This model includes a standardized set of orders and consultant protocols beginning preoperatively and extending from the recovery room to postoperative day 1 and discharge. Another fast-track protocol for hip fractures involving local femoral nerve blocks, early anesthesiologist assessment, preoperative assessment of nutritional, fluid, urinary retention, and oxygen status significantly decreased multiple postoperative complications.[149] Alternatively,

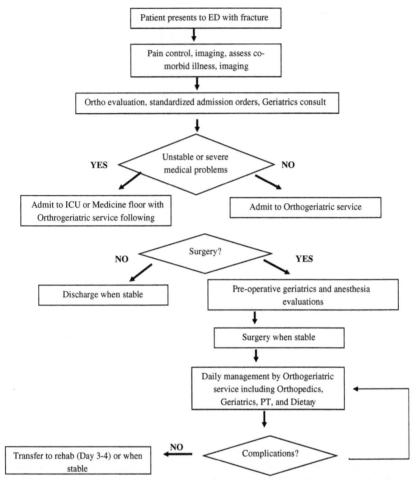

Fig. 4. Multidisciplinary geriatric fracture management model. (*Data from* De Jonge KE, Christmas C, Andersen R, et al. Hip fracture service – an interdisciplinary model of care. J Am Geriatr Soc 2001;49(12):1737–8.)

geriatric and orthopedic comanagement of geriatric patients with a fractured femur has significantly reduced hospital length of stay, surgical delays, complication rates, and mortality.[150]

Pre-and postoperative delirium are common in elderly patients with fractures.[18] Traditionally, the Confusion Assessment Method (CAM) has been used to diagnose delirium,[151] but recently the CAM-ICU has been validated and may be more appropriate for ED-based screening.[152,153] Independent preoperative delirium risk factors include cognitive impairment, indoor injury, fever, and prolonged preoperative waiting time. Risk factors for postoperative delirium include cognitive impairment, indoor injury, and body mass index less than 20 kg/m^2.[24] Most patients who suffer preoperative delirium remain delirious postoperatively.[154]

Five studies have evaluated interventions to reduce delirium.[155,156] Three involved nursing education and routine screening by specially trained nurses.[156–158] The Milisen model also focused on postoperative pain management, but failed to reduce the incidence of delirium.[158] The Lundström model, on the other hand, focused on regional anesthesia, avoiding hypoxia, and early rehabilitation cooperation between anesthesia, orthopedics, and geriatrics demonstrating a reduction of delirium from 61% to 31%.[157] In Lundström and colleagues's[156] subsequent evaluation of postoperative care for femoral neck fractures on a geriatric ward versus a conventional orthopedic floor, staff education emphasized comprehensive geriatric education and routine delirium screening with the duration (5 vs 10 days) and incidence (55% vs 75%) of delirium significantly reduced in conjunction with fewer falls, urinary tract infections, or decubitus ulcers. Marcantonio and colleagues[159] implemented proactive geriatric consults for patients with hip fracture noting a 77% adherence rate for geriatrician recommendations by the managing orthopedic services, but no reduction in delirium. Gustafson and colleagues[160] established an anesthesia and geriatric early collaborative model for femoral neck fractures emphasizing early and routine pre- and postoperative delirium assessments, oxygen therapy, prompt surgical intervention, avoiding hypotension and falls. They demonstrated a reduction in acute confusional states from 61.3% to 47.6% with their intervention along with a reduction in delirium duration, severity, and postoperative complications.

DISPOSITION CONSIDERATIONS

No level I triage criteria exist for geriatric orthopedic trauma.[161] Although not every geriatric fracture patient requires hospital admission or immediate operative intervention, the emergency physician must carefully assess older adults for underlying markers of frailty, baseline functional impairments, socioeconomic constraints, and support system. Although ambulatory assist devices such as canes or walkers may promote functional independence, they can also increase subsequent fall risk. Effective analgesia necessary to facilitate ambulation may precipitate orthostatic hypotension or drug-related cognitive dysfunction. Underlying unrecognized dementia may impair outpatient compliance with orthopedic follow-up, rehabilitation, and pharmacologic pain control.[162] All of these factors should be considered before ED discharge.[163]

When initial plain film imaging is unremarkable following a standing level fall, the ambulatory patient who cannot bear weight represents a challenge to emergency physicians. In ED and postoperative trauma patients, the prevalence of occult hip fractures (negative radiographs, subsequent fracture diagnosed) has been reported as 2.9% to 4.4%.[164–166] In ED settings, the sensitivity of anteroposterior and cross-table lateral projections of the affected hip to identify fractures is 90%, which is lower than in other settings.[164,167] These patients are often admitted for pain control, further imaging, and subsequent physiotherapy if no bony injury is identified (**Fig. 5**).[168]

Several features of the history and physical examination can distinguish older adult trauma patients at increased risk for occult hip fracture. A new inability to bear weight is 73% sensitive for occult fractures in one small series.[169] In addition, pain induced with straight leg raise (sensitivity 50%, specificity 45%) and with passive internal and external rotation (sensitivity 61%, specificity 59%) are not adequate to identify patients with occult hip fracture.[169]

Three imaging modalities are often contemplated when occult hip fracture is suspected. The computerized tomography diagnostic test characteristics for ED patients has not been well described and is generally not supported.[167] Bone scan is rarely used by emergency physicians, but has reported sensitivity of 75% to 97.8% and specificity 94% to 95%.[170,171] Scintigraphy has several disadvantages including inadequate accessibility and inferior spatial resolution resulting in

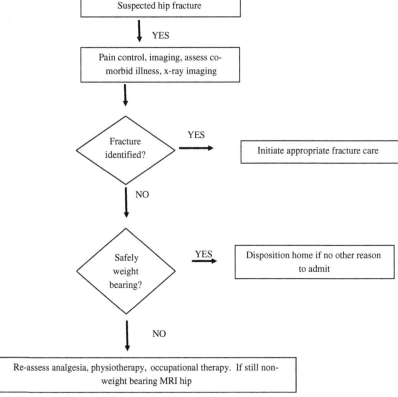

Fig. 5. Pathway for elderly patients with suspected hip fracture. (*Data from* Smith JE, Jenkin A, Hennessy C. A retrospective chart review of elderly patients who cannot weight bear following a hip injury but whose initial x rays are normal. Emerg Med J 2009;26(1):50–1.)

incomplete fracture identification.[167] Magnetic resonance imaging (MRI) is the superior study to identify occult hip fractures with 100% sensitivity, 100% specificity (93% for junior radiologists), and excellent interobserver reproducibility (κ = 0.79).[172] MRI also has the advantage of providing alternative diagnoses that may impede weight bearing such as hematoma, muscle tears, degenerative join disease, and osteonecrosis.[173] Although MRI is not always readily available, early incorporation of MRI into the ED diagnostic armamentarium for occult hip fracture is cost-effective and can save days in reaching the diagnosis.[174,175]

SUMMARY

Multidisciplinary orthogeriatric care can enhance prompt ED diagnosis, optimal pre-and postoperative care, and functional recovery in older adults with bony injuries. Emergency care providers should be cognizant of prevalent geriatric syndromes including delirium and standing level falls to minimize fracture-related morbidity. Recognizing the implications of aging physiology, acute care physicians should be aware of effective efficient alternatives to analgesia, procedural sedation, and definitive imaging to promote early surgical management and postoperative recovery.

REFERENCES

1. Roberts DC, McKay MP, Shaffer A. Increasing rates of emergency department visits for elderly patients in the United States, 1993 to 2003. Ann Emerg Med 2008;51:769–74.
2. Downing A, Wilson R. Older people's use of accident and emergency services. Age Ageing 2005;34:24–30.
3. McNamara RM, Rousseau E, Sanders AB. Geriatric emergency medicine: a survey of practicing emergency physicians. Ann Emerg Med 1992;21:796–801.
4. Lips P. Epidemiology and predictors of fractures associated with osteoporosis. Am J Med 1997;103: 3S–8S.
5. Carter MW, Gupta S. Characteristics and outcomes of injury-related ED visits among older adults. Am J Emerg Med 2008;26:296–303.
6. Cummings SR, Rubin SM, Black D. The future of hip fractures in the United States. Numbers, costs, and potential effects of postmenopausal estrogen. Clin Orthop Relat Res 1990;252:163–6.
7. Wilber ST, Gerson LW, Terrell KM, et al. Geriatric emergency medicine and the 2006 Institute of Medicine reports from the Committee on the Future of Emergency Care in the U.S. Health System. Acad Emerg Med 2006;13:1345–51.
8. Institute of Medicine Committee on the Future of Emergency Care in the U.S. Health System. Hospital-based emergency care: at the breaking point. Washington, DC: National Academies Press; 2006.
9. Potter JF. The older orthopedic patient. Clin Orthop Relat Res 2004;425:44–9.
10. Heyburn G, Beringer T, Elliott J, et al. Orthogeriatric care in patients with fractures of the proximal femur. Clin Orthop Relat Res 2004;425:35–43.
11. Olofsson B, Stenvall M, Lundstrom M, et al. Malnutrition in hip fracture patients: an intervention study. J Clin Nurs 2007;16:2027–38.
12. Duncan DG, Beck SJ, Hood K, et al. Using dietetic assistants to improve the outcome of hip fracture: a randomised controlled trial of nutritional support in an acute trauma ward. Age Ageing 2006;35:148–53.
13. Chao EYS, Inoue N, Koo TK, et al. Biomechanical considerations of fracture treatment and bone quality maintenance in elderly patients and patients with osteoporosis. Clin Orthop Relat Res 2004;425:12–25.
14. Lin JT, Lane JM. Osteoporosis: a review. Clin Orthop Relat Res 2004;425:126–34.
15. Ensrud KE, Ewing SK, Taylor BC, et al. Comparison of 2 frailty indexes for prediction of falls, disability, fractures, and death in older women. Arch Intern Med 2008;168:382–9.
16. Karani R, Meier DE. Systemic pharmacologic postoperative pain management in the geriatric orthopaedic patient. Clin Orthop Relat Res 2004;425:26–34.
17. Carpenter CR. Evidence based emergency medicine/rational clinical examination abstract: will my patient fall? Ann Emerg Med 2009;53:398–400.
18. Bruce AJ, Ritchie CW, Blizard R, et al. The incidence of delirium associated with orthopedic surgery: a meta-analytic review. Int Psychogeriatr 2007;19:197–214.
19. Marcantonio ER, Flacker JM, Michaels M, et al. Delirium is independently associated with poor functional recovery after hip fracture. J Am Geriatr Soc 2000;48:618–24.
20. Pitkala KH, Laurila JV, Strandberg TE, et al. Prognostic significance of delirium in frail older people. Dement Geriatr Cogn Disord 2005;19:158–63.

21. Hustey FM, Meldon SW. The prevalence and documentation of impaired mental status in elderly emergency department patients. Ann Emerg Med 2002;39: 248–53.

22. Wilber ST, Carpenter CR, Hustey FM. The six-item screener to detect cognitive impairment in older emergency department patients. Acad Emerg Med 2008; 15:613–6.

23. Carpenter CR. Does this patient have dementia? Ann Emerg Med 2008;52: 554–6.

24. Juliebo V, Bjoro K, Krogseth M, et al. Risk factors for preoperative and postoperative delirium in elderly patients with hip fracture. J Am Geriatr Soc 2009;57: 1354–61.

25. Feldt KS, Ryden MR, Miles S. Treatment of pain in cognitively impaired compared with cognitively intact older patients with hip-fracture. J Am Geriatr Soc 1998;46:1079–85.

26. Grimes JP, Gregory PM, Noveck H, et al. The effects of time-to-surgery on mortality and morbidity in patients following hip fracture. Am J Med 2002;112: 702–9.

27. Hwang U, Morrison RS. The geriatric emergency department. J Am Geriatr Soc 2007;55:1873–6.

28. Kocher KE. Public health and aging: nonfatal injuries among older adults treated in hospital emergency departments – United States, 2001. JAMA 2003;290: 2657–8.

29. Salter AE, Khan KM, Donaldson MG, et al. Community-dwelling seniors who present to the emergency department with a fall do not receive guideline care and their fall risk profile worsens significantly: a 6-month prospective study. Osteoporos Int 2006;17:672–83.

30. Bloch F, Jegou D, Dhainaut JF, et al. Do ED staffs have a role to play in the prevention of repeat falls in elderly patients? Am J Emerg Med 2009;27:303–7.

31. Carpenter CR, Scheatzle MD, D'Antonio JA, et al. Identification of fall risk factors in older adult emergency department patients. Acad Emerg Med 2009;16: 211–9.

32. Close J, Ellis M, Hooper R, et al. Prevention of falls in the elderly trial (PROFET): a randomised controlled trial. Lancet 1999;353:93–7.

33. Baraff LJ, Lee TJ, Kader S, et al. Effect of a practice guideline for emergency department care of falls in elder patients on subsequent falls and hospitalizations for injuries. Acad Emerg Med 1999;6:1224–31.

34. Gillespie LD, Robertson MC, Gillespie WJ, et al. Interventions for preventing falls in older people living in the community. Cochrane Database Syst Rev 2009;2:CD007146.

35. Barry TB, McNamara RM. Clinical decision rules and cervical spine injury in an elderly patient: a word of caution. J Emerg Med 2005;29:433–6.

36. Bub LD, Blackmore CC, Mann FA, et al. Cervical spine fractures in patients 65 years and older: a clinical prediction rule for blunt trauma. Radiology 2005;234: 143–9.

37. Peddi R, Morley JE. The physiology of aging. In: Meldon SW, Ma OJ, Woolard R, editors. Geriatric emergency medicine. New York: McGraw-Hill; 2004. p. 4–12.

38. Evans R. Physiology of aging. In: Sanders AB, editor. Emergency care of the elder person. St. Louis (MO): Beverly Cracom; 1996. p. 11–28.

39. Inouye SK, Studenski S, Tinetti ME, et al. Geriatric syndromes: clinical, research, and policy implications of a core geriatric concept. J Am Geriatr Soc 2007;55: 780–91.

40. Day S, Karpman R. Geriatric orthopedics. In: LoCicero J, Rosenthal RA, Katlic MR, et al, editors. A Supplement to new frontiers in geriatrics research: an agenda for surgical and related medical specialties. New York: American Geriatrics Society; 2007. p. 289–99.
41. Ganz DA, Bao Y, Shekelle PG, et al. Will my patient fall? JAMA 2007;297:77–86.
42. Close JC, Hooper R, Glucksman E, et al. Predictors of falls in a high risk population: results from the prevention of falls in the elderly trial (PROFET). Emerg Med J 2003;20:421–5.
43. Graafmans WC, Ooms ME, Hofstee HM, et al. Falls in the elderly: a prospective study of risk factors and risk profiles. Am J Epidemiol 1996;143:1129–36.
44. Grisso JA. Prevention of falls in patients with osteoporosis. Rev Rhum Engl Ed 1997;64:75S–7S.
45. Sorock GS, Labiner DM. Peripheral neuromuscular dysfunction and falls in an elderly cohort. Am J Epidemiol 1992;136:584–91.
46. Tinetti ME, Speechley M, Ginter SF. Risk factors for falls among elderly person living in the community. N Engl J Med 1988;319:1701–7.
47. Butler RN, Davis R, Lewis CB, et al. Physical fitness: benefits of exercise for the older patient. 2. Geriatrics 1998;53:49–52, 61–2.
48. Evans WJ. Exercise, nutrition, and aging. Clin Geriatr Med 1995;11:725–34.
49. Province MA, Hadley EC, Hornbrook MC, et al. The effects of exercise on falls in elderly patients. A preplanned meta-analysis of the FICSIT Trials. Frailty and Injuries: Cooperative Studies of Intervention Techniques. JAMA 1995;273:1341–7.
50. Flaherty JH. Who's taking your 5th vital sign? J Gerontol A Biol Sci Med Sci 2001;56:M397–9.
51. Neighbor ML, Honner S, Kohn MA. Factors affecting emergency department opioid administration to severely injured patients. Acad Emerg Med 2004;11:1290–6.
52. Rupp T, Delaney KA. Inadequate analgesia in emergency medicine. Ann Emerg Med 2004;43:494–503.
53. Ferrell BA. Pain evaluation and management in the nursing home. Ann Intern Med 1995;123:681–7.
54. Ferrell BA, Ferrell BR, Rivera L. Pain in cognitively impaired nursing home patients. J Pain Symptom Manage 1995;10:591–8.
55. Herr KA, Garand L. Assessment and measurement of pain in older adults. Clin Geriatr Med 2001;17:457–78.
56. Sloss EM, Solomon DH, Shekelle PG, et al. Selecting target conditions for quality of care improvement in vulnerable older adults. J Am Geriatr Soc 2000;48:363–9.
57. Etzioni S, Chodosh J, Ferrell BA, et al. Quality indicators for pain management in vulnerable elders. J Am Geriatr Soc 2007;55:S403–8.
58. Terrell KM, Hustey FM, Hwang U, et al. Quality indicators for geriatric emergency care. Acad Emerg Med 2009;16:441–9.
59. Duggleby W, Lander J. Cognitive status and postoperative pain: older adults. J Pain Symptom Manage 1994;9:19–27.
60. Lynch EP, Lazor MA, Gellis JE, et al. The impact of postoperative pain on the development of postoperative delirium. Anesth Analg 1998;86:781–5.
61. Duggleby W, Lander J. Patient-controlled analgesia for older adults. Clin Nurs Res 1992;1:107–13.
62. Hurley AC, Volicer BJ, Hanrahan PA, et al. Assessment of discomfort in advanced Alzheimer patients. Res Nurs Health 1992;15:369–77.

63. Brochet B, Michel P, Barberger-Gateau P, et al. Population-based study of pain in elderly people: a descriptive study. Age Ageing 1998;27:279–84.

64. Magni G, Caldieron C, Rigatti-Luchini S, et al. Chronic musculoskeletal pain and depressive symptoms in the general population. An analysis of the 1st National Health and Nutrition Examination Survey data. Pain 1990;43:299–307.

65. Williamson GM, Schulz R. Pain, activity restriction, and symptoms of depression among community-residing elderly adults. J Gerontol 1992;47:367–72.

66. Ferrell BR, Schaffner M. Pharmacoeconomics and medical outcomes in pain management. Semin Anesth 1997;16:152–9.

67. Sengstaken EA, King SA. The problems of pain and its detection among geriatric nursing home residents. J Am Geriatr Soc 1993;41:541–4.

68. Snyder L, Connolly S, Becker B. Pharmacology and adverse drug-related events in elders treated in the emergency department. In: Meldon SW, Ma OJ, Woolard R, editors. Geriatric emergency medicine. New York: McGraw-Hill; 2004. p. 13–21, Chapter 3.

69. Philips A, Polisson R, Simon L. NSAIDs and the elderly. Toxicity and economic implications. Drugs Aging 1997;10:119–30.

70. Elseviers M, De Broe M. Analgesic abuse in the elderly. Renal sequelae and management. Drugs Aging 1998;12:391–400.

71. Blanda MP. Pharmacologic issues in geriatric emergency medicine. Emerg Med Clin North Am 2006;24:449–65.

72. Silverstein FE, Graham DY, Senior JR, et al. Misoprostol reduces serious gastrointestinal complications in patients with rheumatoid arthritis receiving nonsteroidal anti-inflammatory drugs. A randomized, double-blind, placebo-controlled trial. Ann Intern Med 1995;123:241–9.

73. Clive DM, Stoff JS. Renal syndromes associated with nonsteroidal antiinflammatory drugs. N Engl J Med 1984;310:563–72.

74. Deeks DJ, Smith LA, Bradley MD. Efficacy, tolerability, and upper gastrointestinal safety of celecoxib for treatment of osteoarthritis and rheumatoid arthritis: systematic review of randomised controlled trials. BMJ 2002;325:619.

75. Simon LS, Weaver AL, Graham DY, et al. Anti-inflammatory and upper gastrointestinal effects of celecoxib in rheumatoid arthritis: a randomized controlled trial. JAMA 1999;282:1921–8.

76. Mukherjee D, Nissen SE, Topol EJ. Risk of cardiovascular events associated with selective COX-2 inhibitors. JAMA 2001;286:954–9.

77. Beers MH. Explicit criteria for determining potentially inappropriate medication use by the elderly: an update. Arch Intern Med 1997;152:1531–6.

78. Bell GM, Schnitzer TJ. Cox-2 inhibitors and other nonsteroidal anti-inflammatory drugs in the treatment of pain in the elderly. Clin Geriatr Med 2001;17:489–502.

79. Rikans LE. Influence of aging on chemically induced hepatotoxicity: role of age-related changes in metabolism. Drug Metab Rev 1989;20:87–110.

80. Eriksson LS, Broomé U, Kalin M, et al. Hepatotoxicity due to repeated intake of low doses of paracetamol. J Intern Med 1992;231:567–70.

81. Kurtovic J, Riordan SM. Paracetamol-induced hepatotoxicity at recommended dosage. J Intern Med 2003;253:240–3.

82. Corlett AJ. Aids to compliance with medication. BMJ 1996;313:926–9.

83. Gloth FM. Principles of perioperative pain management in older adults. Clin Geriatr Med 2001;17:553–73.

84. Ferrell BA. Pain management. In: Hazzard WR, Blass JP, Ettinger WH, editors. Principles of geriatric medicine and gerontology. New York: McGraw-Hill; 1999. p. 413–33.

85. Levy MH. Pharmacologic management of cancer pain. Semin Oncol 1994;21: 718–39.
86. Collins SL, Edwards JE, Moore RA, et al. Single dose dextropropoxyphene, alone and with paracetamol (acetaminophen), for postoperative pain. Cochrane Database Syst Rev 2000;2:CD001440.
87. Nickander RC, Emmerson JL, Hynes MD, et al. Pharmacologic and toxic effects in animals of dextropropoxyphene and its major metabolite norpropoxyphene: a review. Hum Toxicol 1984;3(Suppl):13S–36S.
88. Ducharme J. Acute pain and pain control: state of the art. Ann Emerg Med 2000; 35:592–603.
89. Knopp JA, Diner BM, Blitz M, et al. Calcitonin for treating acute pain of osteoporotic vertebral compression fractures: a systematic review of randomized, controlled trials. Osteoporos Int 2005;16:1281–90.
90. Parker MJ, Griffiths R, Appadu B. Nerve blocks (subcostal, lateral cutaneous, femoral, triple psoas) for hip fractures. Cochrane Database Syst Rev 2002;1: CD001159.
91. McGlone R, Sadhra K, Hamer DW, et al. Femoral nerve block in the initial management of femoral shaft fractures. Arch Emerg Med 1987;4:163–8.
92. Haddad FS, Williams RL. Femoral nerve block in extracapsular femoral neck fractures. J Bone Joint Surg Br 1995;77:922–3.
93. Finlayson BJ, Underhill TJ. Femoral nerve block for analgesia in fractures of the femoral neck. Arch Emerg Med 1988;5:173–6.
94. Mutty CE, Jensen EJ, Manka MA, et al. Femoral nerve block for diaphyseal and distal femoral fractures in the emergency department. J Bone Joint Surg Am 2007;89:2599–603.
95. Fletcher AK, Rigby AS, Heyes FL. Three-in-one femoral nerve block as analgesia for fractured neck of femur in the emergency department: a randomized, controlled trial. Ann Emerg Med 2003;41:227–33.
96. Gille J, Gille M, Gahr R, et al. Acute pain management in proximal femoral fractures: femoral nerve block (catheter technique) vs. systemic pain therapy using a clinic internal organisation model. Anaesthesist 2006;55: 414–22.
97. Mutty CE, Jensen EJ, Manka MA, et al. Femoral nerve block for diaphyseal and distal femoral fractures in the emergency department. Surgical technique. J Bone Joint Surg Am 2008;90:218–26.
98. Marhofer P, Schrögendorfer K, Koinig H, et al. Ultrasonographic guidance improves sensory block and onset time of three-in-one blocks. Anesth Analg 1997;85:854–7.
99. Reid N, Stella J, Ryan M, et al. Use of ultrasound to facilitate accurate femoral nerve block in the emergency department. Emerg Med Australas 2009;21:124–30.
100. Layzell M. Pain management: setting up a nurse-led femoral nerve block service. Br J Nurs 2007;16:702–5.
101. Vloka JD, Hadzic A, Drobnik L, et al. Anatomical landmarks for femoral nerve block: a comparison of four needle insertion sites. Anesth Analg 1999;89: 1467–70.
102. McGee DL. Local and topical anesthesia. In: Roberts JR, Hedges JR, Chanmugam AS, et al, editors. Clinical procedures in emergency medicine. 4th edition. Philadelphia: Saunders; 2004. p. 533–51.
103. Kendall JM, Allen P, Younge P, et al. Haematoma block or Bier's block for Colles' fracture reduction in the accident and emergency department – which is best? J Accid Emerg Med 1997;14:352–6.

104. Roberts JR. Intravenous regional anesthesia. In: Roberts JR, Hedges JR, Chanmugam AS, et al, editors. Clinical procedures in emergency medicine. 4th edition. Philadelphia: Saunders; 2004. p. 591–5.

105. Singh GK, Manglik RK, Lakhtakia PK, et al. Analgesia for the reduction of Colles fracture. A comparison of hematoma block and intravenous sedation. Online J Curr Clin Trials 1992. Doc no. 23.

106. Dorf E, Kuntz AF, Kelsey J, et al. Lidocaine-induced altered mental status and seizure after hematoma block. J Emerg Med 2006;31:251–3.

107. NIH Consensus Development Panel of Osteoporosis Prevention, Diagnosis, and Therapy. Osteoporosis prevention, diagnosis, and therapy. JAMA 2001;285: 785–95.

108. Dirschl DR, Henderson RC, Oakley WC. Accelerated bone mineral loss following a hip fracture: a prospective longitudinal study. Bone 1997;21:79–82.

109. Gardner MJ, Flik KR, Mooar P, et al. Improvement in the undertreatment of osteoporosis following hip fracture. J Bone Joint Surg Am 2002;84:1342–8.

110. Ross PD. Risk factors for osteoporotic fracture. Endocrinol Metab Clin North Am 1998;27:289–301.

111. Melton LJ, Atkinson EJ, O'Fallon WM, et al. Long-term fracture prediction by bone mineral assessed at different skeletal sites. J Bone Miner Res 1993;8: 1227–33.

112. Genant HK, Cooper C, Poor G, et al. Interim report and recommendations of the World Health Organization Task-Force for Osteoporosis. Osteoporos Int 1999; 10:259–64.

113. Cummings SR, Black DM, Nevitt MC, et al. Bone density at various sites for prediction of hip fractures. The Study of Osteoporotic Fractures Research Group. Lancet 1993;341:72–5.

114. Buchbinder R, Osborne RH, Ebeling PR, et al. A randomized trial of vertebroplasty for painful osteoporotic vertebral fractures. N Engl J Med 2009;361: 557–68.

115. Kallmes DF, Comstock BA, Heagerty PJ, et al. A randomized trial of vertebroplasty for osteoporotic spinal fractures. N Engl J Med 2009;361:569–79.

116. Wardlaw D, Cummings SR, Van Meirhaeghe J, et al. Efficacy and safety of balloon kyphoplasty compared with non-surgical care for vertebral compression fracture (FREE): a randomised controlled trial. Lancet 2009;373:1016–24.

117. Chapuy MC, Arlot ME, Duboeuf F, et al. Vitamin D3 and calcium to prevent hip fractures in the elderly women. N Engl J Med 1992;327:1637–42.

118. Chapuy MC, Arlot ME, Delmas PD, et al. Effect of calcium and cholecalciferol treatment for three years on hip fractures in elderly women. BMJ 1994;308:1081–2.

119. Black DM, Cummings SR, Karpf DB, et al. Randomised trial of effect of alendronate on risk of fracture in women with existing vertebral fractures. Fracture Intervention Trial Research Group. Lancet 1996;348:1535–41.

120. Black DM, Thompson DE, Bauer DC, et al. Fracture risk reduction with alendronate in women with osteoporosis: the Fracture Intervention Trial. FIT Research Group. J Clin Endocrinol Metab 2000;85:4118–24.

121. Chesnut CH III, Silverman S, Andriano K, et al. A randomized trial of nasal spray salmon calcitonin in postmenopausal women with established osteoporosis: the prevent recurrence of osteoporotic fractures study. PROOF Study Group. Am J Med 2000;109:267–76.

122. Martens MG. Risk of fracture and treatment to prevent osteoporosis-related fracture in postmenopausal women. A review. J Reprod Med 2003;48:425–34.

123. Silverman SL. Calcitonin. Endocrinol Metab Clin North Am 2003;32:273–84.

124. Morello KD, Wurz GT, DeGregorio MW. SERMs: current status and future trends. Crit Rev Oncol Hematol 2002;43:63–76.

125. Body JJ, Gaich GA, Scheele WH, et al. A randomized double-blind trial to compare the efficacy of teriparatide [recombinant human parathyroid hormone (1–34)] with alendronate in postmenopausal women with osteoporosis. J Clin Endocrinol Metab 2002;87:4528–35.

126. Dempster DW, Cosman F, Kurland ES, et al. Effects of daily treatment with parathyroid hormone on bone microarchitecture and turnover in patients with osteoporosis: a paired biopsy study. J Bone Miner Res 2001;16:1846–53.

127. Reeve J, Meunier PJ, Parsons JA, et al. Anabolic effect of human parathyroid hormone fragment on trabecular bone in involutional osteoporosis: a multicentre trial. BMJ 1980;280:1340–4.

128. Jilka RL, Weinstein RS, Bellido T, et al. Increased bone formation by prevention of osteoblast apoptosis with parathyroid hormone. J Clin Invest 1999;104: 439–46.

129. Kannus P, Parkkari J, Niemi S, et al. Prevention of hip fracture in elderly people with use of a hip protector. N Engl J Med 2000;343:1506–13.

130. Kiel DP, Magaziner J, Zimmerman S, et al. Efficacy of a hip protector to prevent hip fracture in nursing home residents: the HIP PRO randomized controlled trial. JAMA 2007;298:413–22.

131. Parker MJ, Gillespie LD, Gillespie WJ. Hip protectors for preventing hip fractures in the elderly. Cochrane Database Syst Rev 2004;3:CD001255.

132. Barton BA, Birge SJ, Magaziner J, et al. The Hip Impact Protection Project: design and methods. Clin Trials 2008;5:347–55.

133. Cameron ID, Robinovitch S, Birge SJ, et al. Hip protectors: recommendations for conducting clinical trials – an international consensus statement (part II). Osteoporos Int 2010;21:1–10.

134. Cameron ID, Stafford B, Cumming RG, et al. Hip protectors improve falls self-efficacy. Age Ageing 2000;29:57–62.

135. Kaplan RS, Sinaki M, Hameister MD. Effect of back supports on back strength in patients with osteoporosis: a pilot study. Mayo Clin Proc 1996;71:235–41.

136. Sinaki M, Itoi E, Wahner HW, et al. Stronger back muscles reduce the incidence of vertebral fractures: a prospective 10 year follow-up of postmenopausal women. Bone 2002;30:836–41.

137. Wolf SL, Barnhart HX, Kutner NG, et al. Reducing frailty and falls in older persons: an investigation of Tai Chi and computerized balance training. Atlanta FICSIT Group. Frailty and Injuries: Cooperative Studies of Intervention Techniques. J Am Geriatr Soc 1996;44:489–97.

138. Fanuele J, Koval KJ, Lurie J, et al. Distal radial fracture treatment: what you get may depend on your age and address. J Bone Joint Surg Am 2009;91:1313–9.

139. Koval KJ, Meek R, Schemitsch E, et al. Geriatric trauma: young ideas. J Bone Joint Surg Am 2003;85:1380–8.

140. Egol KA, Strauss EJ. Perioperative considerations in geriatric patients with hip fracture: what is the evidence? J Orthop Trauma 2009;23:386–94.

141. Radcliff TA, Henderson WG, Stoner TJ, et al. Patient risk factors, operative care, and outcomes among older community-dwelling male veterans with hip fracture. J Bone Joint Surg Am 2008;90:34–42.

142. Pioli G, Giusti A, Barone A. Orthogeriatric care for the elderly with hip fractures: where are we? Aging Clin Exp Res 2008;20:113–22.

143. Handoll HH, Cameron ID, Mak JC, et al. Multidisciplinary rehabilitation for older people with hip fractures. Cochrane Database Syst Rev 2009;4:CD007125.

144. Amatuzzi MM, Carelli CD, Leme LEG, et al. Interdisciplinary care in orthogeri-atrics: a good cost-benefit model of care. J Am Geriatr Soc 2003;51:134–6.
145. Vidan M, Serra JA, Moreno C, et al. Efficacy of a comprehensive geriatric inter-vention in older patients hospitalized for hip fracture: a randomized, controlled trial. J Am Geriatr Soc 2005;53:1476–82.
146. De Jonge KE, Christmas C, Andersen R, et al. Hip fracture service – an interdis-ciplinary model of care. J Am Geriatr Soc 2001;49:1737–8.
147. Gilchrist WJ, Newman RJ, Hamblen DL, et al. Prospective randomised study of an orthopaedic geriatric inpatient service. BMJ 1988;297:1116–8.
148. Koval KJ, Chen AL, Aharonoff GB, et al. Clinical pathway for hip fractures in the elderly. Clin Orthop Relat Res 2004;425:72–81.
149. Pedersen SJ, Borgbjerg FM, Schousboe B, et al. A comprehensive hip frac-ture program reduces complication rates and mortality. J Am Geriatr Soc 2008;56:1831–8.
150. Friedman SM, Mendelson DA, Kates SL, et al. Geriatric co-management of prox-imal femur fractures: total quality management and protocol-driven care result in better outcomes for a frail patient population. J Am Geriatr Soc 2008;56:1349–56.
151. Inouye SK, van Dyck CH, Slessi CA, et al. Clarifying confusion: the confusion assessment method. A new method for detection of delirium. Ann Intern Med 1990;113:941–8.
152. Ely EW, Inouye SK, Bernard GR, et al. Delirium in mechanically ventilated patients: validity and reliability of the confusion assessment method for the intensive care unit (CAM-ICU). JAMA 2001;286:2703–10.
153. Han JH, Zimmerman EE, Cutler N, et al. Delirium in older emergency department patients: recognition, risk factors, and psychomotor subtypes. Acad Emerg Med 2009;16:193–200.
154. Edlund A, Lundstrom M, Brannstrom B, et al. Delirium before and after operation for femoral neck fracture. J Am Geriatr Soc 2001;49:1335–40.
155. Bitsch MS, Foss NB, Kristensen BB, et al. Pathogenesis of and management strategies for postoperative delirium after hip fracture: a review. Acta Orthop Scand 2004;75:378–89.
156. Lundström M, Olofsson B, Stenvall M, et al. Postoperative delirium in old patients with femoral neck fracture: a randomized intervention study. Aging Clin Exp Res 2007;19:178–86.
157. Lundström M, Edlund A, Lundstrom G, et al. Reorganization of nursing and medical care to reduce the incidence of postoperative delirium and improve rehabilitation outcome in elderly patients treated for femoral neck fractures. Scand J Caring Sci 1999;13:193–200.
158. Milisen K, Foreman MD, Abraham IL, et al. A nurse-led interdisciplinary intervention program for delirium in elderly hip-fracture patients. J Am Geriatr Soc 2001;49:523–32.
159. Marcantonio ER, Flacker JM, Wright RJ, et al. Reducing delirium after hip fracture: a randomized trial. J Am Geriatr Soc 2001;49:516–22.
160. Gustafson Y, Brannstrom B, Berggren D, et al. A geriatric-anesthesiologic program to reduce acute confusion states in elderly patients treated for femoral neck fractures. J Am Geriatr Soc 1991;39:655–62.
161. Jacobs DG, Plaisier BR, Barie PS, et al. Practice management guidelines for geriatric trauma: the EAST Practice Management Guidelines Work Group. J Trauma 2003;54:391–416.
162. Bryce SN, Han JH. Cognitive impairment and comprehension of emergency department discharge instructions in older patients [abstract #257]. Ann Emerg Med 2009;54:S80–1.

163. Siebens H. The domain management model–a tool for teaching and management of older adults in emergency departments. Acad Emerg Med 2005;12: 162–8.
164. Dominguez S, Liu P, Roberts C, et al. Prevalence of traumatic hip and pelvic fractures in patients with suspected hip fracture and negative initial standard radiographs–a study of emergency department patients. Acad Emerg Med 2005;12:366–9.
165. Pandey R, McNally E, Ali A, et al. The role of MRI in the diagnosis of occult hip fractures. Injury 1998;29:61–3.
166. Lee YP, Griffith JF, Antonio GE, et al. Early magnetic resonance imaging of radiographically occult osteoporotic fractures of the femoral neck. Hong Kong Med J 2004;10:271–5.
167. Cannon J, Silverstri S, Munro M. Imaging choices in occult hip fracture. J Emerg Med 2009;37:144–52.
168. Smith JE, Jenkin A, Hennessy C. A retrospective chart review of elderly patients who cannot weight bear following a hip injury but whose initial x rays are normal. Emerg Med J 2009;26:50–1.
169. Hossain M, Barwick C, Sinha AK, et al. Is magnetic resonance imaging (MRI) necessary to exclude occult hip fracture? Injury 2007;38:1204–8.
170. Evans PD, Wilson C, Lyons K. Comparison of MRI with bone scanning for suspected hip fracture in elderly patients. J Bone Joint Surg Br 1994;76:158–9.
171. Holder LE, Schwarz C, Wernicke PG, et al. Radionuclide bone imaging in the early detection of fractures of the proximal femur (hip): multifactorial analysis. Radiology 1990;174:509–15.
172. Verbeeten KM, Hermann KL, Hasselqvist M, et al. The advantages of MRI in the detection of occult hip fractures. Eur Radiol 2005;15:165–9.
173. Oka M, Monu JU. Prevalence and patterns of occult hip fractures and mimics revealed by MRI. AJR Am J Roentgenol 2004;182:283–8.
174. Lubovsky O, Liebergall M, Mattan Y, et al. Early diagnosis of occult hip fractures MRI versus CT scan. Injury 2005;36:788–92.
175. Rubin SJ, Marquardt JD, Gottlieb RH, et al. Magnetic resonance imaging: a cost-effective alternative to bone scintigraphy in the evaluation of patients with suspected hip fractures. Skeletal Radiol 1998;27:199–204.

Essential Concepts of Wound Management

Carlos F. García-Gubern, MD[a],*, Lissandra Colon-Rolon, MD[a],
Michael C. Bond, MD[b]

KEYWORDS

- Emergency • Wounds • Suture
- Wound documentation and management

The practice of wound care has greatly improved and evolved over the years. Wound care techniques have been documented since 1500 BC in ancient Egypt and Greece where lint was used as a fibrous base, animal grease as a protective barrier, and honey as a topical antibiotic.[1] In 150 AD, the Greek surgeon, Galen of Pergamum, while working with a Roman gladiator's cuts, first addressed the fact that the wound should be kept moist to ensure adequate healing. Honey has been used as both a topical ointment and as an antibacterial for infected wounds.[2] Today the emergency provider (EP) can choose from a wide variety of sutures, adhesives, strips, and surgical staples, and uses proven wound closure techniques to address this common Emergency Department (ED) patient complaint.

It has been reported that lacerations in the United States accounted for approximately 12% of all ED visits in 2005 (115.3 million visits), and almost 40% were related to blunt trauma.[3] The most common anatomic areas for lacerations in decreasing order of frequency are the scalp, face and neck, fingers and toes, lower and upper extremities, and trunk/back.

Many factors contribute to the healing of lacerations. Factors that cannot be controlled by the EP are genetics, shape, and anatomic area. However, bleeding control, inspection, exploration, cleansing, debridement, closure technique, closure materials, dressings, infection control, anesthesia and analgesia, and wound after care can be affected by the EP's actions. The EP must have a good understanding of all these factors to assure that the wounds heal well with a minimum number of complications.

Although patients presenting to the ED with wounds requiring treatment are generally assigned a low acuity level, and often do not have life-threatening injuries, these cases

[a] Department of Emergency Medicine, Ponce School of Medicine/Hospital San Lucas, Ponce, PR 00731, USA
[b] Department of Emergency Medicine, University of Maryland School of Medicine, Baltimore, MD 21201, USA
* Corresponding author. PO Box 195504, San Juan, PR 00919.
E-mail address: prerdoc@yahoo.com

Emerg Med Clin N Am 28 (2010) 951–967
doi:10.1016/j.emc.2010.06.009
0733-8627/10/$ – see front matter © 2010 Elsevier Inc. All rights reserved.

result in a high number of malpractice claims. A study by Karcz, on closed malpractice claims involving EPs in the state of Massachusetts, showed that out of 109 claims, 66% were related to lacerations.[4] Retained foreign bodies, and missed tendon or neurovascular injuries are 2 common issues that result in malpractice claims.

SKIN ANATOMY

The skin is the largest organ in the human body; among its unique functions are heat control, protection against bacteria and trauma, and general environment sensation. Skin (**Table 1**) varies in thickness; from 1 mm found over the eyelids to 4 to 5 mm found over the back, palms, and soles. The skin is composed of the epidermis (outer) and dermis (inner) layers. The epidermis consists of the stratum germinativum where new skin cells develop. The thicker dermis is rich in collagen-producing fibroblasts and is composed of 2 layers: the reticular (deeper) dermis where hair follicles, sweat glands, and vascular plexus are found, and a more superficial layer, the papillary dermis. The papillary dermis is very vascular and is responsible for providing nutrients to the epidermis.

Deep to the skin is the superficial fascia (ie, subcutaneous layer), which is composed of loose connective tissue and fat. Fat provides insulation and acts as a buffer against trauma. At the base lies the deep fascia, which consists of thick, fibrous, white-colored tissue enclosing muscle groups. It forms a barrier against bacterial spread deeper into the muscle compartments.

INJURY AND WOUND HEALING

To adequately evaluate a wound it is important to take a thorough history that includes the circumstances on how and when the wound was inflicted. Specifically, it is important to know if there is a chance of contamination in the wound, whether it is associated with a crushing injury, or if there is a risk of associated injuries (ie, fractures, joint involvement).

Table 1
Skin anatomy and function

Skin Anatomy	Key Facts	Wound Care
Epidermis (skin; cutaneous)	Protection against bacteria, toxic chemicals and electrolytes, and water egress	Cosmetic appearance
Dermis (connective tissue) *Papillary dermis* *Reticular dermis*	Collagen-producing cells Very vascular-nutrient supplier Engulfs skin adnexal structures	The dermis is the key structural layer for adequate wound repair
Superficial fascia (subcutaneous Layer)	Loose connective tissue and Fat for insulation and protection	Always cleanse thoroughly to eliminate contaminants and clots, to decrease risk of infection
Deep fascia	Fibrous, white-colored support layer; protective barrier against infection spread	If lacerated, requires repair

EPs must also understand the basics of the body's normal wound-healing process. The first response after sustaining a laceration is hemostasis. Hemostasis is achieved via vasoconstriction, wound edge retraction, platelet aggregation, and clot formation. The next stage is the inflammatory response. This response occurs with activation of the complement system, which recruits both lymphocytes and granulocytes to suppress bacterial growth. This phase begins within 24 hours of hemostasis, preparing the area for new tissue growth, and builds bridges between the wound edges. Neovascularization ensures oxygenated blood and nutrients are rapidly delivered to the fast-growing epithelial cells. After this complex unit is formed, new collagen is produced underneath it, replacing devitalized or damaged collagen. This process peaks 7 to 10 days after the injury. Wound dehiscence occurs most often during the period of balance between new and old collagen deposits.[5,6] Finally, the remodeling period begins, which can last several months. At the end of the healing process the skin will reach its final strength, which may never be as strong as it was before the injury.

Using the knowledge of skin healing, the EP can make a more informed decision on whether a wound should be closed using primary, secondary, or tertiary intention (**Table 2**). To make a decision on which one to use, the clinician relies on the degree of contamination, devitalized tissue, and the age of the wound.

The final appearance of any wound is affected by numerous factors that can be grouped into the following categories: (1) medications, (2) anatomic location, (3) technical, (4) diseases related, or (5) wound related.[6–11] Not all of these factors are within the control of the clinician. Poor wound outcomes have resulted in malpractice claims, therefore a good knowledge of all these factors can help the EP inform the patient when a poor outcome is predicted and why.[4,11] In a study by Singer and colleagues,[9] these factors were statistically analyzed in a multivariate analysis; the factors most likely associated with poor cosmetic outcomes were tissue trauma, extremity wound location, wider wounds, electrocautery use, and poor wound edge apposition. The medications associated with negative outcomes are corticosteroids, anticoagulants, nonsteroidal anti-inflammatories, colchicine, and antineoplastic pharmacotherapy. These drugs are known to adversely affect the inflammatory response, epithelialization, and neovascularization, which increase the risk for hematoma formation and decreased tensile forces.[12,13] Prolonged shock state, severe anemia, uremia, advanced cancer, hepatic failure, diabetes, and severe cardiovascular disease can adversely affect nutrient delivery and oxygen supply to the wound, leading to poor healing.[12]

Anatomic regions and expression lines (skin tension lines) play an important role in the final appearance of any wound. The extremities and the chest have the greatest chance of evident scar formation as well as oily and pigmented skin.[14,15]

Table 2
Indications and key points to consider for each closure type

Intention (Closure)	Unique Characteristics	Key Points
Primary	Clean, minimally contaminated, mostly shearing forces 6–8 hours old	May close with tape, staplers, and sutures
Secondary	Noncosmetic animal bites Abscess cavities, ulcers	No sutures Delayed skin coverage, graft
Tertiary	Too contaminated to close	Must clean, debride, and observe 4–6 days before suturing

Improper suturing techniques, which can cause increased wound tension leading to ischemia, and poor suture material selection (ie, silk versus nylon) are the most important contributing factors in poor wound healing. In addition, routine hair removal and shaving before suturing can lead to poor outcomes.[15–17] Body hair entangled in sutures and staples or buried inside the wound can alter the healing process and increase the risk of infection. In well-perfused areas such as the scalp, wounds healed without infection in unshaved lacerations.[18] If hair must be removed, scissors or clippers should be used. Shaving causes small dermal wounds that allow bacteria to penetrate into deeper structures and potentially cause an infection. In several studies looking at operative cases, there was an increased risk of infection in those patients who were shaved than in those who were not shaved.[19–21] Although there are no specific studies regarding shaved versus nonshaved wound care in ED patients, the low infection rate of eyebrow lacerations, which are not shaved, supports the practice of not shaving with a razor prior to skin closure.

One of the key factors in preventing wound infections after skin closure is to adequately irrigate the wound. Irrigation decreases bacterial counts in the wound and helps to remove particulate contamination. The major factor in decreasing bacterial counts and contamination is the amount of irrigation. Several prospective studies summarized in a Cochrane review published in 2010 note that tap water irrigation is as good as irrigation with sterile normal saline, and in fact tap water might actually be associated with decreased rates of infection.[22–29] Ideally, the wound should be irrigated with a pressure between 8 and 30 psi[30–33]; this can be achieved with a 20- to 60-mL syringe with an 18- or 19-gauge needle or angiocatheter attached. One article described a technique of breaking off a 19-gauge needle at the hub, while others have described cutting an angiocatheter short so that the stream of water can be aimed.[34] Higher pressures have been shown to cause additional tissue damage in animals, which can lead to poor wound healing.[33] Because tap water irrigation is more cost effective and has similar outcomes, it should be the primary solution used to irrigate wounds in the ED.

Another area where costs can be controlled in the process of dealing with wound repairs is in the use of sterile gloves. A 2004 study compared clean nonsterile gloves with sterile gloves, and demonstrated a higher though not statistically significant rate of infection with sterile gloves (6.1%) than with clean nonsterile gloves (4.4%). With the cost of sterile gloves being about $0.70 and a pair of clean nonsterile gloves $0.10, it is estimated that the average ED seeing approximately 10 noncomplicated lacerations a day could save $2190 per year. Though not conducted in the ED, another study looking at the rate of infection in patients undergoing dressing changes for wound healing by secondary intention had similar outcomes, with no increased rate of infection seen when nonsterile gloves were used.[35,36]

Several studies have shown that many antiseptics have cytotoxic effects on fibroblasts and keratinocytes, as well as on many other key cellular participants of wound healing.[37–40] It has also been shown that the application of local antiseptics to a wound leads to delayed wound healing even at subcytotoxic antiseptic levels.[37] Due to their cytotoxic effects, povidone-iodine–based antiseptics and hydrogen peroxide should no longer be used in any wound to prevent infection. Both solutions alter the migration and proliferation of skin fibroblast, fundamental cells in the proliferative phase of wound healing, and the matrix metalloproteinase release by the dermal fibroblasts, thus making the wound bed a harsh environment for adequate healing. Chlorhexidine is not without its own concerns. First, the required bactericidal concentration varies widely among microorganisms. For example, methicillin-resistant *Staphylococcus aureus* only requires a concentration of 0.002%, while gram-negative organisms might require a bactericidal concentration of 1%.[41] Another disadvantage is the increasing bacterial resistance to antibiotics that is associated with higher antibiotic use.[41,42] The antiseptic solution that least affects the wound-healing process is the silver-containing compounds, which inhibit the growth of *Pseudomonas aeruginosa* even at very low concentrations (10 μmol/L).[43] The mainstay of wound healing is within the fresh wound itself, the natural human healing process. Surgical wound debridement greatly stimulates this natural response.[44–47] Timely and adequate wound margin revisions with debridement of old and necrotic tissue stimulates normal wound healing in the vast majority of lacerations.[46,47]

WOUND ANESTHESIA

There are a wide variety of pharmacologic agents and nerve-blocking techniques to help minimize painful procedures. Some patients will require only topical or local anesthetics whereas others will require procedural sedation and parenteral analgesics. The best choice will depend on the individual. The EP must be aware that the perception of pain is learned and varies between different ethnic groups, age, and prior painful experiences. Cultural differences exist concerning stoicism, expressions, beliefs, and attitudes with respect to pain, which has led to pain being undertreated in some ethnic groups because of cultural and language barriers that may affect the EP's evaluation and understanding of the patient's pain.[48–50]

An understanding of the basic pharmacology of the local anesthetics will help the EP avoid unwanted side effects, toxicity, and complications. Local anesthetic toxicity is related to 2 basic factors: lipid solubility or potency, and the duration of action. The most commonly reported toxic effects of local anesthetics are summarized in **Table 3**.

Topical anesthetic compounds are safe and easy to use, with proven efficacy, and are widely used. When compared with local anesthetic infiltration, topical anesthetics can be applied painlessly, do not affect wound edges, and can help provide hemostasis. These preparations work better in the head and neck region although they have a slower onset of action.[51] The most commonly used and studied formulations are EMLA (lidocaine and prilocaine), LET (lidocaine, epinephrine, and tetracaine), and TAC (tetracaine, adrenaline, and cocaine) (**Table 4**).

Ethyl chloride, a skin refrigerant, has been used in the past as a local anesthetic agent. When it comes in contact with the skin, it vaporizes, causing a drop in skin temperature to −20°C and desensitizing it, thus permitting venipuncture, injections, suturing, and incision and drainage (I&D) with minimum discomfort.

Table 3	
Common toxic effects for local anesthetics listed by organ system	
Respiratory	**Hypoventilation, Respiratory Failure (Arrest)**
Cardiovascular	Hyper-/hypotension, bradycardia, palpitations, vasodilation, ventricular dysrhythmias (bupivacaine), myocardial depression, and cardiovascular collapse
Central nervous system	Severe: seizures, coma Moderate: muscle twitch, slurred speech, drowsiness, excitability, perioral paresthesia Mild: tongue numbness, restlessness, lightheadedness, visual disturbances
Methemoglobinemia (prilocaine and benzocaine)	Cyanosis, dizziness, lethargy, dyspnea (more so in children)

The most common anesthetic techniques used by EPs are local anesthetic infiltration and regional anesthesia. Local anesthesia refers to local infiltration of an agent directly into the wound margins or surrounding the wound or procedural area for either wound repair or for invasive procedural anesthesia (chest tube, lumbar puncture, central line, and so forth). Regional anesthesia consists of peripheral nerve blocks, intravenous blocks (Bier blocks), and hematoma blocks.[52]

The hematoma block is a quick, reliable, and relatively safe procedure to achieve adequate anesthesia for the closed reduction of isolated fractures. After aseptic skin preparation the fracture is palpated, a 10-mL syringe with a 20- to 22-gauge needle is used to aspirate the hematoma for location purposes, and the hematoma is infiltrated with 4 to 10 mL of 1% lidocaine without epinephrine. Adequate anesthesia is achieved in 5 to 15 minutes and lasts several hours.[52]

An intravenous (Bier) block is useful to anesthetize a large area of the distal extremity but it requires special preparation, as the patient should be closely monitored with pulse oximetry, telemetry, and frequent vital signs. A double-cuff constant pressure tourniquet should be used, and the EP must be aware of the proper steps to the procedure in addition to the potential complications and how to deal with them. Some contraindications to performing a Bier block are Raynaud syndrome, hypertension, cardiac conduction abnormalities, overlying cellulitis, age less than 5 years, and sickle cell or peripheral vascular disease.[53]

A Bier block is performed by first diluting 1% lidocaine (10 mg/mL) by half with normal saline to create a 0.5% lidocaine (5 mg/mL) solution for a total dose not to exceed 3 mg/kg (eg, an average 70-kg person can receive 210 mg of lidocaine or 10.5 mL of the 3.33 mg/mL solution). The arm should then be elevated for more than 4 minutes or compressed by the placement of an elastic gauze bandage applied distal to proximal on the arm. The elastic gauze needs to be applied as tight as possible to ensure that the arm is exsanguinated. Cotton Webril can be placed on the proximal arm or leg where the dual tourniquet/blood pressure cuffs will be applied to provide some additional padding. Ideally, blood pressure cuffs should be avoided, as they are not designed to maintain a high pressure for a prolonged period of time, and they also tend to leak, releasing the pressure that is needed to ensure that the lidocaine does not travel centrally. The more proximal tourniquet is inflated to 250 to 300 mm Hg and the lidocaine solution is slowly injected intravenously into a distal vein on the affected side. The lidocaine must be injected distal to the tourniquet on the affected side and not into the patient's other intravenous site, which can be used for intravenous fluids or sedation. If the patient experiences pain from the proximal tourniquet, the distal tourniquet can be inflated to 250 to 300 mm Hg and then the more proximal tourniquet deflated, thus ensuring that the inflated tourniquet is now

Table 4 Common topical anesthetics			
	Topical Agent		
	LET	TAC	EMLA
Mixture %	Lidocaine 4% Epinephrine 0.1% Tetracaine 0.5%	Tetracaine 0.5% Adrenaline 0.05% Cocaine 11.8%	Lidocaine 2.5% Prilocaine 2.5%
AVOID	Mucosa, fingers, toes, ear pinna, penis, and nose tip	Mucosa and in large amounts	Over lacerated skin

overlying a portion of the arm that has been anesthetized. After 30 to 45 minutes the remaining tourniquet can be deflated cyclically (deflated for 5 seconds and then reinflated for 1–2 minutes), as the lidocaine will have bound to the tissue in the extremity and will not be released centrally where it can have toxic side effects such as seizures. The cyclic deflation and reinflation also provides additional safety by ensuring that a large bolus of lidocaine cannot be released into the central circulation.[52,54] A mini-dose of lidocaine has also been described, using 1.5 mg/kg of lidocaine, with a 95% success rate of anesthesia.[55]

Peripheral nerve blocks in general require less medication and are less painful than local infiltration. A neurovascular status must be documented before the procedure, and maximum doses of the anesthetic must be calculated and double-checked to avoid toxicity if inadvertent intravascular injection occurs. The syringe should be aspirated until the proper position is located to ensure that the needle tip is not intravascular. When the patient reports paresthesias in the desired nerve distribution, the needle is in its proper position. Some commonly used regional blocks in the ED are:

1. Upper extremity: radial, ulnar, median, and digital nerve blocks
2. Lower extremity: sural, posterior tibial, deep, and superficial peroneal nerve blocks
3. Facial: supraorbital, infraorbital, and mental nerve blocks.

EXPLORATION AND DEBRIDEMENT

All wounds should be explored and debrided of devitalized tissue or containments. Because of the risk of litigation, good documentation in this area is extremely important. The function and stability of associated structures (ie, tendons and ligaments) must be tested and directly visualized. If a foreign object such as glass, plastic, pencil graphite, metallic fragment, or gravel is suspected, a radiograph should be ordered, reviewed, and documented before any attempt at exploration and closure. If the wound history suggests wood or plant material, it should be explored because these wounds are at high risk for infection due to retained plant matter. Large scalp lacerations should be explored by direct palpation of the skull looking for unrecognized fractures.[56–59]

A thorough neurologic examination of the affected area must be documented and the area anesthetized before conducting a detailed examination. The wound should be explored with blunt objects to avoid any additional tissue damage or the creation of false passages. Often a complete visualization of the underlying structures cannot be achieved with the original wound, and extension of the wound edges might be required. Cosmetic considerations and closing techniques (skin excision or appositional difficulties) must be planned for before extending the wound.

It is imperative that deep lacerations of the hand and forearm be explored to the wound base to ensure that there is no tendon involvement. Patients may only experience a little pain with range of motion and yet have an almost complete tear or laceration of their tendon. Often pain will increase when resistance is applied, though this is not always present. The wound bed should be explored through the fingers' and wrist's full range of motion to ensure that the affected portion of a lacerated tendon has not been pulled more proximally. When the arm or hand is examined on a table or examining table, it is typically flat and extended, which will draw the tendons more proximally as compared with the hand being clenched in a fist.[60]

Bleeding must be controlled. Active bleeding prevents adequate visualization and exploration, and increases the risk of missed injuries. Wound hemostasis can be achieved by direct pressure, application of a tourniquet or blood pressure cuff inflated 20 mm Hg above the patient's systolic blood pressure, or with the use of topical or subcutaneous epinephrine. Epinephrine-moistened gauze (1:100,000) applied directly over the wound for 10 minutes helps to constrict small blood vessels and decrease the bleeding. Pressure should only be applied for 5 minutes when controlling bleeding over the nose tip, mucosa, penis, and earlobe.[10,61] Hemostatic gelatin foam can also be used. Large nondigital vessels can be directly visualized and ligated with clamping or a figure-of-8 suture. The digital arteries should never be ligated or clamped, as they run parallel and in very close proximity to the digital nerve, and clamping both is almost inevitable. The blind clamping of any bleeding wound is strongly discouraged.

Large extremity tourniquets are rarely needed, but when used they must be properly placed. Cotton gauze should be placed on the limb to provide some protection to the skin, and then an inflatable tourniquet or blood-pressure cuff can be inflated to 20 mm Hg higher than the patient's systolic blood pressure, not to exceed 250 mm Hg, to control distal arterial blood flow. The tourniquet should be inflated for no longer than 20 to 30 minutes, before it is deflated for 5 minutes. Total inflation time should not exceed 1 hour. For digital tourniquets, a stretched Penrose drain can be placed at the base of a previously exsanguinated digit or a commercial rubber ring tourniquet can be applied for a maximum of 30 minutes.[10,16]

The axiom "that no finger should be injected with epinephrine because it might lead to necrosis" that has been passed on from one generation of medical clinicians to the next has been disproved. There are sufficient published and reviewed data to verify that the use of epinephrine in digital anesthesia is safe and effective.[61–66]

Epinephrine, which is an effective hemostatic agent, prolongs and improves the effect of digital anesthesia.[62–65] Plastic surgeons have used low-dose epinephrine (1:100,000) in hand and digital procedures as well as in nose and ear surgeries for years, despite the dogma of avoiding this practice. This dogma was based on 48 published cases of digital necrosis that were published from the late 1920s until the early 1950s.[66] A detailed review of the case reports showed that epinephrine was used in only 21 of the 48 cases and procaine in at least 31 cases. Several case reports even reported that there was bleeding or pink color of the finger at the end of the case, which is not compatible with complete vasospasm. A recent study by Altinyazar and colleagues[64] using color Doppler showed that epinephrine used in digital blocks induced a low-flow arterial state but that arterial flow never stopped. The effect of epinephrine also lasted less than 90 minutes, which is well below the ischemic time of a finger. Procaine is the most likely culprit of the necrosis. Procaine degrades with time and heat into para-aminobenzoic acid, creating a very acidic solution. In 1948, the Food and Drug Administration published a recall of procaine in JAMA due to several lots being found that had a pH of 1. No cases of digital necrosis have been published since the 1950s when procaine use was essentially abandoned. Lidocaine came to the market in 1948. Therefore the cause of the necrosis before the 1950s was not vasospasm caused by epinephrine, but rather the injection of highly acidic procaine solution.[62,67,68] The use of low-dose epinephrine with local anesthetics in digital blocks is safe, decreases pain, increases the duration of anesthesia, and improves hemostasis.

CLOSING TECHNIQUES

As with any learned skill, one must become familiarized with the instruments and materials that will be used. Commercial suturing kits can vary in their contents with the exception that they all tend to have a needle holder, scissor, hemostat, and tissue forceps. The other required material is the suture itself; these are divided into absorbable and nonabsorbable materials.

Nonabsorbable sutures are generally used for the outer skin, and absorbable sutures are used for mucosal or subcutaneous suturing. Special attention must be paid when working with absorbable sutures as they tend to break easily, and can get stuck in the tissue and not pull through properly. A small amount of sterile petroleum jelly, or running the complete suture through sterile petrolatum gauze, helps to avoid this complication.

EPs should be familiar with the following suturing techniques (it is not the intention of this article to demonstrate all of them): (1) simple interrupted, (2) continuous, (3) vertical mattress, (4) horizontal mattress, (5) half-buried horizontal mattress, and (6) subcuticular pull-out and running closure.

In addition to these traditional suturing techniques, EPs should be comfortable with using surgical staples, tissue adhesives, and hair apposition techniques. Surgical staplers tend to be favored in noncosmetic wounds because of the ease and quickness of insertion. Both have similar final cosmetic appearance and infection rates.[69] Tissue adhesives have very good cosmetic outcomes and decreased infection rate when used on facial and neck wounds.[70–72]

The hair apposition technique (HAT) and the modified HAT for scalp lacerations should be considered more often for the repair of scalp lacerations that are noncrush injuries less than 10 cm long with regular wound edges, minimal contamination, no evidence of underlying skull fractures, and an intact galea in patients with hair strands longer than 3 cm. These techniques are associated with less scarring, fewer overall complications, shorter procedural time, lower pain scores, and substantially lower costs than standard suturing and stapler techniques. The HAT technique consists of twisting together 3 to 7 strands of hair on either side of the wound. The 2 bundles of hair are then interlocked in a 360° revolution and a small drop of tissue adhesive can be applied to make sure that it does not unravel. The hair is not tied. This same process is repeated as needed for the entire length of the wound. The glue will break down and the hair will unravel by itself after 7 to 10 days.[73–76]

SPECIAL CONSIDERATIONS
Scalp

The scalp is highly vascularized, with the potential to cause hypotension and hypovolemia even with a small laceration. Initial care should consist of direct pressure. If this is not effective, bleeding can normally be controlled by approximating the wound edges. A large needle with 0 or 2-0 nylon suture should be used so that a large wide bite can be taken. Another option for large scalp wounds is to apply surgical scalp clamps (ie, Raney clips) that compress the wound edges and provide hemostasis.

As with all wounds, scalp lacerations need to be adequately debrided and irrigated before closure. However, special attention needs to be made to the galea, a dense fibrous layer covering and protecting the skull. The galea anchors several scalp muscles, and any laceration to it must be repaired to avoid cosmetic abnormalities such as difficulties with facial expressions. Separate absorbable sutures should be placed prior to the skin repair.

In adults and older children, scalp lacerations can be closed with a continuous percutaneous suture using a monofilament nylon suture or staples. Interrupted sutures with absorbable chromic gut can be used in small children, thus avoiding the suture removal process.

Eyebrow and Eyelid

Eyebrows should never be shaved. Eyebrows almost always require some deep suturing, and proper alignment of the margins must be ensured for cosmetic purposes. Special attention must be observed to avoid any hair being sutured into the wound, as this will increase the risk of infection and poor cosmetic closure.

For the eyelids, if the periorbital fat is exposed or a muscle is lacerated, an ophthalmologist should be consulted prior to wound closure in order to ensure good function and cosmetic appearance. An ophthalmologist should also be consulted for suspected intramarginal eyelid lacerations and lacrimal canaliculus or nasolacrimal duct lacerations. These last two should be suspected when there is excessive tearing running down the cheek, and in lacerations that involve the medial canaliculus.

Ears

All perichondral hematomas must be drained to avoid cosmetic complications such as cauliflower ear; drained pressure packs should be applied to avoid reaccumulation of blood. No cartilage should be left exposed; if needed, up to 5 mm of cartilage can be excised before the ear will start to show a deformed appearance. Stitches should not be placed in ear cartilage anchored to overlying skin.

Lips and Oral Cavity

The single most important stitch in lacerated lips is the vermilion border (white line) apposition. If the border is lacerated, the first suture done should carefully align along this border. The second most important suture is the stitch that aligns the transition zone between the dry and wet mucosa of the lip. Both areas must be properly aligned to ensure optimal function and cosmetic appearance.

A buccal wall or through-and-through lacerations should be closed with a minimum of 3 layers (skin, subcutaneous, and mucosal surface); with special care taken to document and repair any muscle lacerations. Tongue lacerations in general do not require repair unless the laceration is bifid, flap-shaped, involving muscle, actively bleeding, or has a significant gap. In general, gaps that are larger than a grain of rice should be repaired.[77]

Bites and Foreign Bodies

EPs must have a high index of suspicion for foreign bodies (FB), as they are commonly encountered.[56–59] All fresh wounds must be explored to rule out any unwanted object. Most of the time the history and physical examination will provide the answer; however, plain radiographs or ultrasound might be needed to exclude FB. Most FB are radiopaque and can be seen on plain radiographs.[56–59] The most commonly encountered FB in wounds that are visible on plain radiographs are glass pieces 2 mm and larger, metal, aluminum, pencil graphite, sand, gravel, fish bones (from red snapper, gray mullet, sole, and cod) and even some plastics. Computed tomography (CT) can visualize FB but has the disadvantage of higher costs and radiation exposure.[78]

Ultrasound detection of FB depends on the anatomic region, material, size, operator ability, and other confounding factors. Several ultrasound findings that suggest the presence of a FB are acoustic shadowing behind the FB and a hypoechoic rim. Once detected by either ultrasound or another radiographic modality; ultrasound can help guide proper removal.[79–82]

Unfortunately, some FB are invisible to visual inspection, plain radiographs, and ultrasound.[83] For this reason liability claims will continue to haunt EPs who take care of wounds and lacerations. The best defense is to inspect the wound in a bloodless field with adequate lighting and then discuss with the patient that you have excluded an FB to the best of your ability. Detailed discharge instructions should then be provided on the possibility of a retained FB and what the patient should look for. Ideally, the patient should follow up with their primary care provider or in the ED within 48 hours for a wound check. The final defense is excellent documentation that should note that the wound was inspected in a bloodless field, so that claims that continued bleeding obscured the field preventing an adequate examination cannot be made at a later date.

Puncture wounds require special consideration, as they are always deeper than they are wide and nearly impossible to explore well, with an estimated infection rate of 6% to 10%.[84–90] These wounds are tetanus prone and have a higher risk for infection and abscess formation, especially if the puncture is through a rubbery shoe and the patient is unable to bear weight 48 hours after the trauma.[86,88–90] Plain radiographs should be ordered to exclude FB, and prophylactic antibiotic therapy started against common skin pathogens (ie, *Staphylococcus aureus* and *Streptococcus* species) if an FB is suspected.[85–90] Plantar puncture wounds through a rubbery sole are at high risk for *Pseudomonas aeruginosa* infection. Patients should be prescribed an antibiotic with antipseudomonas agents such as ciprofloxacin or levofloxicin.[87,89,90]

High-pressure injection injuries represent a less common presentation of small puncture-like wounds. These injuries are commonly seen in middle-aged men and industrial workers, and affect the nondominant arm. The injury occurs due to forceful injection of paint, grease, and liquids through a small high-pressure nozzle. The extent of the damage can be easily overlooked because patients initially do not have significant pain or discomfort, and minimal external injury is seen. Delayed presentation and diagnosis is common. The history should prompt the EP to undertake a very careful examination, as these materials quickly spread along fascia planes and cause widespread inflammation, which leads to severe pain, ischemia, vascular injury, compartment syndrome, and necrosis. Immediate surgical consultation along with pain medications and antibiotic treatment is required.[60,91]

One of the dirtiest, bacteria-containing places on earth is the mouth. Dog, cat, fish, rat, and human oral cavities contain a remarkably high amount of bacteria.[92,93] Cats and dogs are the most common animals that inflict bites to humans, with extremities the most often affected site in adults, and the face and scalp being the most common in children.[94,95] When evaluating children the EP must consider skull penetration. The hand is the most likely site to become infected, and the face the least common. The infection rate for dog bites is less than 6%, whereas cat bites get infected more than 60% of the time.[92–97]

A list of factors that increase the risk for infection from a bite are:

1. Location: Hand, wrist, foot, over large joints, through-and-through oral bites, and the scalp or face in infants
2. Patient history: Patients that are older than 50 years or have the following medical conditions: alcoholism, asplenia, diabetes, peripheral vascular disease, chronic steroid use, prosthetic heart valves or joints
3. Species: Large cat, domestic cat, human, primates, and pigs.

All bites should be copiously irrigated and cleaned. If iodine-based or chlorhexidine antiseptic solutions are used; special precaution must be ensured to avoid the wound margins and the wound itself, as both solutions have been shown to adversely affect adequate wound healing as previously mentioned.[37,39,40,46,98] Tetanus and rabies prophylaxis should be ordered accordingly. Debridement of all devitalized tissue is required.

All noninfected dog bites less than 12 hours old should be sutured. Infection rates in sutured dog bites compared similarly with those in unsutured wounds and nonbite lacerations.[99,100] Cat bites should not be sutured unless cosmetic considerations or tissue coverage is an issue. Closing human bites should be avoided, except for large wounds or facial wounds that are cosmetically necessary.[67,101–103]

ANTIBIOTICS AND TETANUS PROPHYLAXIS

As part of the medical history in any patient, immunization status should be documented. If a patient does not remember or if more than 10 years has elapsed since his or her last tetanus immunization, tetanus toxoid should be given. Although the true incidence of allergy related to tetanus toxoid is low, a known contraindication for the immunization with tetanus toxoid is a previous history of severe systemic reaction.[104,105] If the patient has not been fully immunized against tetanus in the past and has a tetanus-prone wound, 250 units of tetanus immune globulin should be administered along with the tetanus toxoid immunization.[104,106,107]

The routine uses of prophylactic antibiotics remains controversial. The general consensus is that antibiotic prophylaxis should be used in older wounds, in contaminated wounds, in crush injuries, after extensive debridement, over cartilage or involving tendons, in cat and human bites, in puncture wounds through rubbery shoes, in gunshot wounds through clothing, in those with circulatory compromise (ie, peripheral vascular disease or diabetes), and in those who are immunosuppressed. The first dose should be given parenterally as soon as possible, preferably no more than 4 to 6 hours after initial injury.[106]

The antibiotic choice varies based on mechanism and common flora. General wounds will be colonized with *Streptococcus* species and *Staphylococcus aureus* in more than 90% of the cases. If the wound involves salt water, *Vibrio vulnificus* should be suspected; for involvement of lakes or swimming pools, *Aeromonas hydrophila* should be suspected; and in heavily soil-contaminated wounds, *Clostridium* and gram-negative organisms should be suspected.[106,108]

SUMMARY

The management of wounds in the ED is a common occurrence with which all EPs must be comfortable and proficient. Because wound care is responsible for a large number of malpractice claims, EPs need to be aware of practices that can limit bad outcomes and thus decrease their liability risk. EPs should follow a standard examination and ensure that there is no damage to underlying structures (ie, nerves, tendons, and vasculature), and that FB are meticulously looked for and removed if found. Discharge instructions that alert the patient on warning signs of infection, and having all patients return within 48 hours for a wound check are 2 ways to optimize the outcome.

REFERENCES

1. Ovington LG. The evolution of wound management: ancient origins and advances of the past 20 years. Home Healthc Nurse 2002;20:652–6.
2. Sipos P, Gyory H, Hagymasi K, et al. Special wound healing methods used in ancient Egypt and the mythological background. World J Surg 2004;28:211–6.
3. Vital Health Statistics, vol. 386. Advanced data, 2007.

4. Karcz A, Korn R, Burke MC, et al. Malpractice claims against emergency physicians in Massachusetts: 1975–1993. Am J Emerg Med 1996;14:341–5.
5. Dimick AR. Delayed wound closure: indications and techniques. Ann Emerg Med 1988;17:1303–4.
6. Capellan O, Hollander JE. Management of lacerations in the emergency department. Emerg Med Clin North Am 2003;21:205–31.
7. Johnson BW, Scott PG, Brunton JL, et al. Primary and secondary healing in infected wounds. An experimental study. Arch Surg 1982;117:1189–93.
8. Weiss Y. Delayed closure in the management of decontaminated wounds. Int Surg 1982;67:403–4.
9. Singer AJ, Quinn JV, Thode HC Jr, et al. Determinants of poor outcome after laceration and surgical incision repair. Plast Reconstr Surg 2002;110:429–35 [discussion: 436–7].
10. Trott A. Wounds and lacerations: emergency care and closure. St Louis (MO): Mosby; 1997.
11. Pfaff JA, Moore GP. Reducing risk in emergency department wound management. Emerg Med Clin North Am 2007;25:189–201.
12. Howell JM. Current and future trends in wound healing. Emerg Med Clin North Am 1992;10:655–63.
13. Marks JG Jr, Cano C, Leitzel K, et al. Inhibition of wound healing by topical steroids. J Dermatol Surg Oncol 1983;9:819–21.
14. Hollander JE, Blasko B, Singer AJ, et al. Poor correlation of short- and long-term cosmetic appearance of repaired lacerations. Acad Emerg Med 1995;2: 983–7.
15. Singer AJ, Hollander JE, Quinn JV. Evaluation and management of traumatic lacerations. N Engl J Med 1997;337:1142–8.
16. Hollander JE, Singer AJ. Laceration management. Ann Emerg Med 1999;34: 356–67.
17. Edlich R, Rodeheaver G, Thacker J. Technical factors in wound management: fundamentals of wound management in surgery. South Plainfield (NJ): Chirugecon, Inc; 1977.
18. Howell JM, Morgan JA. Scalp laceration repair without prior hair removal. Am J Emerg Med 1988;6:7–10.
19. Seropian R, Reynolds BM. Wound infections after preoperative depilatory versus razor preparation. Am J Surg 1971;121:251–4.
20. Lamas R, Picallos J, Pereira J, et al. [Cranial procedures without shaving. A 1-year experience at the Hospital Sao Joao]. Neurocirugia (Astur) 2003;14: 140–3 [discussion: 143–4] [in Spanish].
21. Celik SE, Kara A. Does shaving the incision site increase the infection rate after spinal surgery? Spine (Phila Pa 1976) 2007;32:1575–7.
22. Bansal BC, Wiebe RA, Perkins SD, et al. Tap water for irrigation of lacerations. Am J Emerg Med 2002;20:469–72.
23. Moscati RM, Mayrose J, Reardon RF, et al. A multicenter comparison of tap water versus sterile saline for wound irrigation. Acad Emerg Med 2007;14:404–9.
24. Cooke M. Irrigation of simple lacerations with tap water or sterile saline in the emergency department did not differ for wound infections. Evid Based Nurs 2007;10:113.
25. Fernandez R, Griffiths R. Water for wound cleansing. Cochrane Database Syst Rev 2008;(1):CD003861.
26. Hall S. A review of the effect of tap water versus normal saline on infection rates in acute traumatic wounds. J Wound Care 2007;16:38–41.

27. Moscati R, Mayrose J, Fincher L, et al. Comparison of normal saline with tap water for wound irrigation. Am J Emerg Med 1998;16:379–81.

28. Moscati RM, Reardon RF, Lerner EB, et al. Wound irrigation with tap water. Acad Emerg Med 1998;5:1076–80.

29. Valente JH, Forti RJ, Freundlich LF, et al. Wound irrigation in children: saline solution or tap water? Ann Emerg Med 2003;41:609–16.

30. Chatterjee JS. A critical review of irrigation techniques in acute wounds. Int Wound J 2005;2:258–65.

31. Draeger RW, Dahners LE. Traumatic wound debridement: a comparison of irrigation methods. J Orthop Trauma 2006;20:83–8.

32. Singer AJ, Hollander JE, Subramanian S, et al. Pressure dynamics of various irrigation techniques commonly used in the emergency department. Ann Emerg Med 1994;24:36–40.

33. Wheeler CB, Rodeheaver GT, Thacker JG, et al. Side-effects of high pressure irrigation. Surg Gynecol Obstet 1976;143:775–8.

34. Lam DG, Rastomjee D, Dynan Y. Wound irrigation: a simple, reproducible device. Ann R Coll Surg Engl 2000;82:346–7.

35. Lawson C, Juliano L, Ratliff CR. Does sterile or nonsterile technique make a difference in wounds healing by secondary intention? Ostomy Wound Manage 2003;49:56–8, 60.

36. Perelman VS, Francis GJ, Rutledge T, et al. Sterile versus nonsterile gloves for repair of uncomplicated lacerations in the emergency department: a randomized controlled trial. Ann Emerg Med 2004;43:362–70.

37. Cooper ML, Laxer JA, Hansbrough JF. The cytotoxic effects of commonly used topical antimicrobial agents on human fibroblasts and keratinocytes. J Trauma 1991;31:775–82 [discussion: 782–4].

38. Wilson JR, Mills JG, Prather ID, et al. A toxicity index of skin and wound cleansers used on in vitro fibroblasts and keratinocytes. Adv Skin Wound Care 2005;18:373–8.

39. McCauley RL, Linares HA, Pelligrini V, et al. In vitro toxicity of topical antimicrobial agents to human fibroblasts. J Surg Res 1989;46:267–74.

40. Damour O, Hua SZ, Lasne F, et al. Cytotoxicity evaluation of antiseptics and antibiotics on cultured human fibroblasts and keratinocytes. Burns 1992;18:479–85.

41. Brooks SE, Walczak MA, Hameed R, et al. Chlorhexidine resistance in antibiotic-resistant bacteria isolated from the surfaces of dispensers of soap containing chlorhexidine. Infect Control Hosp Epidemiol 2002;23:692–5.

42. Koljalg S, Naaber P, Mikelsaar M. Antibiotic resistance as an indicator of bacterial chlorhexidine susceptibility. J Hosp Infect 2002;51:106–13.

43. Fox CL Jr, Modak SM. Mechanism of silver sulfadiazine action on burn wound infections. Antimicrob Agents Chemother 1974;5:582–8.

44. Katz MH, Alvarez AF, Kirsner RS, et al. Human wound fluid from acute wounds stimulates fibroblast and endothelial cell growth. J Am Acad Dermatol 1991;25:1054–8.

45. Bucalo B, Eaglstein WH, Falanga V. Inhibition of cell proliferation by chronic wound fluid. Wound Repair Regen 1993;1:181–6.

46. Stanley AC, Park HY, Phillips TJ, et al. Reduced growth of dermal fibroblasts from chronic venous ulcers can be stimulated with growth factors. J Vasc Surg 1997;26:994–9 [discussion: 999–1001].

47. Broughton G 2nd, Janis JE, Attinger CE. Wound healing: an overview. Plast Reconstr Surg 2006;117:1e-S–32e-S.

48. Lipton JA, Marbach JJ. Ethnicity and the pain experience. Soc Sci Med 1984;19:1279–98.

49. Ortega RA, Youdelman BA, Havel RC. Ethnic variability in the treatment of pain. Am J Anesthesiol 1999;26:429–32.
50. Todd KH, Lee T, Hoffman JR. The effect of ethnicity on physician estimates of pain severity in patients with isolated extremity trauma. JAMA 1994;271:925–8.
51. Singer AJ, Stark MJ. LET versus EMLA for pretreating lacerations: a randomized trial. Acad Emerg Med 2001;8:223–30.
52. Roberts JR, Hedges JR, Chanmugam AS. Clinical procedures in emergency medicine. Philadelphia: W.B. Saunders; 2004.
53. Simpson S. Regional nerve blocks. Part 5—Bier's block (intravenous regional anaesthesia). Aust Fam Physician 2001;30:875–7.
54. Murphy MF. Regional anesthesia in the emergency department. Emerg Med Clin North Am 1988;6:783–810.
55. Farrell RG, Swanson SL, Walter JR. Safe and effective IV regional anesthesia for use in the emergency department. Ann Emerg Med 1985;14:239–43.
56. Russell RC, Williamson DA, Sullivan JW, et al. Detection of foreign bodies in the hand. J Hand Surg Am 1991;16:2–11.
57. Courter BJ. Radiographic screening for glass foreign bodies—what does a "negative" foreign body series really mean? Ann Emerg Med 1990;19: 997–1000.
58. Ellis GL. Are aluminum foreign bodies detectable radiographically? Am J Emerg Med 1993;11:12–3.
59. Chisholm CD, Wood CO, Chua G, et al. Radiographic detection of gravel in soft tissue. Ann Emerg Med 1997;29:725–30.
60. Bond MC, Willis GC. Hand and wrist injuries: diagnostic challenges. Trauma Reports 2010;11:1–11.
61. Newman DH. Truth, and epinephrine, at our fingertips: unveiling the pseudoaxioms. Ann Emerg Med 2007;50:476–7.
62. Thomson CJ, Lalonde DH. Randomized double-blind comparison of duration of anesthesia among three commonly used agents in digital nerve block. Plast Reconstr Surg 2006;118:429–32.
63. Waterbrook AL, Germann CA, Southall JC. Is epinephrine harmful when used with anesthetics for digital nerve blocks? Ann Emerg Med 2007;50: 472–5.
64. Altinyazar HC, Ozdemir H, Koca R, et al. Epinephrine in digital block: color Doppler flow imaging. Dermatol Surg 2004;30:508–11.
65. Sonmez A, Yaman M, Ersoy B, et al. Digital blocks with and without adrenalin: a randomised-controlled study of capillary blood parameters. J Hand Surg Eur Vol 2008;33:515–8.
66. Denkler K. A comprehensive review of epinephrine in the finger: to do or not to do. Plast Reconstr Surg 2001;108:114–24.
67. Donkor P, Bankas DO. A study of primary closure of human bite injuries to the face. J Oral Maxillofac Surg 1997;55:479–81 [discussion: 481–2].
68. Food and Drug Administration. Warning: procaine solution. JAMA 1948;138:599.
69. Hollander JE, Giarrusso E, Cassara G, et al. Comparison of staples and sutures for closure of scalp lacerations. Acad Emerg Med 1997;4:460–1.
70. Easton BT. Tissue adhesive works as well as suturing. J Fam Pract 2002;51:517.
71. Holger JS, Wandersee SC, Hale DB. Cosmetic outcomes of facial lacerations repaired with tissue-adhesive, absorbable, and nonabsorbable sutures. Am J Emerg Med 2004;22:254–7.
72. Parell GJ, Becker GD. Comparison of absorbable with nonabsorbable sutures in closure of facial skin wounds. Arch Facial Plast Surg 2003;5:488–90.

73. Karaduman S, Yuruktumen A, Guryay SM, et al. Modified hair apposition technique as the primary closure method for scalp lacerations. Am J Emerg Med 2009;27:1050–5.
74. Hock MO, Ooi SB, Saw SM, et al. A randomized controlled trial comparing the hair apposition technique with tissue glue to standard suturing in scalp lacerations (HAT study). Ann Emerg Med 2002;40:19–26.
75. Ong ME, Coyle D, Lim SH, et al. Cost-effectiveness of hair apposition technique compared with standard suturing in scalp lacerations. Ann Emerg Med 2005;46:237–42.
76. Aukerman DF, Sebastianelli WJ, Nashelsky J. Clinical inquiries. How does tissue adhesive compare with suturing for superficial lacerations? J Fam Pract 2005;54:378.
77. Bringhurst C, Herr RD, Aldous JA. Oral trauma in the emergency department. Am J Emerg Med 1993;11:486–90.
78. Bodne D, Quinn SF, Cochran CF. Imaging foreign glass and wooden bodies of the extremities with CT and MR. J Comput Assist Tomogr 1988;12:608–11.
79. Graham DD Jr. Ultrasound in the emergency department: detection of wooden foreign bodies in the soft tissues. J Emerg Med 2002;22:75–9.
80. Jacobson JA, Powell A, Craig JG, et al. Wooden foreign bodies in soft tissue: detection at US. Radiology 1998;206:45–8.
81. Blankstein A, Cohen I, Heiman Z, et al. Localization, detection and guided removal of soft tissue in the hands using sonography. Arch Orthop Trauma Surg 2000;120:514–7.
82. Orlinsky M, Knittel P, Feit T, et al. The comparative accuracy of radiolucent foreign body detection using ultrasonography. Am J Emerg Med 2000;18:401–3.
83. Ell SR, Sprigg A, Parker AJ. A multi-observer study examining the radiographic visibility of fishbone foreign bodies. J R Soc Med 1996;89:31–4.
84. Weber EJ. Plantar puncture wounds: a survey to determine the incidence of infection. J Accid Emerg Med 1996;13:274–7.
85. Haverstock BD, Grossman JP. Puncture wounds of the foot. Evaluation and treatment. Clin Podiatr Med Surg 1999;16:583–96.
86. Inaba AS, Zukin DD, Perro M. An update on the evaluation and management of plantar puncture wounds and Pseudomonas osteomyelitis. Pediatr Emerg Care 1992;8:38–44.
87. Schwab RA, Powers RD. Conservative therapy of plantar puncture wounds. J Emerg Med 1995;13:291–5.
88. Miron D, Raz R, Kaufman B, et al. Infections following nail puncture wound of the foot: case reports and review of the literature. Isr J Med Sci 1993;29:194–7.
89. Toohey JS. Pseudomonas osteomyelitis following puncture wounds of the foot. Kans Med 1993;94:325–6.
90. Harrison M, Thomas M. Towards evidence based emergency medicine: best BETs from the Manchester Royal Infirmary. Antibiotics after puncture wounds to the foot. Emerg Med J 2002;19:49.
91. Vasilevski D, Noorbergen M, Depierreux M, et al. High-pressure injection injuries to the hand. Am J Emerg Med 2000;18:820–4.
92. Abrahamian FM. Dog bites: bacteriology, management, and prevention. Curr Infect Dis Rep 2000;2:446–53.
93. Talan DA, Citron DM, Abrahamian FM, et al. Bacteriologic analysis of infected dog and cat bites. Emergency Medicine Animal Bite Infection Study Group. N Engl J Med 1999;340:85–92.
94. Ly N, McCaig LF. National Hospital Ambulatory medical care survey: 2000 outpatient department summary. Adv Data 2002;(327):1–27.

95. Griego RD, Rosen T, Orengo IF, et al. Dog, cat, and human bites: a review. J Am Acad Dermatol 1995;33:1019–29.
96. Morgan M. Hospital management of animal and human bites. J Hosp Infect 2005;61:1–10.
97. Chen E, Hornig S, Shepherd SM, et al. Primary closure of mammalian bites. Acad Emerg Med 2000;7:157–61.
98. Thomas G, Rael L, Bar-Or R, et al. Mechanisms of delayed wound healing by commonly used antiseptics. J Trauma 2009;66:82–90 [discussion: 90–1].
99. Dire DJ, Hogan DE, Riggs MW. A prospective evaluation of risk factors for infections from dog-bite wounds. Acad Emerg Med 1994;1:258–66.
100. Maimaris C, Quinton DN. Dog-bite lacerations: a controlled trial of primary wound closure. Arch Emerg Med 1988;5:156–61.
101. Patil PD, Panchabhai TS, Galwankar SC. Managing human bites. J Emerg Trauma Shock 2009;2:186–90.
102. Stefanopoulos PK, Tarantzopoulou AD. Facial bite wounds: management update. Int J Oral Maxillofac Surg 2005;34:464–72.
103. A bite in the playroom: managing human bites in child care settings. Paediatr Child Health 2008;13:515–26.
104. Jacobs RL, Lowe RS, Lanier BQ. Adverse reactions to tetanus toxoid. JAMA 1982;247:40–2.
105. Zun LS, Downey L. Tetanus immunization shortage in the United States. Am J Emerg Med 2003;21:298–301.
106. Cummings P, Del Beccaro MA. Antibiotics to prevent infection of simple wounds: a meta-analysis of randomized studies. Am J Emerg Med 1995;13: 396–400.
107. Howell JM, Chisholm CD. Outpatient wound preparation and care: a national survey. Ann Emerg Med 1992;21:976–81.
108. Gold WL, Salit IE. *Aeromonas hydrophila* infections of skin and soft tissue: report of 11 cases and review. Clin Infect Dis 1993;16:69–74.

Risk Management and Avoiding Legal Pitfalls in the Emergency Treatment of High-Risk Orthopedic Injuries

Carl A. Germann, MD*, Andrew D. Perron, MD

KEYWORDS

- Emergency providers • Computed tomography
- Open reduction and internal fixation
- Scapholunate advanced collapsed deformity

Orthopedic injuries are seen frequently in the emergency department (ED). Missed fractures and inappropriate management of orthopedic injuries account for a significant proportion of malpractice claims made against emergency providers. This article highlights some of the most frequently missed or mismanaged injuries seen in the ED.

THE UPPER EXTREMITY
Posterior Shoulder Dislocation

The glenohumoral joint of the shoulder is the most commonly dislocated joint in the body. Compared with anterior shoulder dislocation, posterior shoulder dislocation is an infrequent event, with a reported incidence of 1% to 4% of all shoulder dislocations.[1–3] The major clinical significance of posterior dislocation is the frequency of errors in diagnosis and the significant delays in treatment that can result in permanent disability.[4,5] A widely quoted series by Rowe and Zarins[6] found a 79% incidence of missed diagnosis of posterior shoulder dislocation by the initial treating physician. A 1987 review by Hawkins and colleagues[4] showed that nearly all patients with posterior shoulder dislocation have some delay in their diagnosis. Common factors associated with a delayed diagnosis include a late presentation by the patient, inadequate radiologic investigation, elderly patients, and those presenting with multiple injuries.[7–11]

Department of Emergency Medicine, Maine Medical Center, Tufts University College of Medicine, 22 Bramhall Street, Portland, ME 04102, USA
* Corresponding author.
E-mail address: germac@mmc.org

Emerg Med Clin N Am 28 (2010) 969–996
doi:10.1016/j.emc.2010.06.002
0733-8627/10/$ – see front matter © 2010 Published by Elsevier Inc.

emed.theclinics.com

Early recognition requires a high level of suspicion coupled with a careful history and physical examination, and confirmation with appropriate radiographs. The prompt diagnosis and treatment of posterior shoulder dislocation is crucial, because it may prevent the adverse sequelae such as degenerative disease of the shoulder and avascular necrosis of the humeral head.[12] However, neurovascular injuries and rotator cuff tears are less common with posterior dislocations than with anterior dislocations.[13]

Acknowledging the possibility of a posterior glenohumeral dislocation or a fracture-dislocation is the key to making the diagnosis. The classic history for a traumatic posterior dislocation involves a significant blow to the front of the shoulder with internal rotation and a forced adduction or a fall on the outstretched hand with the elbow extended and the humerus internally rotated. Posterior dislocations, however, more commonly result from seizure activity during which contraction of the strong internal rotators of the glenohumeral joint overcome the posterior stabilizers.[8] The physical examination is notable for posterior shoulder prominence, a flattened contour of the anterior shoulder with resultant prominence of the coracoid process, marked inability to externally rotate the arm, and inability to rotate the palm upward. The possibility of bilateral shoulder dislocation should be considered in cases of electrocution or seizure. Approximately 15% of all posterior dislocations are bilateral.[8]

The diagnosis of posterior glenohumeral dislocations depends on the use of appropriate radiograph views and their correct interpretation.[14] A single anteroposterior (AP) view is commonly misinterpreted as looking normal. Often, the inferior third of the glenoid fossa will have no contact with the humeral head. A transscapular view will show the humeral head posterior to the glenoid fossa (**Fig. 1**). The axillary view is the key view, and should always be obtained to rule out this entity if there is clinical suspicion but standard views do not confirm or refute the diagnosis.[4] An axillary-view radiograph will confirm posterior dislocation of the humeral head. If axillary views are difficult to obtain because of pain or physical limitations, axial images of the glenohumeral joint can be obtained with a computed tomography (CT) scan.

The treatment of posterior dislocations depends on timely diagnosis and the size of the anterior impression fracture (the so-called reverse Hills-Sachs lesion). Acute posterior glenohumeral dislocation without any associated fracture is uncommon, and posterior labral detachment is encountered in 10% to 15% of cases.[15] In general, when the humeral defect is less than 20% of the articular surface, closed reduction under conscious sedation is attempted.[2,16] The technique involves gentle traction on an adducted shoulder, with pressure placed posteriorly on the humeral head,

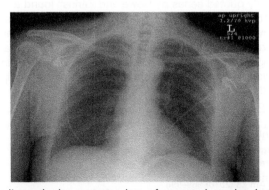

Fig. 1. A chest radiograph demonstrates loss of expected overlap between the (*right*) humeral head and the glenoid fossa characteristic of posterior shoulder dislocation.

pushing it anteriorly. Traction is maintained and the arm is slowly externally rotated. Once reduction is obtained, it is maintained with an immobilization device that holds the arm in external rotation and slight abduction. With larger Hill-Sachs lesions reduction may certainly be attempted, but the joint may not stay reduced. Failure of closed reduction, or chronic posterior dislocation necessitates an operative approach.

Galeazzi-Monteggia Fracture-Dislocation

Monteggia and Galeazzi fracture-dislocations represent 2 important injury patterns that may be missed in patients with forearm fracture. Unfortunately, these associated injuries are frequently subtle and consequently missed on initial ED presentation.[17] Dislocation at the elbow or wrist that accompanies such upper extremity trauma can lead to significant long-term morbidity if left untreated.

Because the radius and ulna have such a close anatomic relationship to one another, injury to either bone will have a direct impact on the other. Although they are in direct contact only at the proximal and distal radioulnar joints, they are joined together along their length by a fibrous interosseous membrane. During supination or pronation, the straight ulna remains in a relatively fixed position, while the anatomically bowed radius rotates around it. When one of the bones suffers a significant trauma, such as a displaced or angulated fracture, it is highly likely that the other will be affected, usually at one or both of the radioulnar joints.

The Monteggia pattern of injury consists of a fracture to the proximal third of the ulna with a concomitant dislocation of the radial head. The Galeazzi pattern of injury consists of a radius fracture, most often at the junction of the middle and distal third of the bone, accompanied by a dislocation at the distal radioulnar joint. This injury is also referred to in medical literature as a "reverse Monteggia fracture" or "the fracture of necessity," because its presence usually necessitates surgery if a good outcome is to be obtained.[18–20]

In the United States, the upper extremity is involved in nearly one-half of all fractures.[21,22] The exact incidence of Galeazzi and Monteggia fracture-dislocation in an ED population is unknown, but these so-called double injuries in forearm fracture are thought to be relatively common. One orthopedic series reported that Galeazzi fractures account for 3% to 7% of all forearm fractures seen.[23] Cited incidences of dislocation accompanying fracture range from 10% to 60%.[7,22,24]

Monteggia and Galeazzi fracture-dislocations can be caused by either low-energy trauma, such as a fall from standing, or high-energy mechanisms, such as motor vehicle crashes or a fall from a height. The Galeazzi lesion is 3 times more common than the Monteggia pattern of injury.[25] Older series reported an initial "miss rate" of up to 50% in the diagnosis of these 2 lesions, with most injuries not diagnosed until more than 4 weeks after the trauma.[26] More recent series have not specifically reported rates of delay in diagnosis, but it is generally thought to be less than this quoted figure of 50%.[27,28]

The most common mechanism for a Monteggia fracture-dislocation (**Fig. 2**) is a fall on an outstretched and hyperpronated hand, resulting in an ulnar shaft fracture and anterior radial head dislocation.[29–31] It can also result from a direct blow to the ulna, or hyperextension injuries. The radial head will dislocate anteriorly in 60% of the cases,[29,30] with anterolateral and posterolateral dislocations also a possibility.[30–32]

On presentation, patients with a Monteggia fracture-dislocation demonstrate pain and swelling at the elbow with extremely limited, if any, range of motion at that joint. Some, however, may not have impressive pain at rest, but elbow flexion and forearm supination will be limited and painful.[33] The dislocated radial head may be palpable in an anterior, anterolateral, or posterolateral location. With Monteggia

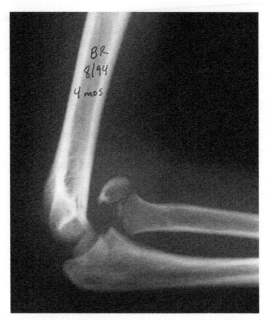

Fig. 2. A lateral elbow radiograph in Monteggia fracture-dislocation.

fracture-dislocation, the deep branch of the radial nerve (the posterior interosseous nerve) can be injured, because it is intimately associated with the radial head at the elbow.[28,29,34] Injury to this nerve is manifested as weakness or paralysis of extension in the fingers or thumb. The sensory branch is not typically involved.[34]

With the Monteggia fracture-dislocation, the ulna fracture is usually clearly visible on a radiograph (see **Fig. 2**). Unfortunately, the presence of the fracture frequently overshadows the less obvious radial head dislocation. One simple technique the emergency practitioner can use to avoid missing a proximal dislocation is to draw a line through the long axis of the radius at the elbow. This line should intersect the capitellum regardless of the degree of elbow flexion or extension. Comparison films of the contralateral elbow have been advocated, but have not been shown to be consistently helpful.[35] If the ulnar fracture is angulated, the apex of the angulation will point in the same direction of the radial head dislocation.[28,32]

The treatment of Monteggia injuries differs in adults and children. These injuries have been successfully treated in children with closed reduction and supinated long-arm splinting.[36] Monteggia fracture-dislocation is usually considered a more severe injury in adults, who most often require open reduction and internal fixation (ORIF).[30,31,36] If the radial head dislocation is missed and the injury treated as a simple fracture, chronic unreducible radial head dislocation can occur, resulting in painful and limited supination and pronation.[30,31,37] Late discovery of the dislocation is usually treated with radial head excision.

Like Monteggia injuries, Galeazzi fracture-dislocations are usually the result of a fall on an outstretched hand in forced pronation.[20,21,25] A direct blow is also a frequently cited mechanism, especially when the blow is to the dorsolateral wrist.[38] The fracture is diaphyseal, at the distal one-third of the radius. Fracture to the proximal radius is more uncommon, as it is protected from direct trauma by both the ulna and the surrounding mass of musculature of the forearm. The fracture in Galeazzi injury occurs distal to the bicipital tuberosity, and proximal to an area 4 cm from the distal articular surface of the radius. With displaced radial shaft fractures distal radioulnar joint disruption is common, but frequently subtle.[28,39] The injury at the distal radioulnar joint can be purely ligamentous (eg, a tear in the triangular fibro-cartilage) or can involve fracture to the ulnar styloid process in association with the ligamentous injury.[20,40]

With Galeazzi fracture-dislocation, patients will usually resist any attempts at pronation or supination owing to pain. If the dislocation is of enough severity, the ulnar styloid process may be prominent and palpable. Although the wrist is typically tender to palpation with this injury, in nondisplaced fractures the only swelling or deformity may be at the site of the fracture, and the patient may not complain of significant wrist pain. As opposed to the Monteggia injury, distal neurovascular injury is rare with Galeazzi fracture-dislocation.[20,39] The radius fracture is usually plainly evident on a radiograph, with the radius appearing shortened (relative to the ulna) due to the proximal pull of the pronator quadratus muscle. An associated fracture of the ulnar styloid may also be seen. On the posteroanterior (PA) view the radius will appear shortened, with an increase in the space between the distal radius and ulna where they articulate. The distal radioulnar joint is normally not wider than 1 to 2 mm, so a gap greater than this suggests ligamentous injury.[37] On the lateral view the fractured radius is usually angulated dorsally, and the distal ulna will be seen to be dorsally displaced. In a normal lateral view the ulna is seen to directly overlie the radius, or be no more than 3 mm dorsal to the radius.[37] Inability of the technician to obtain an adequate lateral film should trigger the suspicion of this injury, as it is difficult to obtain a true lateral in this condition.

Galeazzi fracture-dislocation is even more prone to poor outcome if missed than the Monteggia lesion. Older reported series of Galeazzi injuries treated with closed reduction and cast immobilization reported poor outcomes in greater than 90% of patients.[41] This injury is almost always now treated with ORIF of the radius fracture and open or pin fixation of the distal radioulnar joint. If this injury is missed, progressive subluxation of the distal radioulnar joint and dorsal angulation of the radius fracture usually occur.[40,41] If not treated definitively within 10 weeks, the dislocation can lead to limitation of supination and pronation, chronic pain, and weakness.[18,20,40]

Lunate/Perilunate Injury

The wrist is a complex structure with multiple bones and joints that result in the possibility of a nearly infinite combination of positions and motions. The effects of trauma on the wrist can be both subtle and complex. The morbidity of wrist injury is tied, in part, to the frequently missed diagnosis of lunate or perilunate dislocation in the ED.[42-46] One multicenter study reported a missed diagnosis in 25% of patients with perilunate dislocations and fracture-dislocations.[44] Unfortunately, missed injuries to the wrist are associated with a high incidence of long-term pain, dysfunction, and disability.[45,47,48] Often, patients are not diagnosed with these injuries until weeks following the initial injury.[44,47-49]

In the United States, wrist injuries are estimated to account for 2.5% of all ED visits.[42,50] The exact incidence of lunate and perilunate injury in an ED population is unknown, but these specific injuries are estimated to account for 10% of all carpal injuries.[51,52]

Perilunate and lunate dislocations result from similar hyperextension mechanisms, with perilunate dislocations being more common and lunate dislocations being more severe. Perilunate and lunate dislocations generally are the result of high-energy trauma to the wrist, with the most common mechanism being a fall on the outstretched hand, followed by motor vehicle and motorcycle crashes.[43,44,51] The hallmark and defining feature of perilunate dislocation is a dislocation of the head of the capitate from the distal surface of the lunate. Most often this occurs in a dorsal direction, but can also occur anteriorly. The defining feature of lunate dislocation is disruption of the association between the lunate and the lunate fossa of the distal radius. Originally described by Mayfield, perilunate and lunate dislocations are thought to be progressions of the same pathologic process.[53]

The mechanism of carpal dislocations is a progressive pattern of carpal ligamentous injuries caused by wrist hyperextension and ulnar deviation.[53–55] Mayfield's study of the pathomechanics of these injuries led to the classification of carpal dislocations into 4 distinct stages with each stage representing a sequential intercarpal injury, beginning with scapholunate joint disruption and proceeding around the lunate, creating progressive ligamentous injury and progressive carpal instability.[53] Each stage of dislocation may also be associated with specific bony fractures which, if present, should alert the physician to the possibility of an occult perilunate ligamentous injury. These associated fractures include fractures of the radial styloid, scaphoid, capitate, and triquetrum.[53,54]

A stage I injury, also called scapholunate dissociation, results in a characteristic widening of the scapholunate joint on the PA view, which has been given the eponym the "Terry Thomas sign," after the British comedian with a gap between his front teeth.[56] A gap of 2 mm or less between the scaphoid and lunate is considered normal on the PA view. Scapholunate dissociation can be associated with a rotatory subluxation of the scaphoid, where the scaphoid is seen on its end with the cortex of the distal pole appearing as a ring shadow superimposed over the scaphoid; this is known as the "signet ring sign."[57] Standard radiographs are usually normal, so when a scapholunate ligament injury is suspected clinically, additional stress views can be obtained. Views taken in ulnar deviation with a clenched fist (the clenched-fist AP view) will accentuate widening of the scapholunate joint.

A stage II injury, or perilunate dislocation, is seen best on the lateral view of the wrist. Although the lunate remains in normal position in relation to the distal radius, the capitate is dislocated, usually in a dorsal direction (**Fig. 3**). The PA view often will show overlap of the distal and proximal carpal rows and may also demonstrate an associated scaphoid fracture or subluxation.

A stage III injury appears similar to a stage II injury but with the addition of a dislocation of the triquetrum, best seen on the PA view, with overlap of the triquetrum on the lunate. The stage III injury is frequently associated with a volar fracture of the triquetral bone.

A stage IV injury, or lunate dislocation, results in a characteristic triangular appearance of the lunate on the PA view, also known as the "piece of pie sign", caused by the rotation of the lunate in a volar direction. The triangular appearance of the lunate with dislocation is in contradistinction to its normal quadrangular appearance. This rotation is also visible on the lateral view of the wrist, where the lunate looks like a teacup tipped in a volar direction that has spilled its contents into the palm. This latter sign is called the "spilled teacup sign" (**Fig. 4**).[58] On the lateral view, the capitate will lie posterior to the lunate and can even migrate proximally and make contact with the distal radius.

Complications of carpal dislocation include median nerve injury from lunate dislocation with an acute or subacute carpal tunnel syndrome. Other complications include chronic carpal instability with resultant degenerative arthritis, chronic pain, and limitation in range of motion. Scapholunate advanced collapsed deformity (so-called SLAC wrist) is the end-stage result for many patients.[59]

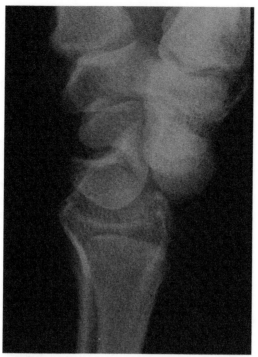

Fig. 3. A lateral radiograph of a perilunate dislocation. The lunate has maintained its normal relationship with the distal radius, but the capitate has dislocated dorsally, relative to the lunate.

Patients with these carpal dislocation injuries typically have a history of a high-energy mechanism, such as a fall from a height on the outstretched hand or a motor vehicle crash. The mechanism of injury is ulnar deviation of the wrist coupled with dorsiflexion. The patient will complain of pain and swelling over either the dorsum or volar aspect of the wrist, with limited range of motion. On physical examination there will likely be palpable tenderness over the dorsum of the wrist, particularly in the region of the scapholunate ligament, located just distal to Lister's tubercle. With palpation alone it is often difficult to distinguish one source of wrist pain from other causes, including scapholunate strain, scaphoid fracture, triangular fibrocartilage complex tears, and other disorders.

Plain radiographs of the wrist, both PA and lateral views, are essential to diagnose wrist dislocations (as well as other carpal instabilities). The PA view should be obtained with the wrist in a neutral position. The scaphoid is viewed in an oblique projection in this view, and scaphoid fractures can be obscured. A constant 2-mm intercarpal joint space should be seen on a normal PA view. An increase in this distance suggests ligamentous interruption or a stage I injury (scapholunate dissociation).

On the AP view, 3 arcs should be identified. The first arc consists of the radiocarpal row, which should be both smooth and continuous. Disruption of this arc is suggestive of a lunate dislocation. The second arc consists of the midcarpal row, which should similarly be smooth and continuous. Disruption of this arc is suggestive of a perilunate dislocation. The third arc outlines the proximal surface of the distal carpal row. Disruption of any of these arcs is a sign of carpal dislocation or fracture.

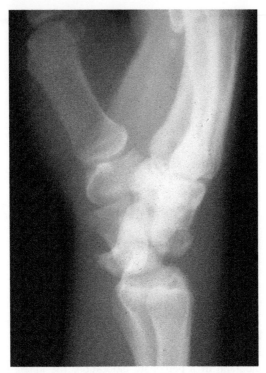

Fig. 4. A lateral radiograph of the wrist in lunate dislocation. The lunate has dislocated in a volar direction and has tipped anteriorly. This is the "spilled teacup" sign.

On the lateral view the radius, lunate, and capitate should all line up in a row. The lunate should lie within the radius cup and the capitate should rest within the lunate cup. Loss of this normal column configuration implies lunate or perilunate dislocation. Stress radiographs obtained with radial and ulnar deviation of the hand may demonstrate scapholunate dissociation.

Carpal dislocation injuries usually mandate the consultation of a hand surgeon in the ED for reduction and stabilization. It is obvious that open fractures and open dislocations need operative intervention. These patients should be given analgesia, be splinted, receive intravenous antibiotics, and be kept without oral food or water for the anticipated procedure.

Closed reduction and long-arm splint immobilization may be attempted but is frequently not successful. If attempted, it is more likely to be successful with perilunate rather than lunate dislocations, owing to the extent of ligamentous disruption in the latter. If the dislocation is irreducible or the result is unstable, open reduction with internal fixation will be required. Many investigators think immediate open reduction with internal fixation is the treatment of choice, citing the extensive ligamentous injury inherent in such injuries, and frequent unstable results that come with closed reduction.[44,46,53–56] A lunate or perilunate injury with median nerve symptoms requires immediate operative reduction, carpal tunnel release, and ligamentous reconstruction.

Scaphoid Fracture

Of all the wrist injuries encountered in the ED, fracture of the scaphoid is one of the most commonly missed.[57–59] Scaphoid fractures account for 60% to 70% of all diagnosed carpal injuries,[60–63] making them the most common wrist bone fracture.[61,62,64] Radiographic findings can be subtle or even absent, rendering the diagnosis even more difficult to make. In such cases, a thorough history and well-performed physical examination, coupled with a high index of suspicion, are necessary to make the diagnosis. Accurate early diagnosis of scaphoid fracture is critical as the morbidity associated with a missed or delayed diagnosis is significant, and can result in long-term pain, loss of mobility, and decreased function.[58,61,64]

The propensity for nonunion and avascular necrosis (AVN) of the scaphoid is due entirely to its blood supply, which arises distally from small branches off of the radial artery and the palmar and superficial arteries.[65–67] The proximal portion of the scaphoid is completely dependent on this distal blood supply, and hence most at risk for AVN following fracture. In general, the more proximal, oblique, or displaced the fracture, the greater the risk of interrupting the blood supply.[58,59,65,67]

Snuff box tenderness is classically cited as the most common finding,[43,61,68] although the sensitivity of this test has been disputed.[64,69] Many investigators believe that a better physical examination test for scaphoid injury is axial compression of the thumb along its longitudinal axis.[69,70] Described by Chen,[69] this test translates force directly across the scaphoid, and should elicit pain if there is a fracture.

The emergency physician (EP) should remain vigilant for associated injuries that can be found on physical examination. Common associated injuries include fractures of the distal radius, lunate, or radial head at the elbow. Median nerve injury has also been described in association with scaphoid fracture.[71]

Even with appropriate films, fractures of the scaphoid can be subtle and difficult to visualize. Conservative estimates suggest that 10% to 20% of these fractures will not be visible on any view in the acute setting.[64,72,73] One prospective trial estimated found the sensitivity of initial radiographs for diagnosing scaphoid fracture to be 86%.[74] A typical wrist series includes a PA and lateral of the wrist (**Fig. 5**). These films are as important for ruling out other concomitant injuries as they are for accurately diagnosing the scaphoid fracture itself.

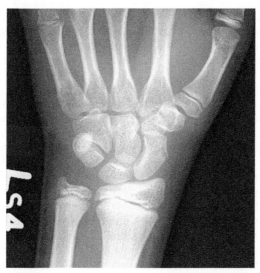

Fig. 5. A PA radiograph of the wrist demonstrates a subtle scaphoid fracture.

In cases where there is a high clinical suspicion, a scaphoid view of the wrist can also be obtained. This image reduces the foreshortening of the scaphoid that occurs on a normal PA view, and displays the length of the scaphoid. Again, however, even with excellent radiographic technique, a fracture may not be visualized. Magnetic resonance imaging (MRI) and CT scanning can both make the diagnosis of scaphoid fracture when plain films are negative.[59,75–78] However, this is not routinely done in the ED, as it would not affect initial treatment of immobilization and orthopedic follow-up for clinically suspected scaphoid injury.[79]

Treatment of scaphoid fracture in the ED can be divided into 2 clinical scenarios. The first is when a scaphoid fracture is suspected, but radiographs are negative. The second is when fracture has been confirmed with diagnostic radiographs.

The most common complication of scaphoid fracture is nonunion. Because of the precarious nature of the blood supply and potential for movement at the fracture line, nonunion has an overall occurrence rate of 8% to 10%.[58,59,64] The rate of nonunion varies with the actual fracture site. Nonunion complicates up to 20% to 30% of proximal third fractures and 10% to 20% of middle third fractures. Nonunion of distal third fractures is relatively rare.[58,59,80,81]

Besides nonunion, patients are also at risk to develop AVN of the scaphoid. This outcome occurs in approximately 10% of proximal pole fractures and 5% of middle third fractures.[59,71,80] SLAC wrist is a late complication of scaphoid fracture, scapholunate dissociation, or lunate injury.[68,82] The proximal pole of the scaphoid and the lunate undergo AVN with collapse.

Closed-Fist Injury: "Fight Bite"

Closed-fist injuries result from the patient's practice of striking another individual in the mouth region with the fist; such blunt impact on the aggressor's hand likely produces soft tissue and bony injury to the hand. When the soft-tissue injury includes a break in the integrity of the skin on the dorsum of the hand, infection may complicate the original injury. As such, these "fight bite" injuries should be approached with thoroughness and great respect.

These injuries are common but frequently mismanaged. Mismanagement results from several factors. The patients who suffer these injuries are often intoxicated, making an adequate history and thorough examination difficult. Patients are also frequently reluctant to admit to the cause of the injury, providing misleading histories. The physician must have a high index of suspicion for any injury where there are lacerations, abrasions, or bruising over the metacarpophalangeal (MCP) joints.

Human saliva contains as many as 42 species of bacteria with a microbe concentration of 1×10^8 organisms per milliliter.[83,84] Fist-to-mouth contact is perhaps the most common cause of human bite wounds. These "fight bite" wounds have the highest incidence of complications of any closed-fist injury and of any type of bite wound.[85] These injuries usually occur over the dorsal aspect of the third, fourth, or fifth MCP joints, an area that is susceptible to deep infection because the thin skin overlying the joint provides little protection to the underlying ligaments, synovium, and cartilage.[86] Joint space infections resulting from a human bite wound are aggressive and rapidly destructive. Such infections usually occur in young people, and the resulting destructive changes of the MCP joint can be devastating, as there is no good surgical option to reconstruct the MCP joint of a young person. For these reasons, it is a commonly accepted axiom in the world of hand surgery that all open wounds over the MCP joints are considered to be probable "fight bites"; such an approach will ensure that patients will receive appropriate therapy.

The wound must be thoroughly explored to rule out joint capsule violation as well as retained foreign body, such as a tooth fragment or piece of jewelry. Exploration must be done throughout a full range of motion, because the injury may only be noted when the hand is flexed, as with a fist.[83,86] The wound should be copiously irrigated. If the joint space was violated, this area should be thoroughly irrigated as well. After aggressive care has been completed, the wound should be left open—that is, no primary closure should be attempted in that such an approach will increase the possibility of infection. Prophylactic antibiotics should be initiated in the ED in all but the most superficial wounds. For patients with a delayed presentation and clinically obvious infection, a hand surgeon should be consulted and consideration given to bringing the patient to the operating room for open irrigation and debridement with subsequent admission for intravenous antibiotics.

If careful exploration in the ED demonstrates no tendon or joint involvement and there are no signs of infection, outpatient treatment and follow-up may be appropriate. Unless the wound is superficial, this patient population should receive a parenteral, broad-spectrum antibiotic in the ED (ie, ampicillin/sulbactam) with continued outpatient oral antimicrobial agents (ie, amoxicillin/clavulanate). Early follow-up—24 to 48 hours—with a physician skilled in the management of such injuries is encouraged. If the patient appears to be noncompliant, consideration should be made for initial inpatient care. Early range of motion is initiated, and the wound is allowed to heal in secondary or closed as a delayed primary closure.

THE LOWER EXTREMITY
Knee Dislocation

Knee dislocation can represent a true vascular emergency resulting in profound consequences for the patient. Therefore, clinicians must maintain a high degree of suspicion for arterial injury following significant knee trauma. Knee dislocation can result from high- or low-velocity injuries such as motor vehicle crashes, martial arts, or water skiing. The most common mechanism of injury is motor vehicle crashes, which is responsible for two-thirds of cases.[87] Dislocation may occur in an anterior, posterior, medial, lateral, or rotatory fashion. However, most knee dislocations are anterior (**Fig. 6**). Nearly 30% of high-velocity knee dislocations will have associated life-threatening injuries.[88] Up to 60% of patients will have an associated fracture and 41% will have multiple fractures present.[87–90]

The popliteal artery is tethered as it passes behind the knee at the adductor hiatus (above) and the soleus (below), predisposing the vessel to injury during joint dislocation. The incidence of associated popliteal artery injury in patients with knee dislocation has been reported to be between 21% and 40%.[89–92] With vascular injury, ischemic time is the single most important predictor of amputation.[87–89,91–93] An amputation rate of 85% is reported in patients who have no surgery or a delay to arterial repair longer than 8 hours, compared with an amputation rate of 15% in patients who have restored blood flow in less than 8 hours.[87–89,91,92]

The literature is consistent regarding the value of a thorough physical examination.[94–97] An abnormal vascular examination mandates angiography. Hard signs of a vascular lesion include a diminished dorsalis pedis or posterior tibial pulse, active hemorrhage, and expanding or pulsatile hematoma. However, patients with a normal examination often have either no injury or inconsequential vascular injury.

Traditional teaching recommends angiography for all patients with documented or suspected knee dislocation (**Fig. 7**). Recently, serial clinical examinations and other noninvasive testing have been supported in the literature as an alternative to

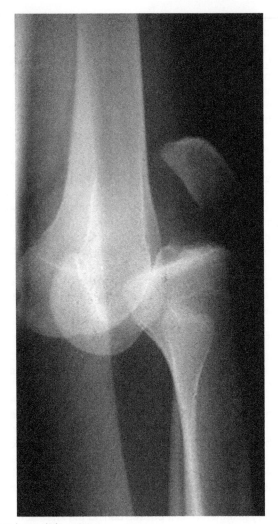

Fig. 6. An anterior knee dislocation.

angiography. Duplex Doppler ultrasonography has a reported sensitivity of 95% and a specificity of 99%.[98] However, ultrasonography may miss intimal tears and is operator dependent. At present, there are few data regarding the utility of CT angiography in assessing vascular injury from knee dislocation.

The utility of the ankle-brachial index (ABI; defined as the ratio of the blood pressure in the lower legs to the blood pressure in the arms) for assessing chronic arterial insufficiency is well established. Its role in assessing acute arterial injury is supported for both upper and lower extremity trauma. Patients with good pulses, ABIs greater than 0.9, and no hard signs of ischemia can likely be watched as inpatients and undergo serial examinations. Patients with normal examinations and ABI measurements should be observed for a 24-hour period.[99] Traditionally, an ABI less than 0.9 indicates vascular injury, whereas an ABI greater than 0.9 is highly predictive of the lack of vascular injury or inconsequential injury. Mills and colleagues[100] performed a prospective study that enrolled 38 patients with knee dislocation to evaluate for

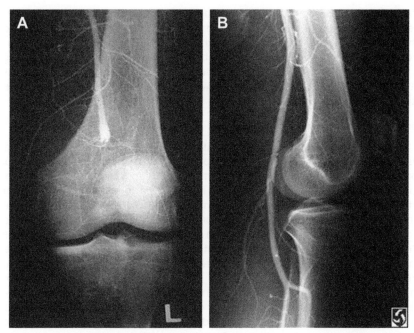

Fig. 7. (*A, B*) Angiographic evidence of popliteal artery disruption following a motor vehicle accident. This patient suffered a posterior dislocation from a dashboard type of injury on a flexed knee. Note the abrupt vessel cut-off.

potential arterial injury using clinical pulse examination and ABI. All patients with an ABI lower than 0.9 underwent arteriography. Those with an ABI of 0.9 or higher were immobilized and admitted for serial examination and delayed arterial duplex evaluation. Of the 38 patients, 11 (29%) had an ABI lower than 0.9. All 11 had arterial injury requiring surgical treatment. Of the remaining 27 patients with an ABI of 0.9 or higher, none had vascular injury detectable by serial clinical examination or duplex ultrasonography.

Achilles Tendon Rupture

The Achilles tendon is a frequently ruptured structure, accounting for 40% of all surgically repaired tendon ruptures,[101] yet the diagnosis is initially missed in about 25% of cases.[102,103] An overlooked rupture can lead to chronic weakness and loss of function.

Achilles tendon rupture occurs when stress is applied to the previously contracted muscle/tendon. A rapid push off with the knee extended, or a sudden unexpected dorsiflexion have been suggested as the mechanisms of injury. These injuries occur most frequently (81%) while playing sports, most often during sporting activity requiring sudden acceleration or jumping.[102] Rarely does the rupture occur from a direct blow to the tendon. The injury typically occurs in middle-aged men who are occasional athletes (the "weekend warrior"). Although patients may describe symptoms related to Achilles tendinitis before the injury, this prodromal complaint is generally not the case. Histologically, however, virtually all patients with acute Achilles tendon rupture have preexisting degenerative changes in their tendon.[104]

Both steroids and fluoroquinolones have been associated with Achilles tendon rupture.[105–107] Van der Linden and colleagues[106] found a relative risk of 1.9 for Achilles tendon disorders among fluoroquinolone users, and also that this risk was further increased among those 60 years or older and those concurrently taking corticosteroids.

The history of the injury frequently is pathognomonic. In general, the diagnosis of ruptured Achilles tendon is made based on history and physical examination findings, and radiographic examination serves to rule out other possible injuries to the ankle joint.[108] MRI may be of benefit for patients with chronic complaints or in cases where partial tear of the tendon is suspected.[109]

Lisfranc Fracture-Dislocation

The articulation between the tarsal and metatarsal bones in the foot is named after Jacques Lisfranc, a French physician in Napoleon's army who first described amputations through this joint. Injuries to this region commonly result from falls and motor vehicle or industrial accidents, and can range from mild sprains to severe dislocations and fracture-dislocations. Because Lisfranc joint fracture-dislocations and sprains carry such a high risk of chronic pain and functional disability if they go unrecognized and hence untreated,[110–113] EPs should maintain a high index of suspicion for these injuries.

Historically, Lisfranc injuries were thought to be a rare problem accounting for less than 1% of all orthopedic trauma; the overall incidence, however, is increasing and more common than initially recognized.[110,114,115] It is estimated that this diagnosis is missed on initial presentation to the ED in approximately 20% of cases.[110,114–117]

Lisfranc injuries can be caused by either direct or indirect trauma. Direct or crush injuries to the dorsum of the foot are rare and are often complicated by contamination, vascular compromise, and compartment syndrome.[114] The displacement of the metatarsal bases may occur in either the plantar or dorsal direction depending on the direction of force at the time of injury; and no distinctive pattern of injury exists for this mechanism. Indirect forces constitute the vast majority of injuries, resulting from either rotational forces or axial loading on a plantar flexed foot. The longitudinal force results in metatarsal dislocation dorsally at the site of least resistance while the rotational force causes dislocation medially or laterally. In that tremendous energy is required for dislocation, these injuries are frequently associated with multiple other fractures and significant soft-tissue injury.[118] Common causes of indirect trauma include falls from a height, motor vehicle accidents or motorcycle accidents, equestrian accidents, and athletic injuries.[110,115]

Lisfranc injuries range from mild, undetectable subluxations to obvious fracture-dislocations. Following a significant tarsometatarsal injury, patients generally present with complaints of midfoot pain, swelling, and difficulty with weight bearing. With milder injuries, the patient may be able to bear weight acutely and be surprisingly active despite the pain. Tenderness along the Lisfranc joint is common and passive pronation with abduction of the forefoot with the hindfoot held fixed will elicit pain; this maneuver is specific for tarsometatarsal injuries.[118] The foot may appear normal or markedly deformed depending on the severity of the injury. Plantar ecchymosis may be noted, and if found should prompt aggressive search for Lisfranc joint injury.[119] If the mechanism of injury is severe or deformity is obvious, manipulation of the foot should be kept to a minimum to prevent further displacement. A broadened foot, shortening in the anteroposterior plane, and a pathologic range of motion suggest severe fracture dislocation.[116] Serial vascular examinations are important when this injury is suspected. Tense swelling of the foot with diminished pulses suggests compartment syndrome, and in these cases immediate surgical intervention is necessary to save the extremity.[114,118] In a multiply injured, unconscious patient, the injury is easily missed because more life-threatening issues preclude full evaluation of the extremities.

Proper radiographic evaluation and interpretation of the foot is the key to diagnosis of Lisfranc injuries. Knowledge of the normal anatomic relationships at the Lisfranc joint is vital to radiographic interpretation (**Fig. 8**). The tarsometatarsal trauma series should include 3 views of the injured foot: AP, lateral, and oblique views. Major fracture-dislocations are easily recognized and rarely missed on a roentgenogram.[120] Sprain injuries without dislocation, however, are difficult to diagnose radiographically even though physical examination findings are highly suggestive of tarsometatarsal involvement. Weight-bearing stress views (AP and lateral) can be obtained if the diagnosis is suspected, but the plain film series is not diagnostic.[110,115,121–123] Roentgenograms of the tarsometatarsal joint may be daunting at first glance because of confusion caused by overlapping bony articulations. The second metatarsal base should always be carefully evaluated for fracture, avulsions, and displacement. On AP and oblique radiographs, the medial border of the second metatarsal base and the middle cuneiform as well as the medial border of the fourth metatarsal base and cuboid should form straight, unbroken lines. Any disruption of these lines or fracture fragments around the base of the second metatarsal or along the lateral border of the cuboid indicates significant tarsometatarsal injury. On the lateral film, a metatarsal shaft should never be more dorsal than its respective tarsal bone.[115] A fracture of the cuboid, cuneiforms, navicular, or metatarsal shafts is suggestive of disarticulation of the tarsometatarsal joint. In minor subluxation injuries, the key to diagnosis is the mortise configuration of the second metatarsal. Separation between the base of the first and second metatarsal or between the medial and middle cuneiforms is strongly

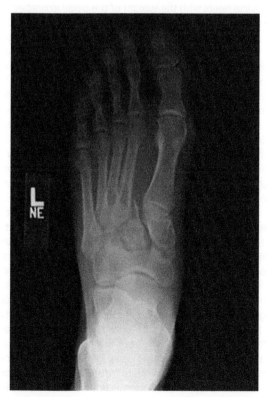

Fig. 8. A PA radiograph of the foot demonstrating a Lisfranc fracture-dislocation.

suggestive of subluxation.[116,118] If plain radiographs and weight-bearing radiographs do not yield the diagnosis, MRI or CT can be used to definitively rule the diagnosis in or out.[121,122,124]

Early diagnosis of a Lisfranc joint injury is imperative for proper management, and can contribute to the prevention of a poor functional outcome.[110,111,115,117] The definitive treatment of these fractures usually involves surgical intervention, although there is some controversy in the literature.[111,118,125] The EP's responsibility in the ED is to suspect the diagnosis, confirm the injury radiographically, and to recognize the potential compartment syndrome, which may be associated with the fracture. If orthopedic consultation is not immediately available, the EP can attempt closed reduction by hanging the foot by the toes using finger traps.[126] If reduced, a bulky compressive dressing is then applied with a posterior splint. These injuries almost always warrant acute orthopedic evaluation. The ultimate goal in treating this injury is to reestablish a painless, stable, and functional joint. To do this, precise anatomic reduction is necessary, which usually requires operative intervention.[111,116,125]

Fractures of the Calcaneus

The calcaneus is the largest and most commonly fractured tarsal bone, accounting for approximately 60% of all foot fractures.[19,127–130] Intra-articular fractures, accounting for 75% of calcaneus fractures, are the most common and potentially morbid of the fractures to this bone. This injury virtually always results from a fall from a height and is often associated with other fractures, particularly involving the spine.[131,132] The patient lands on the heels with the weight of the body absorbed by the calcaneus. The severity of the injury is more dependent on the exact location of the point of impact than on the height of the fall. It is critical to appreciate that these injuries have a significant potential for soft-tissue problems if not recognized and properly treated in the acute setting. Twenty percent of patients with calcaneal fractures may be totally incapacitated for up to 3 years and partially impaired for up to 5 years.[128,129,133,134]

The patient will present with varying degrees of heel pain and swelling. The powerful forces required in a calcaneal fracture can cause considerable damage to the surrounding soft tissue of the foot itself. This injury is associated with other lower extremity injuries in 70% of the cases and spine fractures in 10%[131,132]; the associated injuries can be painful enough to overshadow the foot injury, and the patient may not even complain of significant heel pain. All patients who have suffered a fall from a height should be suspected of having such an injury, with examination directed from the heel to the thoracic spine.

These patients will have tenderness, swelling, and ecchymosis of the tissues surrounding the calcaneus. The normal contour of the heel is lost and the heel appears widened and shortened. Open fractures are common, and the skin should be carefully examined for small puncture wounds. The basic radiographic series for a suspected calcaneus fracture includes AP, lateral, and Harris axial views of the foot. The lateral view demonstrates most intra-articular fractures. Bohler's angle, measured on the lateral view, is used to assess the degree of compression of the calcaneus; it also is useful in detecting a radiographically occult calcaneal compression fracture as well as in determining the congruity of the posterior facet of the subtalar joint. The angle itself is obtained by drawing 2 lines: one from the posterior tuberosity to the apex of the posterior facet and the other from the apex of the posterior facet to the apex of the anterior process. Bohler's angle may vary from 20° to 40°[132]; a compression fracture is suggested with an angle of less than 20°. The axial view of the foot demonstrates the amount of widening of the heel. The AP of the foot will show extension of the fracture into the calcaneocuboid joint or associated subluxation of the talona-vicular joint.

The ED treatment of these fractures revolves mostly around the appropriate handling of the soft tissues. Immediate application of a bulky, compressive dressing with a posterior splint, combined with elevation and ice application, can prevent fracture blisters, skin slough, and the ultimate delay of surgical intervention when it is necessary. Intra-articular fractures often require ORIF, whereas the less common extra-articular fractures are usually treated conservatively with casting under the supervision of an orthopedic surgeon.

OTHER ORTHOPEDIC PITFALLS
Compartment Syndrome

Compartment syndrome is a serious life- and limb-threatening complication of extremity trauma. A delay in diagnosis or treatment can result in significant morbidity for the patient. Fractures, crush injuries, burns, and arterial injuries all can result in an acute compartment syndrome.[134,145] Compartment syndrome develops when there is increased pressure within a closed tissue space, such as muscle compartments bound by dense fascial sheaths. This increased pressure compromises the flow of blood through vessels supplying the contained muscles and nerves. Those compartments in the arm and leg are most vulnerable to this syndrome, but virtually any muscle mass surrounded by fascia is at risk. Frequently sited locations for compartment syndrome other than the lower leg include the hand, forearm, arm, shoulder, back, buttocks, thigh, and foot.[49,135,136]

The exact incidence of compartment syndrome in the ED is unknown. It is known that approximately three-quarters of cases are associated with fractures,[137] and that tibia fracture has the highest association.[136,138] Early diagnosis and treatment of acute compartment syndrome is of the utmost importance, as delay can lead to tissue necrosis and ultimately severe, permanent disability, as with Volkmann ischemic contracture.

Compartment syndrome results when there is increased pressure within a closed tissue space that compromises the flow of blood to muscles and nerves. The increase in compartmental pressure can result from (1) external compression of the compartment, for example, by a circumferential cast or burn eschar, and (2) volume increase within the compartment secondary to edema or hematoma formation.

The pathophysiology of compartment syndrome involves hydrostatic and osmotic pressure conditions within the myofascial compartment. When the intracompartmental pressure increases to above a specific level owing to the aforementioned factors, perfusion to the compartment is impaired, resulting in disruption of skeletal muscle metabolic processes. Cell wall membrane integrity is compromised, leading to cytolysis with the release of osmotically active cellular contents into the compartment; this draws additional fluid from plasma into the interstitial space.[139] The net effect is increased intracompartmental pressure and further impairment of perfusion to the closed space of the myofascial compartment, as well as to distal structures in that vascular distribution. This process can ultimately lead to a compromise of the circulation and/or nerve conduction as well as irreversible muscle injury, contractions, loss of limb, myoglobinuria, renal failure, and even death.[140,141]

Common fractures associated with compartment syndrome are tibial fractures, supracondylar fractures of the humerus and humoral shaft, and forearm fractures. Crush injuries to the hand or foot, with or without associated fractures, are also at risk. The potential for compartment syndrome should also be considered with multiple meta-carpal or metatarsal fractures, Lisfranc fracture-dislocations, and calcaneal fractures.

Each limb contains several compartments that are at risk for compartment syndrome. The anterior compartment of the lower leg is most frequently involved in this syndrome, and contains the tibialis muscle and the extensors of the toes.

A very high suspicion remains the cornerstone of diagnosing acute compartment syndrome. A traditional hallmark element in the history of a patient presenting with compartment syndrome is pain disproportionate to the mechanism of injury. However, this assumes an awake, neurologically intact patient. Unfortunately, many patients at risk for compartment syndrome are severely injured or impaired, and cannot relate whether they are experiencing pain.

The clinical signs of compartment syndrome are often remembered by using the mnemonic of the 5 Ps: pain, paresthesia, paresis, pallor, and pulses. Pain, especially disproportionate pain, is often the earliest sign, but the loss of normal neurologic sensation is most reliable.[140,142,143] On physical examination, palpation of the compartment may or may not demonstrate swelling or a tense compartment. In the awake, intact patient, pain on active or passive range of motion in the affected limb will elicit significant pain. Decrease or loss of 2-point discrimination can also be an early finding of compartment syndrome.[140,142] Clinical findings can also include shiny, erythematous skin overlying the involved compartment (described as a "woody" feeling), and excessive swelling. A thready or diminished pulse is not a reliable sign. Intracompartmental tissue pressure is usually lower than arterial blood pressure, making peripheral pulses and capillary refill poor indicators of blood flow within the compartment. Patients with a very low diastolic blood pressure are more susceptible to compartment syndrome.[144–146]

The diagnosis of compartment syndrome is primarily based on determinations of the intracompartmental pressure. There is some debate in the literature regarding what pressure level mandates fasciotomy. Some investigators base recommendations on absolute compartment pressure,[140,147,148] whereas others believe the intracompartmental pressure is meaningful only as it relates to the mean blood pressure or diastolic blood pressure.[138,146] Most literature and recommendations, however, are based on absolute pressures within the compartment.

Normal tissue pressure ranges between 0 and 10 mm Hg. Capillary blood flow within the compartment may be compromised at pressures greater than 20 mm Hg. Muscle and nerve fibers are at risk for ischemic necrosis at pressures greater than 30 to 40 mm Hg. Several techniques are available for intracompartmental pressure determinations, each with advantages and disadvantages. These methods include the Stryker (Stryker Instruments, Kalamazoo, MI, USA) or Ace (Ace Medical Company, Los Angeles, CA, USA) pressure monitors, the needle technique, the wick catheter, and the slit catheter. The Stryker and Ace monitors are used most frequently, and have largely replaced the other methods owing to their ease of use and reproducible results. These monitors are self-contained, battery-powered pressure transducers. Compartment pressures are measured after careful aseptic preparation of the site. An 18-gauge needle is attached to the monitor and is inserted into the suspect compartment. A small (<1 mL) amount of saline is injected and the pressure, in mm Hg, is determined. The needle and wick methods are also well described in the literature, but their use is infrequent because of the advantages of the aforementioned devices.

Pulse oximetry has been advocated as a simple noninvasive indicator of vascular compromise. Mars and Hadley[149] investigated the reproducibility of pulse oximetry and the effect on arterial hemoglobin saturation of raising intracompartmental pressure by compression bandaging. At clinically significant pressures, the test had a sensitivity of approximately 40%. With a greater than 50% risk of a false-negative result, pulse oximetry is not recommended in the detection of elevated intracompartmental pressure.

Several recent trials have supported the use of infrared imaging as a noninvasive means of diagnosing compartment syndrome.[150,151] However, this is not considered a conventional diagnostic tool, as further studies are needed to validate its utility.

The goal of treatment of compartment syndrome is to decrease tissue pressure, restore blood flow, and minimize tissue damage and related functional loss. External pressure from casts or dressings should be removed immediately. It has been shown that if a cast is bivalved, the compartment pressures may decrease as much as 55%, and if a cast is completely removed, the pressure may decrease as much as 85%.[136,145] The effected limb should be elevated to the level of the heart to promote arterial blood flow and not decrease venous return. Elevation above the heart can result in decreased perfusion. Ice is contraindicated because it may compromise the microcirculation. Steroids and vasodilating agents have been proposed to be useful in the past, but have not been shown to be of benefit when subject to clinical trials.

Acute compartment syndrome is a surgical emergency. Fasciotomy is the definitive therapy and should be performed as soon as possible. Delays of more than 24 hours can have devastating consequences, including significant muscle mass damage resulting in myoglobinuria, renal failure, metabolic acidosis, hyperkalemia, and ultimately contracture formation or loss of the limb.[136,142,145] According to Mabee,[134] absolute indications for fasciotomy are (1) clinical signs of acute compartment syndrome, (2) raised tissue pressure greater than 30 mm Hg in a patient with the clinical picture of compartment syndrome, and (3) interrupted arterial circulation to an extremity for greater than 4 hours. If performed within 12 hours of symptom onset, fasciotomy can prevent most ischemic myoneural deficits.[152] Most studies report that between 1% and 10% of patients with acute compartment syndrome go on to develop Volkmann ischemic contracture.[136]

Pediatric Growth Plate Fracture

The epiphyseal plate (physis) is the growth cartilage of the long bones of children. Injuries to the physis are a cause for concern, as bone growth can be slowed or stopped after a physeal injury. Physeal injuries have been reported to account for 15% to 30% of all skeletal injuries in children.[153–155] Approximately 80% of physeal injuries will occur between the ages of 10 and 16 years, with the median age being 13 years.[156–158] Injuries to the physis occur much more frequently in boys than girls, reflective of the overall increased incidence of musculoskeletal injury in this population, as well as the late development of skeletal maturity in boys as opposed to girls.[156,157,159] When unrecognized and improperly treated, Salter and Harris[160] found that 15% of these injuries resulted in physeal arrest. Proper therapy for these injuries, however, has reduced the incidence of physeal arrest to 1% to 2%.[154]

Anteroposterior and lateral radiographic views are the basic diagnostic tools for growth plate injuries; comparison views of the contralateral bone may often assist in determining the difference between an irregular physis and a fracture. Complex fractures may require plain tomography, CT, or MRI to fully define the extent of the fracture.[161]

Type I fractures are most frequently seen in infants and toddlers. The prognosis for ensuing growth is good unless there has been damage to the arterial supply of the epiphysis, which is seen with injuries involving displacement of the capital femoral epiphysis or the epiphysis of the head of the radius. Type II (**Fig. 9**) injuries occur most often in children older than 8 years and involve a fracture line that passes through

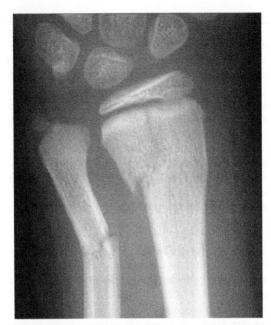

Fig. 9. A PA radiograph of the wrist demonstrates a Salter-Harris type II growth plate injury, with a fracture of the metaphysis extending up into the physis.

the epiphyseal plate; the epiphysis is laterally displaced, tearing the periosteum on one side while leaving it intact on the side of the metaphyseal fracture. Type II fractures are easily reduced because of the intact periosteum on the fracture side. Because the circulation to the epiphysis remains intact, the prognosis for growth is good. Type III (**Fig. 10**) fractures are uncommon, generally occurring at the upper or lower tibial physis. Intra-articular shearing forces cause the injury, with the fracture line passing

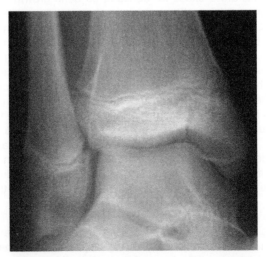

Fig. 10. A PA radiograph of the ankle demonstrates a Salter-Harris type IV growth plate injury, with a fracture of metaphyseal and epiphyseal portions of the bone.

through the epiphysis. Accurate reduction of a type III fracture is essential to restore the joint surface. Prognosis for growth is good provided that the blood supply to the fractured epiphysis remains intact. More than 2 mm of displacement suggests the need for surgery with open reduction. Type IV injuries are seen most commonly at the lower end of the humerus with the fracture line passing through the metaphyseal and epiphyseal portions of the bone. Unless the fracture is nondisplaced, open reduction is always necessary to restore the smooth joint surface. The physis must be perfectly aligned to prevent premature closure of the growth plate. Type V fractures are severe crush injuries through the epiphysis damaging a portion of the physis, with movement of the epiphyseal and metaphyseal segments toward one another. These injuries are uncommon but can lead to severe growth reduction problems. Because of minimal displacement, this fracture is often occult radiographically. As the prognosis for continued bone growth is poor, localized physeal tenderness should influence the examiner to suspect a Type V fracture. Maintaining non–weight bearing for 3 weeks can reduce the risk of premature growth arrest.

SUMMARY

Although the diagnosis and management of most orthopedic injuries is straightforward, there are distinct pitfalls to be avoided. The common theme among those high-risk, pitfall injuries discussed here, besides a thorough history and careful physical examination coupled with appropriate radiographs, is a high suspicion for their presence. EPs may limit potential legal risk by being knowledgable about these orthopedic pitfalls and being vigilant for these injuries in their clinical practice.

REFERENCES

1. Rowe CR. Prognosis in dislocations of the shoulder. J Bone Joint Surg Am 1956; 38:957–77.
2. Samilson RL, Prieto V. Posterior dislocation of the shoulder in athletes. Clin Sports Med 1983;2(2):369–78.
3. Schultz TJ, Jacobs B, Patterson RL. Unrecognized dislocations of the shoulder. J Trauma 1969;9:1009–23.
4. Hawkins RJ, Neer CS, Pianta RM, et al. Locked posterior dislocation of the shoulder. J Bone Joint Surg Am 1987;69:9–18.
5. Neviaser TJ. Old unreduced dislocations of the shoulder. Orthop Clin North Am 1980;11:287–94.
6. Rowe CR, Zarins B. Chronic unreduced dislocations of the shoulder. J Bone Joint Surg Am 1982;64:494–505.
7. Andreson LD, Meyer FN, Lippincott JB. Fractures of the shafts of the radius and ulna. In: Bucholz RW, Heckman JD, Court-Brown CM, et al, editors. Rockwood and Green's fractures in adults. 3rd edition. Philadelphia (PA): Lippincott-Raven; 1991. p. 679–737.
8. Kowalsky MS, Levine WN. Traumatic posterior glenohumeral dislocation: classification, pathoanatomy, diagnosis, and treatment. Orthop Clin North Am 2008; 39:519–33.
9. Jensen KL, Rockwood CA. X-ray evaluation of shoulder problems. In: Rockwood CA, Matsen FA, Wirth MA, editors. The shoulder, vol. 1. 3rd edition. Philadelphia (PA): Saunders; 2004. p. 187–222.
10. O'Connor SJ, Kacknow AJ. Posterior dislocation of the shoulder. J Bone Joint Surg Am 1955;37:1122.

11. Meadows T, Wallace WA. Missed posterior dislocation of the shoulder. J Bone Joint Surg Br 1987;69:152.

12. Ogawa K, Yoshida A, Inokuchi W. Posterior shoulder dislocation associated with fracture of the humeral anatomic neck: treatment guidelines and long-term outcome. J Trauma 1999;46:318–23.

13. Matsen FA, Thomas SC, Rockwood CA. Anterior glenohumeral instability. In: Rockwood CA, Matsen FA, editors. The shoulder. Philadelphia: W.B. Saunders; 1990. p. 526–622.

14. Rockwood CA. Subluxations and dislocations about the shoulder. In: Rockwood CA, Green DP, editors. Fractures in adults. Philadelphia: J.B. Lippincott; 1984. p. 722–860.

15. Pollock RG, Bigliani LU. Recurrent posterior shoulder instability: diagnosis and treatment. Clin Orthop 1993;291:85–96.

16. Green A, Norris TR. Glenohumeral dislocations. In: Browner BD, Jupiter JB, Levine AM, et al, editors. Skeletal trauma. Philadelphia: W.B. Saunders; 1992. p. 1639–56.

17. Perron AD, Hersh RE, Brady WJ, et al. Orthopedic pitfalls in the ED. Galeazzi and Monteggia fracture-dislocation. Am J Emerg Med 2001;19:225–8.

18. Bhan S, Rath S. Management of the Galeazzi fracture. Int Orthop 1991;15(3): 193–6.

19. Bruckner JD, Lichtman DM, Alexander AH. Complex dislocations of the distal radioulnar joint: recognition and management. Clin Orthop 1992;275:90–103.

20. Kraus B, Horne G. Galeazzi fractures. J Trauma 1985;25(11):1093–5.

21. Morgan WJ, Breen TF. Complex fractures of the forearm. Hand Clin 1994;10(3): 375–90.

22. Zautcke JL. Forearm injuries. In: Hart RG, Rittenberry TJ, editors. Handbook of orthopaedic emergencies. Philadelphia (PA): Lippincott Williams & Wilkins; 1999. p. 222–32.

23. Faierman E, Jupiter JB. The management of acute fractures involving the distal radio-ulnar joint and distal ulna. Hand Clin 1998;14(2):213–29.

24. Goldberg HD, Young JW, Reiner BI, et al. Double injuries of the forearm: a common occurrence. Radiology 1992;185(1):223–7.

25. Khaldun JS, Gore RJ. Forearm fracture. In: eMedicine [serial online]. Available at: http://emedicine.medscape.com/article/824949-overview. Accessed December 2009.

26. Speed JS, Boyd HB. Treatment of fractures of ulna with dislocation of the head of the radius. JAMA 1940;115(20):1699–704.

27. Brunswick JE, Ilkhanipour K, Seaberg DC, et al. Radiographic interpretation in the emergency department. Am J Emerg Med 1996;14(4):346–8.

28. Thompson E, Cordas M. Fracture-dislocations you can't afford to miss. Phys Sportsmed 1996;24(6):36–42.

29. Boyd HB, Boals JC. The Monteggia lesion. A review of 159 cases. Clin Orthop 1969;66:94–100.

30. Ring D, Jupiter JB. Current concepts review. Fracture-dislocation of the elbow. J Bone Joint Surg Am 1998;80(4):566–80.

31. Ring D, Jupiter JB, Waters PM. Monteggia fractures in children and adults. J Am Acad Orthop Surg 1998;6(4):215–24.

32. Ring D, Jupiter JB, Simpson SN. Monteggia fractures in adults. J Bone Joint Surg Am 1998;80(12):1733–44.

33. Stoll TM, Willis RB, Paterson DC. Treatment of the missed Monteggia fracture in the child. J Bone Joint Surg Br 1992;74(3):436–40.

34. Jessing P. Monteggia lesions and their complicating nerve damage. Acta Orthop Scand 1975;46:601–9.
35. Chacon D, Kissoon N, Brown T, et al. Use of comparison radiographs in the diagnosis of traumatic injuries of the elbow. Ann Emerg Med 1992;21(8):895–9.
36. Oveson O, Brok KE, Arreskov J, et al. Monteggia lesions in children and adults: an analysis of etiology and long-term results of treatment. Orthopedics 1990; 13(5):529–34.
37. Mital RC, Beeson M. The wrist and forearm. In: Schwartz DT, Reisdorf E, editors. Emergency radiology. New York (NY): McGraw Hill; 2000. p. 47–76.
38. Simon RR, Koenigsknecht SJ, Stevens C. Emergency orthopedics: the extremities. 2nd edition. New York (NY): Appleton & Lange; 1987.
39. Freed HA, Shields NN. Most frequently overlooked radiographically apparent fractures in a teaching hospital emergency department. Ann Emerg Med 1984;13:900–4.
40. Mikic ZD. Galeazzi fracture-dislocations. J Bone Joint Surg Am 1975;57:1071–8.
41. Hughston JC. Fracture of the distal radial shaft: mistakes in management. J Bone Joint Surg Am 1957;39:249–64.
42. Beeson MS. Wrist dislocations. In: eMedicine [serial online]. Available at: http://emedicine.medscape.com/article/823944-overview. Accessed December 2009.
43. Chin HW, Uehara DT. Wrist injuries. In: Tintinalli JE, Kelen GD, Stapczynski JS, editors. Emergency medicine. New York: McGraw-Hill; 2000. p. 1772–83.
44. Herzberg G, Comtet JJ, Linscheid RL, et al. Perilunate dislocations and fracture dislocations: a multicenter study. J Hand Surg Am 1993;18:768–79.
45. Rockwood CA Jr, Green DP, Bucholz RW. Fractures and dislocations of the wrist. In: Rockwood CA Jr, Green DP, editors. Fractures in adults, vol. 1. New York: Lippincott Williams & Wilkins Publishers; 1996. p. 745–867.
46. Perron AD, Brady WJ, Keats TE, et al. Orthopedic pitfalls in the ED: lunate and perilunate injuries. Am J Emerg Med 2001;19:157–62.
47. Inoue G, Kuwahata Y. Management of acute perilunate dislocations without fracture of the scaphoid. J Hand Surg Br 1997;22(5):647–52.
48. McCue FC, Bruce JF. The wrist. In: DeLee JC, Drez D, editors. Orthopedic sports medicine. Philadelphia: W.B. Saunders; 1994. p. 913–44.
49. Bednar JM, Osterman AL. Carpal instability: evaluation and treatment. Am Acad Ortho Surg 1993;1(1):10–5.
50. Cooney WP, Linscheid RL, Dobyns JH. Fractures and dislocations of the wrist. In: Rockwood CA, Green DP, Bucholz RW, et al, editors. Rockwood and Green's fractures in adults. 3rd edition. Philadelphia: Lippincott-Raven; 1996. p. 745–867.
51. Larsen CF, Lauritsen J. Epidemiology of acute wrist trauma. Int J Epidemiol 1993;22(5):911–6.
52. Meldon SW, Hargarten SW. Ligamentous injuries of the wrist. J Emerg Med 1995;13(2):217–25.
53. Watson HK, Weinzweig J, Zeppieri J. The natural progression of scaphoid instability. Hand Clin 1997;13(1):39–49.
54. Adkinson JW, Chapman MW. Treatment of acute lunate and perilunate dislocations. Clin Orthop Relat Res 1982;164:199–207.
55. Rettig ME, Raskin KB. Long-term assessment of proximal row carpectomy for chronic perilunate dislocations. J Hand Surg Am 1999;24(6):1231–6.
56. Watson HK, Weinzweig J, Guidera PM, et al. One thousand intercarpal arthrodeses. J Hand Surg Br 1999;24(3):307–15.
57. Duncan DS, Thurston AJ. Clinical fracture of the carpal scaphoid-an illusory diagnosis. J Hand Surg Br 1985;10:375–6.

58. Ring D, Jupiter JB, Herndon JH. Acute fractures of the scaphoid. J Am Acad Orthop Surg 2000;8:225–31.
59. Ritchie JV, Munter DW. Emergency department evaluation and treatment of wrist injuries. Emerg Med Clin North Am 1999;17(4):823–42.
60. Berger RA. The ligaments of the wrist: a current overview of anatomy with consideration of their potential functions. Hand Clin 1997;13(1):63–82.
61. Eisenhauer MA. Wrist and forearm. In: Rosen P, Barkin R, editors. Emergency medicine: concepts and clinical practice. St Louis (MO): CV Mosby; 1998. p. 669–83.
62. Nguyen DT, McCue FC, Urch SE. Evaluation of the injured wrist on the field and in the office. Clin Sports Med 1998;17(3):421–32.
63. Zemel MP, Stark HH. Fractures and dislocations of the carpal bones. Clin Sports Med 1986;5:709–23.
64. Wackerle JF. A prospective study identifying the sensitivity of radiographic findings and the efficacy of clinical findings in carpal navicular fractures. Ann Emerg Med 1987;16:733–7.
65. Barber H. The intraosseous arterial anatomy of the adult human carpus. Orthopedics 1972;5:1–20.
66. Lindstrom G, Nystrom A. Natural history of scaphoid non-union, with special reference to "asymptomatic" cases. J Hand Surg Br 1992;17:697–700.
67. Taleisnik J, Kelly PJ. The extraosseous and intraosseus blood supply of the scaphoid bone. J Bone Joint Surg Am 1966;48:1125–37.
68. Cooney WP, Bussey R, Dobyns JH, et al. Difficult wrist fractures: perilunate dislocations of the wrist. Clin Orthop Relat Res 1987;214:136–47.
69. Chen SC. The scaphoid compression test. J Hand Surg Br 1989;14:323–5.
70. Waizenegger M, Barton NJ, Davis TR, et al. Clinical signs in scaphoid fractures. J Hand Surg Br 1994;19:743–7.
71. Schubert HE. Scaphoid fracture: review of diagnostic tests and treatment. Can Fam Physician 2000;46:1825–32.
72. Leslie IJ, Dickson RA. The fractured carpal scaphoid. J Bone Joint Surg Br 1981;63:225–30.
73. Murphy D, Eisenhauer M. The utility of a bone scan in the diagnosis of clinical scaphoid fracture. J Emerg Med 1994;12:709–12.
74. Tiel-van Buul MM, van Beek EJ, Borm JJ, et al. The value of radiographs and bone scintigraphy in suspected scaphoid fracture. A statistical analysis. J Hand Surg Br 1993;18:403–6.
75. Cook PA, Yu JS, Wiand W, et al. Suspected scaphoid fracture in skeletally immature patients. Application of MRI. J Comput Assist Tomogr 1997;21:511–5.
76. Pennes RD, Jonsson K, Buckwalter KA. Direct coronal CT of the scaphoid bone. Radiology 1989;171:870–1.
77. Biodetti PR, Vannier MW, Gilula LA, et al. Wrist: coronal and trans-axial CT scanning. Radiology 1987;163:149–51.
78. Hunter JC, Escobedo EM, Wilson AJ, et al. MR imaging of clinically suspected scaphoid fractures. Am J Roentgenol 1997;168:1287–93.
79. Perron AD, Brady WJ, Keats TE, et al. Orthopedic pitfalls in the ED: scaphoid fracture. Am J Emerg Med 2001;19:310–6.
80. Amadio PC, Berquist TH, Smith DK, et al. Scaphoid malunion. J Hand Surg Am 1989;14:679–87.
81. Verdan C, Narakas A. Fractures and pseudoarthrosis of the scaphoid. Surg Clin North Am 1968;48:1083–95.

82. Moritomo H, Tada K, Yoshida T, et al. The relationship between the site of nonunion of the scaphoid and scaphoid nonunion advanced collapse (SNAC). J Bone Joint Surg Br 1999;81(5):871–6.
83. Faciszewski T, Coleman DA. Human bite wounds. Hand Clin 1989;5:561–9.
84. Rayan GM, Flournoy DJ. Hand infections. Contemp Orthop 1990;20:41–54.
85. Perron AD, Miller MD, Brady WJ. Orthopedic pitfalls in the ED: fight bite. Am J Emerg Med 2002;20:114–7.
86. Mann RJ, Hoffeld TA, Farmer CB. Human bites of the hand: twenty years' experience. J Hand Surg Am 1977;97(2):104–11.
87. Perron AD, Brady WJ, Sing RF. Orthopedic pitfalls in the ED: vascular injury associated with knee dislocation. Am J Emerg Med 2001;19:583–8.
88. Wascher DC. High velocity knee dislocation with vascular injury. Clin Sports Med 2000;19:457–78.
89. Varnell RM, Coldwell DM, Sangeorzan BJ, et al. Arterial injury complicating knee disruptions. Am J Surg 1989;55:699–704.
90. Kendall RW, Taylor DC, Salvian AJ, et al. The role of arteriography in assessing vascular injuries associated with dislocations of the knee. J Trauma 1993;35: 875–9.
91. Green NE, Agel BL. Vascular injuries associated with dislocation of the knee. J Bone Joint Surg Am 1977;59:236–9.
92. Roberts DM, Stallard TC. Emergency department evaluation and treatment of knee and leg injuries. Emerg Med Clin North Am 2000;18:67–84.
93. Patterson BM, Agel J, Swiontkowski MF, et al. Knee dislocations with vascular injury: outcomes in the Lower Extremity Assessment Project (LEAP) study. J Trauma 2007;63:855–8.
94. Miranda FE, Dennis JW, Veldenz HC, et al. Confirmation of the safety and accuracy of physical examination in the evaluation of knee dislocation for injury of the popliteal artery: a prospective study. J Trauma 2002;52:247–51.
95. Stannard JP, Sheils TM, Lopez-Ben RR, et al. Vascular injuries in knee dislocations: the role of physical examination in determining the need for arteriography. J Bone Joint Surg Am 2004;86:910–5.
96. Treiman GS, Yellin AE, Weaver FA, et al. Examination of the patient with a knee dislocation. The case for selective arteriography. Arch Surg 1992; 127:1056–62.
97. Barnes CJ, Pietrobon R, Higgins LD, et al. Does the pulse examination in patients with traumatic knee dislocation predict a surgical arterial injury? A meta-analysis. J Trauma 2002;53:1109–14.
98. Fry WR, Smith RS, Sayers DV. The success of duplex ultrasound arterial scanning in diagnosis of extremity vascular trauma. Arch Surg 1993;128: 1368–72.
99. Nicandri GT, Chamberlain AM, Wahl CJ. Practical management of knee dislocations: A selective angiography protocol to detect limb-threatening vascular injuries. Clin J Sport Med 2009;19:125–9.
100. Mills WJ, Barei DP, McNair P. The value of the ankle-brachial index for diagnosing arterial injury after knee dislocation: a prospective study. J Trauma 2004;56:1261–6.
101. Jozsa L, Kvist M, Balint BJ, et al. The role of recreational sport activity in Achilles tendon rupture. A clinical, pathoanatomical, and sociological study of 292 cases. Am J Sports Med 1989;17:338–43.
102. Hooker CH. Rupture of the tendo calcaneus. J Bone Joint Surg Br 1963;45(2): 360–3.

103. Leppilahti J, Puranen J, Orava S. Incidence of Achilles tendon rupture. Acta Orthop Scand 1996;67:277–9.

104. Kvist H, Kvist M. The operative treatment of chronic calcaneal paratendinitis. J Bone Joint Surg Br 1980;62:353–6.

105. Melhus A, Apelqvist J, Larsson J, et al. Levofloxacin-associated Achilles tendon rupture and tendinopathy. Scand J Infect Dis 2003;35:768–70.

106. Van der Linden PD, Sturkenboom MC, Herings RM, et al. Fluoroquinolones and risk of Achilles tendon disorders: case control study. Br Med J 2002;324:1306–7.

107. Ufberg J, Harrigan RA, Perron AD, et al. Orthopedic pitfalls in the ED: Achilles tendon rupture. Am J Emerg Med 2004;22:596–600.

108. Cetti R, Andersen I. Roentgenographic diagnoses of ruptured Achilles tendons. Clin Orthop Relat Res 1993;286:215–21.

109. Haims AH, Schweitzer ME, Patel RS, et al. MR imaging of the Achilles tendon: overlap of findings in symptomatic and asymptomatic individuals. Skeletal Radiol 2000;29:640–5.

110. Burroughs KE, Reimer CD, Fields KB. Lisfranc injury of the foot: a commonly missed diagnosis. Am Fam Physician 1999;58(1):118–24.

111. Buzzard BM, Briggs PJ. Surgical management of acute tarsometatarsal fracture dislocation in the adult. Clin Orthop 1998;353:125–33.

112. Mulier T, Reynders P, Sioen W, et al. The treatment of Lisfranc injuries. Acta Orthop Belg 1997;63(2):82–90.

113. Rabin SI. Lisfranc dislocation and associated metatarsophalangeal joint dislocations. A case report and literature review. Am J Orthop 1996;25(4):305–9.

114. Arntz CT, Hansen ST. Dislocations and fracture dislocations of the tarsometatarsal joints. Orthop Clin North Am 1987;18:105–14.

115. Englenhoff G, Anglin D, Hutson HR. Lisfranc fracture dislocation: a frequently missed diagnosis in the emergency department. Ann Emerg Med 1995;26:229–33.

116. Goosens M, DeStoop N. Lisfranc's fracture dislocations: etiology, radiology, result of treatment. Clin Orthop 1983;176:154–62.

117. Vuori JP, Aro HT. Lisfranc joint injuries: trauma mechanisms and associated injuries. J Trauma 1993;35:40–5.

118. Myerson M. The diagnosis and treatment of injuries to the Lisfranc joint complex. Orthop Clin North Am 1989;20:655–64.

119. Margolis M, McLennan MK. Radiology rounds. Tarsometatarsal fracture dislocation (also called a fracture dislocation of Lisfranc's joint). Can Fam Physician 1994;40(1103):1108–10.

120. Potter HG, Deland JT, Gusmer PB, et al. Magnetic resonance imaging of the Lisfranc ligament of the foot. Foot Ankle Int 1998;19(7):438–46.

121. Lu J, Ebraheim NA, Skie M, et al. Radiographic and computed tomographic evaluation of Lisfranc dislocation: a cadaver study. Foot Ankle Int 1997;18(6):351–5.

122. Ross G, Cronin R, Hauzenblas J, et al. Plantar ecchymosis sign: a clinical aid to diagnosis of occult Lisfranc tarsometatarsal injuries. J Orthop Trauma 1996;10(2):119–22.

123. Chiodo CP, Myerson MS. Recent developments and advances in the diagnosis and treatment of injuries to tarsometatarsal joint. Orthop Clin North Am 2001;32:11–20.

124. Wartella J, Cohen R, Schwartz DT. The foot. In: Schwartz DT, Reisdorff E, editors. Emergency radiology. New York: McGraw-Hill; 2000. p. 135–56.

125. Preidler KW, Peicha G, Lajtai G, et al. Conventional radiography, CT, and MR imaging in patients with hyperflexion injuries of the foot: diagnostic accuracy

in the detection of bony and ligamentous changes. Am J Roentgenol 1999; 173(6):1673–7.

126. Perron AD, Brady WJ, Keats TE. Orthopedic pitfalls in the ED: Lisfranc fracture-dislocation. Am J Emerg Med 2001;19:71–5.

127. Germann CA, Perron AD, Miller MD, et al. Orthopedic pitfalls in the ED: calcaneal fractures. Am J Emerg Med 2004;22:607–11.

128. Lowery RB, Claxon JH. Fractures of the calcaneus: part 1: anatomy, injury, mechanism, and classification. Foot Ankle Int 1996;17:230–5.

129. Weedier IS, Charted J. Emergency department evaluation and treatment of ankle and foot injuries. Emerg Med Clin North Am 2000;18:85–113.

130. Fitzgibbons TC, McMullen ST, Mormino MA. Fractures and dislocations of the calcaneus. In: Bucholz RW, Heckman JD, editors. Rockwood and Green's fractures in adults. Philadephia: Lippincott-Raven; 2001. p. 2133–79.

131. Cave EF. Fracture of the os calcis—the problem in general. Clin Orthop 1963;30: 64–6.

132. Juliano P, Nguyen HV. Fractures of the calcaneus. Orthop Clin North Am 2001; 32(1):35–51.

133. Paley D, Hall H. Calcaneal fracture controversies: can we put humpty-dumpty together again? Orthop Clin North Am 1989;20:665–7.

134. Mabee JR. Compartment syndrome: a complication of acute extremity trauma. J Emerg Med 1994;12:651–6.

135. Foster RD, Albright JA. Acute compartment syndrome of the thigh: case report. J Trauma 1990;30:108–10.

136. Hoover TJ, Siefert JA. Soft tissue complications of orthopedic emergencies. Emerg Med Clin North Am 2000;18(1):116–39.

137. Blick SS, Brumback RJ, Poka A, et al. Compartment syndrome in open tibial fractures. J Bone Joint Surg Am 1986;68:1348–53.

138. McQueen MM, Christie J, Court-Brown CM. Acute compartment syndrome in tibial diaphyseal fractures. J Bone Joint Surg Br 1996;78:95–8.

139. Linjen P, Hespel P, Eynde EV, et al. Biochemical variables in plasma and urine before and after prolonged exercise. Enzyme 1985;33:134–42.

140. Mars M, Hadley GP. Raised intracompartmental pressure and compartment syndromes. Injury 1998;29(6):403–11.

141. Matsen FA. Compartment syndrome: an unified concept. Clin Orthop 1975;113: 8–14.

142. Matsen FA, Winquist RA, Krugmire RB. Diagnosis and management of compartment syndromes. J Bone Joint Surg Am 1980;62:286–91.

143. Perron AD, Brady WJ, Keats TE. Orthopedic pitfalls in the ED: acute compartment syndrome. Am J Emerg Med 2001;19:413–6.

144. Finkelstein JA, Hunter GA, Hu RW. Lower limb compartment syndrome: course after delayed fasciotomy. J Trauma 1996;40:342–4.

145. Van Essen GJ, McQueen MM. Compartment syndrome of the lower limb. Hosp Med 1998;59(4):294–7.

146. Whitesides TE, Haney TC, Morimoto K, et al. Tissue pressure measurements as a determinant for the need for fasciotomy. Clin Orthop 1975;113:43–51.

147. Heckman MM, Whitesides TE, Grewe SR, et al. Histologic determination of the ischemic threshold of muscle in the canine compartment syndrome model. J Orthop Trauma 1993;7(3):199–210.

148. Matsen FA, Wyss CR, King RV, et al. Factors affecting the tolerance of muscle circulation and function for increased tissue pressure. Clin Orthop 1981;155: 224–30.

149. Mars M, Hadley GP. Failure of pulse oximetry in the assessment of raised limb intracompartmental pressure. Injury 1994;25(6):379–85.

150. Gianotti G, Cohn SM, Brown M, et al. Utility of near-infrared spectroscopy in the diagnosis of lower extremity compartment syndrome. J Trauma 2000;48:396–401.

151. Katz LM, Nauriyal V, Nagaraj S, et al. Infrared imaging of trauma patients for detection of acute compartment syndrome of the leg. Crit Care Med 2008;36: 1756–61.

152. Lagerstrom CF, Reed RL, Rowlands BJ, et al. Early fasciotomy for acute clinically evident posttraumatic compartment syndrome. Am J Surg 1989;158:36–9.

153. Mann DC, Rajmaira S. Distribution of physeal and nonphyseal fractures in 2,650 long bone fractures in children aged 0-16 yrs. J Pediatr Orthop 1990;10:713–6.

154. Mizuta T, Benson WM, Foster BK, et al. Statistical analysis of the incidence of physeal injuries. J Pediatr Orthop 1987;7:518–23.

155. Ogden JA. Skeletal growth mechanism injury patterns. J Pediatr Orthop 1982;2: 371–7.

156. Perron AD, Miller MD, Brady WJ. Orthopedic pitfalls in the ED: pediatric growth plate injuries. Am J Emerg Med 2002;20:50–4.

157. Rogers L. Children's fractures. Philadephia: Lippincott Co; 1970.

158. Peterson CA, Peterson HA. Analysis of the incidence of injuries to the epiphyseal growth plate. J Trauma 1872;12:275–81.

159. Musharafieh RS, Macari G. Salter-Harris I fractures of the distal radius misdiagnosed as wrist sprain. J Emerg Med 2000;19:265–70.

160. Salter RB, Harris WR. Injuries involving the epiphyseal plate. J Bone Joint Surg Am 1963;45:587–622.

161. Rogers LF, Poznanski AK. Imaging of epiphyseal injuries. Radiology 1994; 191(2):297–308.

Index

Note: Page numbers of article titles are in **boldface** type.

Emerg Med Clin N Am 28 (2010) 997–1003
doi:10.1016/S0733-8627(10)00098-2
0733-8627/10/$ – see front matter © 2010 Elsevier Inc. All rights reserved.

emed.theclinics.com

United States Postal Service

Statement of Ownership, Management, and Circulation
(All Periodicals Publications Except Requestor Publications)

1. Publication Title	2. Publication Number	3. Filing Date
Emergency Medicine Clinics of North America	0 0 0 - 7 1 1 4	9/15/10

4. Issue Frequency	5. Number of Issues Published Annually	6. Annual Subscription Price
Feb, May, Aug, Nov	4	$247.00

7. Complete Mailing Address of Known Office of Publication (Not printer) (Street, city, county, state, and ZIP+4®)

Elsevier Inc.
360 Park Avenue South
New York, NY 10010-1710

Contact Person
Stephen Bushing
Telephone (Include area code)
215-239-3688

8. Complete Mailing Address of Headquarters or General Business Office of Publisher (Not printer)

Elsevier Inc., 360 Park Avenue South, New York, NY 10010-1710

9. Full Names and Complete Mailing Addresses of Publisher, Editor, and Managing Editor (Do not leave blank)

Publisher (Name and complete mailing address)

Kim Murphy, Elsevier, Inc., 1600 John F. Kennedy Blvd. Suite 1800, Philadelphia, PA 19103-2899

Editor (Name and complete mailing address)

Patrick Manley, Elsevier, Inc., 1600 John F. Kennedy Blvd. Suite 1800, Philadelphia, PA 19103-2899

Managing Editor (Name and complete mailing address)

Catherine Bewick, Elsevier, Inc., 1600 John F. Kennedy Blvd. Suite 1800, Philadelphia, PA 19103-2899

10. Owner (Do not leave blank. If the publication is owned by a corporation, give the name and address of the corporation immediately followed by the names and addresses of all stockholders owning or holding 1 percent or more of the total amount of stock. If not owned by a corporation, give the names and addresses of the individual owners. If owned by a partnership or other unincorporated firm, give its name and address as well as those of each individual owner. If the publication is published by a nonprofit organization, give its name and address.)

Full Name	Complete Mailing Address
Wholly owned subsidiary of	4520 East-West Highway
Reed/Elsevier, US holdings	Bethesda, MD 20814

11. Known Bondholders, Mortgagees, and Other Security Holders Owning or Holding 1 Percent or More of Total Amount of Bonds, Mortgages, or Other Securities. If none, check box ☐ None

Full Name	Complete Mailing Address
N/A	

12. Tax Status (For completion by nonprofit organizations authorized to mail at nonprofit rates) (Check one)
The purpose, function, and nonprofit status of this organization and the exempt status for federal income tax purposes:
☐ Has Not Changed During Preceding 12 Months
☐ Has Changed During Preceding 12 Months (Publisher must submit explanation of change with this statement)

PS Form 3526, September 2007 (Page 1 of 3 (Instructions Page 3)) PSN 7530-01-000-9931 PRIVACY NOTICE: See our Privacy policy in www.usps.com

---

13. Publication Title	14. Issue Date for Circulation Data Below
Emergency Medicine Clinics of North America	August 2010

15. Extent and Nature of Circulation			Average No. Copies Each Issue During Preceding 12 Months	No. Copies of Single Issue Published Nearest to Filing Date
a. Total Number of Copies (Net press run)			1779	1645
b. Paid Circulation (By Mail and Outside the Mail)	(1)	Mailed Outside-County Paid Subscriptions Stated on PS Form 3541. (Include paid distribution above nominal rate, advertiser's proof copies, and exchange copies)	826	871
	(2)	Mailed In-County Paid Subscriptions Stated on PS Form 3541 (Include paid distribution above nominal rate, advertiser's proof copies, and exchange copies)		
	(3)	Paid Distribution Outside the Mails Including Sales Through Dealers and Carriers, Street Vendors, Counter Sales, and Other Paid Distribution Outside USPS®	223	263
	(4)	Paid Distribution by Other Classes Mailed Through the USPS (e.g. First-Class Mail®)		
c. Total Paid Distribution (Sum of 15b (1), (2), (3), and (4))	▶		1049	1134
d. Free or Nominal Rate Distribution (By Mail and Outside the Mail)	(1)	Free or Nominal Rate Outside-County Copies Included on PS Form 3541	97	84
	(2)	Free or Nominal Rate In-County Copies Included on PS Form 3541		
	(3)	Free or Nominal Rate Copies Mailed at Other Classes Through the USPS (e.g. First-Class Mail)		
	(4)	Free or Nominal Rate Distribution Outside the Mail (Carriers or other means)		
e. Total Free or Nominal Rate Distribution (Sum of 15d (1), (2), (3) and (4))	▶		97	84
f. Total Distribution (Sum of 15c and 15e)	▶		1146	1218
g. Copies not Distributed (See instructions to publishers #4 (page #3))	▶		633	427
h. Total (Sum of 15f and g)	▶		1779	1645
i. Percent Paid (15c divided by 15f times 100)			91.54%	93.10%

16. Publication of Statement of Ownership
If the publication is a general publication, publication of this statement is required. Will be printed ☐ Publication not required
in the November 2010 issue of this publication.

17. Signature and Title of Editor, Publisher, Business Manager, or Owner

Stephen R. Bushing (signature)
Date: September 15, 2010
Stephen R. Bushing – Fulfillment/Inventory Specialist

I certify that all information furnished on this form is true and complete. I understand that anyone who furnishes false or misleading information on this form or who omits material or information requested on the form may be subject to criminal sanctions (including fines and imprisonment) and/or civil sanctions (including civil penalties).

PS Form 3526, September 2007 (Page 2 of 3)

Moving?

Make sure your subscription moves with you!

To notify us of your new address, find your **Clinics Account Number** (located on your mailing label above your name), and contact customer service at:

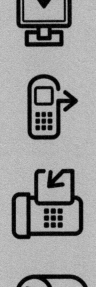

Email: journalscustomerservice-usa@elsevier.com

800-654-2452 (subscribers in the U.S. & Canada)
314-447-8871 (subscribers outside of the U.S. & Canada)

Fax number: 314-447-8029

Elsevier Health Sciences Division
Subscription Customer Service
3251 Riverport Lane
Maryland Heights, MO 63043

*To ensure uninterrupted delivery of your subscription, please notify us at least 4 weeks in advance of move.

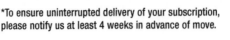
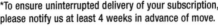

Printed and bound by CPI Group (UK) Ltd, Croydon, CR0 4YY

03/10/2024

01040460-0007